THE PATH TO LONGEVITY

THE PATH TO LONGEVITY

HOW TO REACH 100 WITH THE HEALTH AND STAMINA OF A 40-YEAR-OLD

LUIGI FONTANA
MD, PhD, FRACP

Hardie Grant

BOOKS

The information contained in this book is provided for general purposes only. It not intended as a substitute for the advice and care of your physician. The author and publisher expressly disclaim responsibility for any specific health needs that may require medical supervision. The diet, nutrition, exercise and health regimes described in this book should be followed only after consulting with your physician to make sure that they are appropriate to your individual circumstances.

Published in 2020 by Hardie Grant Books, an imprint of Hardie Grant Publishing

Hardie Grant Books (Melbourne)
Building 1, 658 Church Street
Richmond, Victoria 3121

Hardie Grant Books (London)
5th & 6th Floors
52–54 Southwark Street
London SE1 1UN

hardiegrantbooks.com

A catalogue record for this book is available from the National Library of Australia

The Path to Longevity
ISBN 978 1 74379 596 5

10 9 8 7 6 5 4 3 2 1

Cover design by Luke Causby, Blue Cork
Typeset in 11/14 pt Garamond by Kirby Jones
Printed in Spain

The paper this book is printed on is certified against the Forest Stewardship Council® Standards. FSC® promotes environmentally responsible, socially beneficial and economically viable management of the world's forests.

CONTENTS

ABOUT THE AUTHOR

An internationally recognised physician scientist, Professor Luigi Fontana is a world leader in the field of nutrition, physical exercise and healthy longevity in humans. His pioneering studies on the effects of dietary restriction, fasting and diet composition have opened a new area of nutrition-related research that holds tremendous promise for the prevention of age-related chronic illnesses and for the understanding of the biology of human ageing. He is credited with the foundational research that gave rise to the hugely popular 5:2 diet.

Trained under Professor John Holloszy, a leading scientist in exercise physiology and preventative medicine, Professor Fontana has worked in some of the great medical institutions around the world. These include two Nobel-laureate producing institutions: Washington University in St Louis, one of the top medical schools in the United States, where he was Professor of Medicine and the co-director of the Longevity Research Program, and the Italian National Institute of Health in Rome, where he was Director of the Division of Nutrition and Healthy Aging. He was also a Professor of Nutrition in the Department of Clinical and Experimental Sciences at Brescia University Medical School in Italy.

His career move to Australia came about thanks partly to the $21 million sale of a 1935 Pablo Picasso painting, *Jeune fille endormie*. The masterpiece was donated to the University of Sydney by an anonymous American philanthropist in 2010 on condition that it be sold, with the proceeds directed to fund four new medical research chairs. In 2018, Professor Fontana was appointed as the fourth and final Leonard P. Ullmann Chair of Translational Metabolic Health and Director of the Healthy Longevity Research and Clinical Program at the Charles Perkins Centre at the University of Sydney. He is also a Clinical Academic in the Department of Endocrinology at Royal Prince Alfred Hospital in Sydney, where he continues his clinical practice and research into health, wellbeing and disease prevention.

Professor Fontana has published over 130 highly-cited academic papers in prestigious journals, including *Science, Nature, Cell, New England Journal of Medicine, JAMA, Cell Metabolism, Circulation, Journal of the American College of Cardiology,* and *PNAS*, among others. He has presented his work at more than 250 international conferences and top medical schools and research institutes around the world, including Harvard University, Cambridge University, Yale University, Université Paris 'Pierre et Marie Curie', Baylor College of Medicine, Spanish National Cancer Research Centre, and National University of Singapore.

He is the recipient of three prestigious awards: the 2009 American Federation for Aging Research (AFAR) Breakthroughs in Gerontology Award; the 2011 Glenn Award for Research in Biological Mechanisms of Aging; and the 2016 American Federation of Aging Research Vincent Cristofalo Rising Star Award. Fontana is also the Editor in Chief of the scientific journal *Nutrition and Healthy Aging*.

As one of the few physician scientists active in the fields of healthy ageing, nutrition, exercise and metabolism, interacting with patients both in the clinic and in the experimental trials that he designs and conducts, Professor Fontana understands not just the practical effects of changing behaviours, but the physiological and molecular mechanisms underlying those changes. He is interested in empowering people to maximise their health and wellbeing. He also has a keen interest in the role of nutrition in promoting the ecological health of the world. In 2013, he wrote an influential article with Daniel Kammen (a coordinating lead author for the Intergovernmental Panel on Climate Change which won the 2007 Nobel Peace Prize) on the beneficial role of efficient use of food and energy in promoting human, environmental, and planetary health, and sustainable economic development.

Professor Fontana believes that it is urgent that as a society, we begin to take a *prevention-based* approach to health, not a *disease-based* one. People can make choices that will set themselves up for long, healthy and happy lives, while contributing to the protection of the environment. Those already suffering from chronic conditions, such as obesity, hypertension, diabetes, heart disease, cancer, autoimmune and allergic disorders, and emotional and psychological distress, can also make positive changes that will have a beneficial influence on their lives now.

In this book, Professor Fontana shares information and knowledge that has proven invaluable to him, his family and friends, and to the patients he has treated. Perhaps the changes that must be made to health and economic systems around the world could be made more easily if individuals were aware of just how much control each of us has in preventing a wide range of physical, mental and spiritual afflictions that cause so much suffering in later life. What Professor Fontana illustrates here is what each of us wants to be: disease-free, pain-free, and capable of doing what we enjoy for as long as possible, ideally for our entire lives.

PREFACE

Every day I see people who are suffering, and who mistakenly believe that their chronic diseases and emotional distress are due to bad genes or an unlucky roll of the dice. It's very sad, because we now know that many chronic illnesses are preventable.

Thanks to major advances in public health and medicine, life expectancy in the Western world has nearly doubled since 1850. Improvements in sanitation, better animal health and pest control, water chlorination, national vaccination programs, and the advent of antibiotics, vitamins, insulin, cortisone and chemotherapy drugs – among many other scientific innovations – have made it possible for humans to survive illnesses that would have killed their grandparents.

Men and women can now live longer. But, unfortunately, too many individuals are troubled by multiple chronic illnesses such as heart disease, stroke, cancer, liver and kidney diseases, dementia, frailty and a wide range of mental disorders. Modern medicine makes it possible for patients to live with these conditions for decades, but these years are characterised not by joy, freedom, action and independence, but by suffering, anxiety, depression, debility and dependence on increasingly costly medical systems.

Of the many trillions of dollars spent on medical care in Western countries, the majority is used to treat chronic diseases. For instance, in the US, 90 per cent of the 3.3 trillion dollars spent on medical care in 2017 went to treating people after they had fallen ill.[1] This extremely expensive 'sick-care' medical system is unsustainable and won't last. The future will be a 'pay for prevention' health system that will reward care that keeps people out of hospitals in the first place. Beyond health-cost savings, preventing diseases would yield immeasurable gains in other essential aspects such as quality of life and extended access to the wisdom that comes with healthy ageing.

In 1948, the World Health Organization (WHO) defined health as 'a state of complete physical, mental, and social wellbeing, and not merely the absence of disease or infirmity'. Since I began to practise medicine – and, indeed, even as a youth – I have searched for ways to achieve a state of complete physical, mental and spiritual health, and deep satisfaction in life. My clinical practice and research have focused not only on increasing longevity, but also on understanding the precise mechanisms by which nutrition, exercise and other lifestyle interventions can lead to a healthy old age, and a creative, successful and fulfilling life.

As I will discuss in this book, studies of longevity in animal and clinical models and in human centenarians have shown that it is possible for people to live past the age of 100 *without* developing major chronic illnesses. I believe that this kind of healthy longevity is not a matter of genetics or chance, though those factors do play a role. The WHO estimates that by amending lifestyle factors including poor diet, physical inactivity, smoking and excess body weight, we could prevent at least 80 per cent of cases of cardiovascular disease, stroke and type 2 diabetes and more than 40 per cent of cancers.[2] I think these numbers are conservative.

It is essential that more people know how they can prevent disease, improve their quality of life and reduce suffering from the chronic conditions they have. The time has come to take control of our own health. Instead of dealing with the long-term consequences of chronic diseases, we need to modify our behaviours, because to do so will have a cascading effect on many fatal and disabling illnesses, and on ecosystems and planetary health as well.

What I hope to show in this book is how nutrition, physical exercise and brain training can lead to a long life, free of diseases, and why these factors have the influence on health that they do. I believe that, if people can understand the physiological, biochemical and molecular mechanisms, they can make informed choices that will help them live longer, and also be happier and healthier. Additionally, I explain other practices and interventions that promote wellbeing and happiness, such as mindfulness, meditation, healthy sleeping patterns, some breathing techniques and the importance of social relationships and environmental health. These, too, have scientific backing.

WHERE THIS ALL BEGAN

My interest in the topic of preventive medicine, healthy longevity, mindfulness and personal empowerment started many years ago. When I was about five years old, my maternal uncle Francesco persuaded my mother to change our family's diet. In the 1960s, Francesco was one of the first people in Italy to buy 'organic' whole grains and beans straight from the biodynamic farm.

We had not been eating poorly – my family always had a garden and grew vegetables – but in Trento, in Northern Italy where I was born, the cuisine was dominated by meat, cheese, milk, refined carbohydrates and sweets. My mother did the cooking and was in charge of what my two sisters, my father, and I ate. After Francesco convinced her to modify our diet, we began eating a greater variety of leafy vegetables, minimally processed whole grains, beans, nuts, seeds, and fish and shellfish as the main sources of vitamin B12 and zinc. Now, along with my wife Laura and son Lorenzo, we eat in a similar way and we are free of maladies and take no medications.

Not only did my family's diet change, but also my perception of the inter-relationship of man with nature. From childhood, I have been taught to consider the body as a temple in which our mind, our inner soul can thrive, grow and empower itself. When I became a teenager, Uncle Francesco began introducing me to philosophical and traditional medicinal books from China and India, including the *Tao Te Ching*, the *Chuang Tzu*, the *I Ching*, the *Upanishads*, the *Yellow Emperor's Classic of Medicine* and the *Yoga Sutra of Patañjali*. He also led me to more modern interpretations, such as the *Manual of Zen Buddhism* by DT Suzuki, *Total Freedom* by Jiddu Krishnamurti, and the *Art of Yoga* by B.K.S. Iyengar.

I remember long discussions with my uncle, over games of ping-pong, about the importance of cultivating the whole person, an entity that is not only physical, but also affective, imaginative, intuitive, psychic and spiritual. Although I was still enjoying time with my friends, I set aside a considerable amount of time to read, think and meditate. I also began to practise hatha yoga.

Empowered with this holistic approach, I advanced through six years of medical school, five years of residency in internal medicine, and four years of a PhD in metabolism. But it became increasingly obvious to me that the teaching, and also the standard medical practice itself, were both exclusively focused on disease diagnosis and treatment. Unfortunately, medical training was more about caring for the sick than health care. We were trained – as the great majority of physicians still are – to recognise the signs of diseases and treat established medical conditions (which normally develop over many decades of unhealthy lifestyle) with either drugs or surgery.

During my first 11 years of medical training, we learned almost nothing about the role of nutrition, physical exercise, cognitive training, mindfulness, meditation, sleep hygiene, and the many other interventions in the prevention and treatment of the most typical chronic diseases that now overwhelm our hospitals. Nobody told us anything about the importance of emotions, compassion and warm-heartedness in dealing with our distressed and fearful patients.

I knew I did not want to be that kind of doctor, merely spending the rest of my life prescribing the latest anticancer or antidepressant medicine, a better wheelchair or incontinence device. But at the same time, I was not interested in embracing alternative medicine either, because its scientific basis was weak on evidence, or had no science at all. So, with the support of my beloved mother Antonietta, I embarked on a scientific career to explore, with rigorous experiments, the mechanisms regulating ageing and the interventions that could promote healthy longevity.

Over the years, I began to address some key questions that had long fascinated me:

- What biological factors regulate ageing and longevity?
- What are the roles of nutrition and exercise in promoting health and in preventing some of the most common chronic illnesses?

Ageing and age-related diseases, especially in humans, are complex processes, regulated by an intricate network of metabolic and molecular mechanisms still only minimally known and understood. I realised that it was illusionary to believe that we could successfully intervene in these sophisticated metabolic and molecular networks with drugs or gene therapies, without risking disrupting a delicate balance.

But, as I will try to illustrate, the quantity, quality and frequency of the foods we eat, in combination with a range of physical and cognitive activities, can be the key to slowing the ageing process and maintaining or regaining our health, strength and vigour. Additionally, by working with research volunteers and patients affected by various chronic medical conditions, I came to understand that knowledge does not always translate immediately into action.

In science, we are forced to design studies analysing one intervention at the time. However, my personal experience as a physician suggested that linking nutritional and exercise interventions together with motivational, awareness and meditation exercises could bring about surprisingly positive modifications in behaviour where changes were rooted in a new mind-set.

I also understood that to foster the creation of this new mind-set, we must learn to open our minds and our hearts. Altruism, compassion and warm-heartedness are essential tools to reduce all those negative feelings and behaviours that are so harmful for our own health and for the environment. The cultivation of these three qualities is also instrumental to building our *inner strength,* so we can walk with confidence and trust in this world, make many friends and fulfil our goals, whatever they are, which will bring a deep sense of satisfaction in life.

INFORMATION IS POWER

I understand that many readers are confused by the contradictory and potentially biased information provided by the mass media, food companies and some non-profit health organizations. For instance, the American Society for Nutrition, which is the main nutritional association in North America, acknowledges in its official scientific journal, *The American Journal of Clinical Nutrition,* the 'generous support' of many food and pharmaceutical companies. Here is a full list.* Similarly, the European Food

---

* The full list of the 2019 Sustaining Partners of the American Society for Nutrition are: Ajinomoto Health and Nutrition North America, Almond Board of California, Bayer HealthCare, Biofortis Clinical Research,

Information Council (EUFIC), a non-profit organisation that has as one of its main goals to 'communicate science-based information on nutrition and health, food safety and quality, to help consumers to be better informed when choosing a well-balanced, safe and healthful diet' is governed by a Board of Directors which is elected from member companies, including Bunge, Cargill, Cereal Partners, Coca-Cola, Corteva Agriscience, DSM, Ferrero, General Mills, Mars, Nestlé, PepsiCo, Tereos, Ülker and Unilever.[5]

It is little wonder people are confused and desperate to find reliable, unbiased and science-based advice on nutrition and health. One of my goals, as someone who is at the centre of Western academic medicine, is to share the latest scientific information, and clarify the biological mechanisms through which nutrition and other lifestyles can maximise health and wellbeing. This draws on knowledge I have acquired and mastered during 25 years of medical practice and scientific research studies, and primarily the interventions and techniques that I have studied, practised and experienced myself.

In this book, I hope to empower readers to understand the immense benefits of making comprehensive changes to their lifestyle, attitude and personal growth. You will find:

- practical suggestions on how to make positive changes to your lifestyle and behaviour

- easy-to-understand, science-based explanations of the mechanisms that make this effective

- specific parameters to measure your progress towards health

- examples of interventions that have improved health and wellbeing – not just in Western cultures, but in cultures around the world

- information on 'whole person' development and what aspects of your personality you should cultivate in order to boost your emotional, creative and intuitive intelligence, your self-confidence, self-esteem and life satisfaction

- how, ultimately, improving your dietary and lifestyle choices can reduce global warming, pollution and environmental degradation.

California Walnut Commission, Cargill, Inc., Corn Refiners Association, Council for Responsible Nutrition, Distilled Spirits Council, DSM Nutritional Products, LLC, Dupont Nutrition & Health, Egg Nutrition Center, General Mills Bell Institute of Health and Nutrition, Hass Avocado Board, Herbalife Nutrition, Ingredion, Kellogg Company, Kyowa Hakko U.S.A., Inc., Mars Inc., Mondelez International, National Cattlemen's Beef Association, a contractor to The Beef Checkoff, National Dairy Council, Nestle Nutrition, PepsiCo, Pfizer, Inc., Pharmavite LLC, Tate & Lyle, The Dannon Company, Inc., The Sugar Association, The Wonderful Company and Unilever.[3] In the past, sustaining partners included McDonald's, The Coca-Cola Company, Kraft Foods, The Procter & Gamble Company, Monsanto Company, GlaxoSmithKline Consumer Healthcare.[4]

I hope my readers will be inspired by the stories I tell. I experience so much joy in life that it saddens me to see others suffering. I hope that you can adopt some of the practices that I have found so fulfilling. However, success in transforming your life and implementing these comprehensive lifestyle changes depends on your ability to change the way you think and live, which can be part of a profound cultural revolution.

Luigi Fontana

PART I

THE BEGINNING OF WISDOM

CHAPTER ONE

ARE YOU READY TO ENJOY YOUR LIFE?

Life is beautiful. Being born on this spectacular planet, and being able to travel, experience and enjoy the marvels around us and, most importantly, inside us, is a gift. The most important one!

However, too many people do not appreciate how crucial it is to maintain or regain health in order to fully enjoy this amazing and transformative voyage in the company of our beloved relatives and dear friends. Too often, people are so busy accumulating money and material goods that they cannot find time to take care of themselves, their family and the environment around them. They forget to live and most importantly 'to be'. The Dalai Lama says in this regard:

> *Man sacrifices his health to make money. Then he sacrifices his money to treat the diseases. He is so anxious for the future that he does not enjoy the present, with the result that he does not live either in the present or in the future. He lives as if he is never going to die, and then dies having never really lived.*

The truth is that to maximise our chances of living a long, happy, creative and meaningful life, we need to address both our physical and our mental health. We need to balance and care for both. If our body is not kept in good shape, it is unlikely that we will be able to deal with life's challenges and sometimes perils. At the same time, a healthy and resilient body without an attentive, curious, intuitive and compassionate mind would be incapable of exploring and sharing the wonders of this planet and of enjoying the rich depths of our inner selves.

> Are you doing everything you can to keep your body in good shape, or to regain your health?
>
> Do you know and understand what is required to keep your body and mind strong and healthy?
>
> Do you know how to empower your life and make the best of yourself?

These are crucial questions. The art of living a long, healthy, empowered and happy life is not simple and straightforward. There are no shortcuts. No magic pills or expensive procedures that can replace the beneficial effects of a healthy diet, exercise and mindfulness, or of a regenerating night's sleep. Moreover, we have to bear in mind that what we eat, think and do influence not only our wellbeing and degree of success in life, but also the health of the environment, which in a vicious circle impacts our risk of becoming sick and miserable. Everything is interconnected.

Beware of snake oil salesmen who swoop in and promise to make you healthy, smart and happy with something requiring little effort and producing a 'quick fix'. If someone were to tell you that by taking a pill or a couple of lessons, you would become an accomplished concert violinist or a black-belt Aikido Sensei, would you believe him? It's easy to take someone's word for it when you're not knowledgeable.

To guard against being taken advantage of, you need to understand the mechanisms of how things work and how you can measure the results. If you master these things, you will be in a better position to protect yourself. I hope that by reading this book, you may acquire some of this knowledge, but most importantly, you will start to examine your own rational and subconscious expectations for the future. You might discover that they are uncomfortably in conflict both in what you do and how you do it. I hope that by understanding this divergence you will unlock a profoundly felt need for transformation.

ARE YOU READY TO EMBARK ON THE MIRACULOUS VOYAGE THAT IS YOUR LIFE?

Typically, before we head out for a long road journey, we make sure that our car is up to the task. Nothing can ruin a trip faster than car trouble, especially if it could have been prevented. Keeping up with our regularly scheduled car maintenance, and understanding the car's basic requirements, can help keep our journey from becoming a nightmare, complete with costly repair bills, and the disruption of our long-awaited trip.

Would you feel safe driving a car that had not undergone its regular servicing and inspections, had not been supplied with the appropriate types of oil and fuel or had dangerously low tyre pressure? So then, shouldn't we show the same concern for our body, that we take on a journey lasting many decades, and for some, more than a century? Are you really doing everything you can to keep your body in good shape? Do you maintain it with the best energy sources, or to keep up the analogy, do you use the cheapest fuel, lowest grade transmission oil and not bother to check that everything is running smoothly?

WHAT DO YOU REALLY KNOW ABOUT YOUR HEALTH?

Are you metabolically healthy and fit? For instance, what is your body weight and waist circumference? How much weight have you gained since you were 18 years old? Do you lead a sedentary life, smoke or drink? Do you have issues with blood pressure, cholesterol, glucose, insulin, testosterone, insulin-like growth factor-1 (IGF-1) and C-reactive protein levels, a marker of systemic inflammation? All these, as I will illustrate in this book, are some of the most important predictors of our risk of developing chronic illnesses. If they are not kept in order, they will spoil our journey, and most importantly will dramatically *shorten* it.

Unfortunately, due to unhealthy diets and sedentary lifestyle, the present average values for many of these risk factors in both men and women are far from optimal.[1,2,3] We must also bear in mind that some of the classical risk factors for the build-up of hard 'calcified' plaques around the arteries that can lead to a heart attack, a stroke and heart failure do not explain the full risk. At least 25 per cent of patients with cardiovascular disorders lack any of the conventional risk factors,[4] implying that other elements play a role, such as physical inactivity, abdominal obesity, insulin resistance, mental stress, and, as we will see later, the type of bacteria living in our gut. The same applies to the risk of developing cancer, dementia and many other inflammatory and autoimmune diseases.

IT'S NEVER TOO LATE

Adopting a healthy lifestyle can drastically improve your health at any age, even if you are already suffering from one or more diseases. Of course, the sooner you start the better, but it is never too late to turn back the clock. The benefits of improving your diet quality and engaging in regular exercise and cognitive training (keeping your mind active and engaged) don't accrue only to people who have been doing this all along. You can make changes in your 50s, 60s and 70s that result in a healthier, longer life.

In some of our studies, we have seen dramatic and rapid health gains in middle-aged and elderly people affected by chronic illnesses, including obesity, type 2 diabetes, cardiovascular disease, and diabetic kidney disease. Also, a growing body of evidence strongly suggests that changing lifestyle can reduce the risk of cancer recurrence, improve cognitive function in persons with early dementia, and influence mental health in people affected by depression, anxiety and other mental health conditions.

WHO IS IN CHARGE?

Would you ever get in a car driven by someone who is insecure, confused, or, even worse, depressed? Similarly, if you were planning an extraordinary adventure, such as climbing Mount Everest, wouldn't you seek a guide or instructor who is not only knowledgeable about the risks, but also focused, resourceful and confident?

It has been shown that Sherpas, who climb Everest and the tallest mountains in the world, have developed some of these unique traits, including lower levels of guilt and anxiety coupled with superior levels of mental toughness, independence and emotional stability.[5] In a personality study of Sherpa climbers, it was shown that these men not only are unbelievably skilled, but also possess key qualities such as leadership, trust, loyalty, calmness, spirituality, kindness and compassion.

Wouldn't it be fantastic to have these Sherpa traits? The good news is we can develop and enhance our own levels of mental energy, enthusiasm and positivity and be ready to embark on new experiences with enthusiasm too. It is within our power to develop these traits, so that we can empower our life and fully enjoy our journey.

WHO ARE YOU?

Are you full of vigour, with high levels of mental energy, enthusiasm and positivity, or do you feel powerless, insecure, bored or awkward? Are you creative, imaginative and ready to embark with zeal on new experiences or are you confused and fearful? Are you agreeable, conscientious and kind-hearted or are you stubborn, selfish and overly competitive?

Do you know that negative emotions have a powerful influence on health and wellbeing? If you are anxious, bored, depressed, angry or unhappy, do you know why? Is there a particular reason for these distressing feelings? Is something missing in your life? What is it? Are you aware of your emotions?

LISTEN AND LEARN

First, it is important to learn to 'listen'. Very few of us really know how to listen, because we are too often caught up in our own opinions, preconceived ideas, prejudices, and dogmas. Our social, cultural and religious upbringing influences our world view, so that we cannot see our physical and psychological problems as they really are.

Many people are also too busy seeking approval or concerned that they will attract disapproval. People think they no longer need to listen or ask questions. But, by asking some of these questions, you can discover a new path that can take you in a fresh and unexpected direction. Smart people never stop learning, because they know that this is the way to deeper insights and revolutionary changes.

During the Japanese Meiji era (1868-1912) there was a famous Zen master, called Nan-in. One day he received a university professor who came to inquire about Zen philosophy. Nan-in started pouring tea into the professor's cup until full, and then kept on pouring. The professor watched the tea overflowing out of the cup for a moment, until he no longer could restrain himself. 'It is overfull. No more will go in!' he exclaimed. Gently, Nan-in replied 'Like this cup, you are full of your own opinions and speculations. How can I show you what is Zen, unless you first empty your cup?'[6]

BE YOUR OWN LIGHT: SELF-AWARENESS IS KEY

Our thoughts, actions and habits are critical in creating a healthy, happy and fulfilling life. What we eat and what we do shapes not only our metabolic health, but also our emotions, and how our brain processes information and creates thoughts and ideas. Our thinking and ideas influence our actions that in time become our habits. A collection of habits forms a large portion of our personality. We don't have to reach far to see that our habits, health and personality ultimately decide our success in life and our degree of freedom and happiness.

In the coming chapters, I will illustrate how healthy nutrition, fasting, physical exercise, cognitive training for the mind, deep sleep, and meditation can maximise our physical and mental health and wellbeing, and our performance and success in life. However, the cultivation of our inner strength and resilience should be our ultimate goal. If we can learn how to travel the paths of life with confidence, if we can master how to experience life without anxiety or fear, but with curiosity, creativity, trust, serenity, kindness and compassion we can achieve our true potential.

The Book of Changes (better known as the *I Ching*), one of the oldest and most important Chinese classic texts, says:

As long as a man's inner nature remains stronger and richer than anything offered by external fortune, as long as he remains inwardly superior to fate, fortune will not desert him.[7]

The plan

CHAPTER TWO

HEALTHY CENTENARIANS: THE QUEST FOR HEALTHY LONGEVITY

The percentage of nonagenarians (90-year-olds) and centenarians has increased dramatically in the past few decades.

In 1950, the chance of survival from the age of 80 to 90 years old in most developed countries was 15–16 per cent for women and 12 per cent for men. In 2002, the chance of survival improved to 37 per cent and 25 per cent, respectively, and in Japanese women today it is greater than 50 per cent.[1] This is an extraordinary and unprecedented achievement in human history. Yet, even today, only 1 per cent of newborns will reach 100 years of age.

Of these exceptionally long-lived individuals, only 19 per cent enjoy the fruits of such success in health: they do not develop any age-associated medical condition before age 100. All the rest reach 100 years of age affected by many chronic conditions: 43 per cent are what we call delayers (that is they develop age-associated disease after the age of 80 years) and 38 per cent are what we call survivors (that is they develop age-associated disease before the age of 80 years but survive).[2] Similar results have been found among most centenarians.[3]

Indeed, the large increase in the number of nonagenarians and centenarians is probably the consequence of medical and technological advances available to an increasing proportion of sick and frail individuals into old age. This has enormous societal and financial costs.[4] In my clinical practice, I had met some of them. It is sad to see these old, tired and exhausted human beings. They have multiple chronic conditions and are taking a long list of medications that make their life painful and complicated. Some of them have severe dementia; others have had a stroke that has confined them to a wheelchair; many are frail and depressed.

Our goal, I hope, is not to become an old diseased, frail, sad and maybe demented nonagenarian or centenarian, but to understand how we can live a long, but most importantly healthy, creative and successful life. We should be able to fully enjoy, for as long as possible, this amazing journey in the company of our treasured family and friends.

Observational data from happy and long-living populations are pointing us in the right direction and there are many scientific studies underway to understand this. We already know that genetics plays a small role in longevity. Analyses on identical twins (siblings that share the same DNA) clearly show that no more than 25 per cent of the probability of living a long or short life, and of the risk of developing cancer, depends on inherited genes.[5,6,7] A new study published in *Genetics*, which analysed data from Ancestry public trees, including hundreds of millions of people, shows that the true heritability of human longevity is much lower, probably less than 10 per cent.[8]

My colleagues, Professors Paola Sebastiani and Tom Perls of Boston University, estimate that even in families with a centenarian, no more than 33 to 48 per cent of longevity is due to genetic inheritance.[9] The rest is due to several environmental factors that my lab and others around the world are trying to explain. Nutrition and physical activity play crucial roles, but as we will see, there are other important contributing factors as well.

SECRETS SHARED BY WORLD'S MOST LONG-LIVING POPULATIONS

There are a growing number of randomly distributed centenarians living predominantly in the most industrialised countries, but only a few regions of the world where populations as a whole seem to live much longer than average. Examples are the inhabitants of Okinawa in Japan and those of some areas of Sardinia, Cilento and Calabria in Italy. The observational data collected by local researchers show that the inhabitants of these regions not only enjoy the longest life expectancy on Earth, but live many of those years in excellent health. These people seem to have certain characteristics in common: a frugal diet based mainly (but not exclusively) on plant foods; constant physical activity, but without excesses; strong attachment to family, friends and community; and a noble purpose in life driven by a set of spiritual values.

OKINAWA: 'LAND OF THE IMMORTALS'

The beautiful and lush island of Okinawa is located about 640 km south of mainland Japan, between the East China Sea and the Pacific Ocean. Its inhabitants are the oldest in the world: a 2006 census determined that the island had 54.4 centenarians for every 100,000 people, amounting to about 650 centenarians; this is four to five times more than in many other developed countries.[10] In 2010 on mainland Japan there were 36.8 centenarians for every 100,000 people, in Italy 26.8, in France 25.8, in the UK 20.3, in Canada 17.4, in the US 17.3, in Germany 15.1, and in Russia 3.8.

Not only do these Okinawan centenarians live much longer, but they suffer a fraction of the ailments that usually kill people. Almost two-thirds of them live independently until the age of 97. In a 1995 survey, it was estimated that the total mortality, in those older than 60 years was half that observed elsewhere in Japan.[11]

Okinawan women compared with American women:

- Death from cardiovascular disease was 12 times lower in Okinawa
- Death from breast cancer and colon cancer was three to six times lower in Okinawa

Okinawan men compared with American men:

- Death from heart attack was six times lower in Okinawa
- Death from prostate cancer was seven times lower in Okinawa

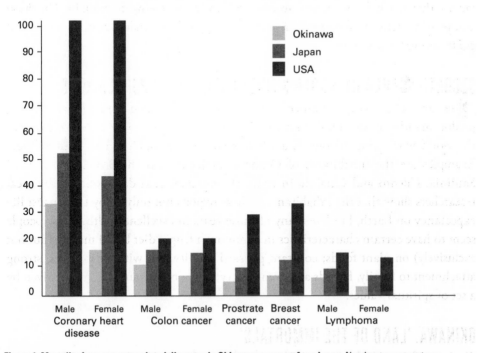

Figure 1: Mortality from age-associated diseases in Okinawans versus Americans. Numbers represent age-adjusted mortality rate in deaths per hundred thousand persons per year for 1995. Coding was according to ICD-9 codes; populations were age-adjusted to World Standard Population. These data show markedly lower mortality risk from age-related diseases in Okinawans compared to other Japanese and Americans.[12]

Food diaries collected by American researchers in 1950 at the end of World War II revealed that the inhabitants of Okinawa consumed, on average, 1785 calories per day; that is, about 14 per cent less than other Japanese back then (who consumed around 2070 calories) and 43 per cent less than the average man in the US in the 1950s (around 3100 calories).[13,14] Protein intake was also much lower in Okinawa than elsewhere in Japan and the US; on average 39 g per day, which is equivalent to 9 per cent of calories from protein sources.[15] In mainland Japan in 1950, the average consumption of protein was approximately 68 g per day, while in the United States it was 90 g, which corresponds to 13 per cent of total calories. This is quite the opposite of current popular fads that advocate a high-protein, low-carb diet. The source of proteins was also very different. Okinawans ate mostly beans, some whole grains and fish, while Americans' protein source derived primarily from meat, eggs and dairy. The intake of animal products in Okinawa was on average only 19 g per day (of which 15 g was from fish).

The dietary staple of Okinawans prior to the arrival of the Americans at the end of World War II was sweet potatoes, which provided approximately 50 per cent of daily calories. Purple (*Beni Imo*) or yellow orange (*Satsuma Imo*) sweet potatoes are extremely rich in vitamin A, vitamin C, vitamin B6, manganese and other antioxidants like anthocyanins – the same pigments that give blueberries their colour. Elsewhere in Japan, about 78 per cent of dietary calories came from cereals, especially rice.

In 2009, I was invited by Professor Craig Willcox, who has been studying the Okinawan centenarians for many years, to visit this amazing and peaceful island. With Craig and Professor Eiji Takeda we travelled to the village of Ogimi to meet some of these centenarians, who spoke about their diet and lifestyle.

I was told that every meal starts with a miso soup, charged with tofu and seaweed, and accompanied by enormous amounts of leafy green vegetables, cabbage, onions, bitter melon and yellow and orange roots (carrots, squash, daikon, turmeric), gathered from the large gardens that each family has in their backyards.

When I asked if the consumption of fish was plentiful, the answer was a definite 'no'. Although the island is surrounded by ocean, fish was eaten only once or twice a week; most proteins were from legumes and soy products like tofu and miso. Pork was a luxury dish, consumed in very small portions a few times a year. The dessert, typically, was based on local fruits, accompanied by a hot cup of jasmine tea.

Unfortunately, even in Okinawa in recent decades, with the advent of fast food chains imported by American soldiers (who still have a large military base on the island), eating habits have become Westernised and people have gained weight. The average body mass index (BMI), a simple physical measurement of body fat, has increased from 21 to 24 kg/m^2, just under the 25 considered overweight. In line with this increase, mortality from cardiovascular disease and cancer has increased dramatically.[16] (See page 32 for more information on the importance of BMI and how to calculate your own.)

Their diet, however, is not the only factor that distinguishes the lifestyle of Okinawan centenarians. Because of the constantly warm and sunny weather, men and women on this marvellous island tend to spend a lot of time outdoors, walking and working in the fields. They believe that growing and harvesting the fruits of Mother Earth is important for health.

The elderly visit their gardens, which they like to see grow and flourish, at least three times a day. I still remember this beautifully happy and serene 95-year-old Okinawan woman, still living alone and growing her own vegetables in a perfectly kept garden at the back of her house. At the end of the field, luxuriant crops of pineapples mangoes and papayas merged with the forest, populated by hundreds of joyfully singing birds.

Most of the Okinawans I met participate regularly in a local form of dance and practise martial arts, such as karate and kobudo, which were both invented on this island. For them karate is not a simple exercise, but an art that serves to strengthen the body, mind and spirit. Gichin Funakoshi, the founder of the style of Shotokan karate, which was born in Naha, the capital of Okinawa, believed that:

Just like the surface of a clean mirror reflects images without distortion,
so the student of karate must purge himself from selfish and wicked
thoughts, because only with a clear mind and conscience, can we
understand the meaning of life and absorb everything that we will meet
during our journey on this spectacular planet.

Spiritual life represents a key aspect of Okinawan daily life. Everyone has a small home altar, where they pray each morning and thank the ancestors. According to Professor Makoto Suzuki, a local cardiologist and geriatrician, 'these prayers help to reduce stress and soothe the mind'.

Residents of Okinawa are very calm and friendly; they take life easy. One of their typical sayings, *'Nan kuru nai'*, means 'Don't worry, everything will be fine'. They are convinced that whatever happens in life has a positive meaning and helps us grow and become stronger and wiser. Probably, this attitude is the result of philosophical concepts that have been circulating for centuries in many Eastern societies. In the *I Ching*, which has deeply influenced the Okinawan culture, it is written:

The superior man focuses his attention on himself, and by doing so he
shapes his character. Difficulties and obstructions throw a man back

upon himself. While the inferior man seeks to put the blame on other persons, bewailing his fate, the superior man seeks the error within himself, and through this introspection the external obstacle becomes for him an occasion for inner enrichment and education.[17]

Finally, in their villages you can feel a strong sense of social connection. The family comes first and the elderly are respected and protected. '*Tusui ya takara*' in Okinawan means: 'The elderly represent a treasure for us'. In return, the old look after the children with kindness and love. This feeling is well represented by the motto: '*Shikinoo chui shiihii shiru kurasuru*', which means: 'We live in this world by helping one another'. For the elders, seeing their children, grandchildren and great-grandchildren grow is one of the most rewarding experiences of life. Unlike in many Western countries, this tight-knit family and community life also helps the inhabitants to retain an active social life into old age. Solitude and isolation have been shown to impair health. Some studies suggest that loneliness is as bad as smoking 15 cigarettes a day.[18]

It is said that in the village of Ogimi, in the northwest of the island, there is a stone on the beach with a medieval inscription:

> *At 70 years you're just a child, to 80 barely a youngster, and at 90, if your ancestors invite you to the Heaven, ask them to wait until you have 100 years ... only then maybe you can think about it.*

SARDINIA AND SOUTH ITALY: KINGDOM OF METHUSELAHS

Another fascinating part of the world where the number of nonagenarians and centenarians seem to be on average much higher is South Italy, and in particular, Sardinia and the Cilento region of Campania. According to the 2015 census, there were about 50 centenarians living in the mountainous villages of Ogliastra province on the Italian island of Sardinia for every 100,000 residents; an extremely high number. These super long-lived people are residents of several villages, including Villagrande, Strisaili, Arzana, Baunei, Urzulei and Talana.

An interesting fact is that this part of the world is home to the world's longest-living men. Usually female centenarians outnumber male centenarians by a ratio of four to one; in Sardinia, the ratio is one to one. I met a few of them in the small town of Perfugas in Sardinia. These centenarians struck me because, despite their venerable age, each was still in excellent physical shape; lean, with sharp minds and contagious smiles – the smile of a human being who has lived a long, healthy, challenging but rewarding life. Two words well summarise the impression that talking with them has left in my heart: simplicity and harmony.

The scientific data collected so far on the lifestyles on these 'exceptional' human beings have several limitations, but it would seem that the residents of these areas have certain characteristics in common:

- a mainly plant-based diet comprising vegetables, whole grains, legumes and small quantities of local goat cheese

- occasional consumption of meat, typically only on Sunday and special occasions

- a very physically active outdoor life, with long walks looking after grazing sheep and manual work in the field

- a quiet and compassionate temperament, sensitive to the natural flow of life

- an untroubled life characterised by very strong family ties with extended families composed of great-grandparents, grandparents, parents, children and grandchildren who take care of each other.

Longevity is not limited to Sardinia. In Southern Italy there are many other villages – such as Acciaroli in Cilento and Molochio in Calabria – where the number of 'golden agers' appears considerably higher than in other parts of Italy and the world. In all these picturesque small towns, for centuries people have consumed the traditional Mediterranean diet, which is predominantly plant-based.

IS VEGETARIANISM THE MAIN SECRET TO A LONG HEALTHY LIFE?

If a predominantly plant-based diet is one of the secrets of healthy centenarians, what happens if we take it to the extreme by eliminating meat, or even better all animal products altogether? Would this lead to a longer and illness-free life?

To answer this question, we need to observe the populations of vegetarians and vegans around the world. Take for instance people living in the Indian subcontinent. A great percentage of them have been vegetarians for many generations, for religious reasons, of course. According to Hinduism, killing a cow – the incarnation of the divine – is equivalent to murder, but the same is true for other animals, which may be a close relative reincarnated as an animal because of wrongdoing in a previous life.

If you look at the health status of Indians, data show that they do not fare so well. Not so much because of infectious diseases, which are still a huge problem in India, but because there is an unprecedented epidemic of abdominal obesity and type 2 diabetes mellitus.[19] This preventable disease is a powerful risk factor for heart disease or kidney failure (the terrible diabetic nephropathy); leg amputation following the closure of the peripheral vessels (diabetic microangiopathy); or blindness (diabetic retinopathy). The long silent stages preceding overt diabetes also increases the risk of developing some of the most common cancers, as I will explain in Chapter 3, because of hyperinsulinemia – higher than normal levels of insulin in the blood –, systemic inflammation and other hormonal alterations.

In India there is a very high prevalence of type 2 diabetes, with approximately 12 people out of 100 are affected, while in the United States it is only 8 out of 100. Why? Probably because the Indian cuisine is rich in refined carbohydrates (white rice, naan, chapati, sweets and sugary drinks), and copious quantities of vegetable oil are used in cooking. Vegetarianism is not bad at all, but it depends on what foods we consume, how much exercise we do, whether we smoke or drink too much alcohol, and many other things.

FACTS, NOT MYTHS ON VEGETARIAN DIETS: THE RESULTS OF THE SCIENTIFIC STUDIES

There are an estimated 375 million vegetarians in the world. In Australia 12 per cent of the population are estimated to be vegetarians, in Europe 10 per cent, while in the United States only 3 per cent claim to be vegetarian.

A 2008 survey showed that a large proportion of the vegetarians in Europe and the US are young women, who care about animal welfare. There are different kinds of vegetarians, depending on what they eat. Vegans are those that have eliminated all animal products from their diet, excluding meat, fish, milk, cheese, eggs, and the more conservative even honey. Lacto-ovo vegetarians, consume dairy products and eggs but no meat or fish. Pesco-vegetarians eat some fish.

The American and Canadian Dietetic Associations state that vegetarian diets, if properly balanced, are nutritionally adequate and have beneficial health effects.[20,21] The results of scientific studies suggest that vegetarians tend to have a lower risk of cancer and cardiovascular death compared to omnivores eating typical Western diets. Not a great surprise! Any diet is better than the usual Western diet.

But let's dive deeper into the data. A joint analysis of five prospective studies has shown that the mortality for ischemic heart disease in vegetarians was significantly lower than in omnivores: 34 per cent less in lacto-ovo-vegetarians and pesco-vegetarians, and 26 per cent less in vegans.[22] However, subsequent studies have found that the protective effect against heart disease of vegetarian diets is almost exclusively limited to the Seventh-day Adventists, who, as we will see, don't smoke, don't drink alcohol, do regular physical activity and are socially connected.[23]

Other studies, such as those on English and German vegetarians, show only a modest effect on cardiovascular mortality.[24] The same happens for total mortality (all causes), which is lower in the Seventh-day Adventists, but not in other groups of German and British vegetarians.[25] A German study on vegetarians, for instance, has shown that there is no difference in mortality among vegetarians and a control group of health-conscious individuals, eating meat from time to time. In addition, it was noted that cigarette smoking, the amount of exercise, obesity and alcohol intake explain most of the differences in cancer and cardiovascular mortality among these different groups.

Generally, however, well-educated vegetarians who consume balanced diets have a lower body weight than non-vegetarians[26] and have lower levels of cholesterol, glucose and blood pressure.[27] A recent meta-analysis has confirmed that people who eat vegetarian diets have lower levels of total cholesterol, about 14 mg/dl (0.36 mmol/L) less than omnivores. But unfortunately they also have less of the good type of cholesterol (HDL-cholesterol), which is lower by an average of 4 mg/dl (0.1 mmol/L).[28]

For cancer, data are less clear and more heterogeneous. Vegetarians seem to have a reduced incidence of cancer compared to the general population, but many factors beyond the vegetarian diet probably explain this association. Lung cancer is much lower in vegetarians, but this is due almost entirely to the reduced smoking habit in this population. Vegetarians who smoke are not protected! The incidence of bowel cancer is reduced by 22 per cent among Seventh-day Adventist vegetarian community members, but not in British vegetarians. In the latter group, for example, it seems that vegans have an even higher risk of colon cancer, while in pesco-vegetarians there is a 33 per cent reduction, even after correcting for body weight.[29]

Breast cancer risk is no different between vegetarian and non-vegetarian women; and some studies in the Adventist and British women suggest vegans, but not lacto-ovo vegetarians, may have an increased risk.[30] The same is true for prostate cancer, with the risk no different among lacto-ovo-vegetarians and omnivores, but 34 per cent lower in the Adventists vegans.[31] In these instances, the explanation could be partly linked to the consumption of dairy and milk, which seem to increase the circulating levels of the powerful growth factor IGF-1,* a risk factor for prostate cancer, breast and colon cancer.[32]

THE SEVENTH-DAY ADVENTIST VEGETARIANS

With more than 25 million adherents, Seventh-day Adventists live in many parts of the world. In Loma Linda, a town of about 23,000 inhabitants located in San Bernardino County in California, one-third of the residents are members of the Seventh-day Adventist community. Men of this religious community reportedly live an average of 7.3 years longer than other Californians, while Seventh-day Adventist women have an advantage of 4.4 years. Mortality from cardiovascular disease, lung

---

*   Insulin-like growth factor 1 (IGF-1) is one of the most powerful growth factors. It is similar in molecular structure to insulin and participates in the growth and function of every tissue and organ of our body. Recent studies indicate that IGF-1 play a key role in cancer and ageing. Nutrition affects serum IGF-I concentrations.

cancer (given the smoking ban imposed by their faith) and colon cancer is much lower, but there is no difference in the risk of developing breast and prostate cancer.[33]

What is so different about these people? Their faith instructs them to treat the body as a temple. In particular, a Bible passage educates them to prefer plant to animal food. Genesis (1.29) says:

> *Behold, I have given you every plant yielding seed that is on the face of all the earth, and every tree with seed in its fruit. You shall have them for food.*

The result is that about 30 per cent of the Adventists are lacto-ovo vegetarians, 8 per cent vegans, 9 per cent pesco-vegetarians, 6 per cent semi-vegetarian (eat meat three to four times a month) and only 44 per cent are omnivores.

A larger study, which followed 73,000 American Adventists over six years, confirmed that compared to omnivores their mortality was lower by 9 per cent in lacto-ovo vegetarians, by 15 per cent in vegans and by 19 per cent in pesco-vegetarians.[34] In the same cohort, the risk of developing colon cancer was 6 per cent lower in vegans, 18 per cent in lacto-ovo vegetarians, and 43 per cent in pesco-vegetarians.[35]

It is important to note that nearly half of the Seventh-day Adventists practise 15 minutes or more of physical activity at least three times a week, and no one is drinking alcohol or smoking cigarettes (although some were smokers before entering this congregation). Members of the Seventh-day Adventist Church, finally, are very religious, with a strong sense of attachment to their family and community.

To summarise, being a vegetarian in itself does not mean much to one's health. A vegetarian can decide not to consume meat, but still overindulge in sweets, sweetened beverages, white bread, and many other energy-dense foods loaded with trans fatty acids, vegetable oil and salt, and spend all day in front of the TV in complete solitude, smoking cigarettes and drinking wine, beer and spirits.

A recent analysis of the American Adventists found that the mean BMI of their vegans was 24.1 (the upper limit of normal), lacto-ovo-vegetarians and pesco-vegetarians were overweight with a BMI of 26, while semi-vegetarians had a BMI of 27.3 and omnivores 28.3 respectively.[36] This demonstrates that most of these people, even vegans, consume far more calories than is optimal for staying healthy.

Let's remember that Okinawan centenarians, when they were young adults, had a BMI of 21, which is considerably lower than the 24 of vegans in this study. Excessive calorie intake, as I will explain, plays a major role in driving all sorts of chronic disease and in accelerating ageing.

IS THE HUNTER-GATHERER LIFESTYLE THE ANSWER FOR A LONG AND HEALTHY LIFE?

If orthodox vegetarians rank A+ in dietary fervency, 'Paleo diet' practitioners follow with an A-. The followers of these paleo diets claim that the transition from the nomadic life of the hunter-gatherers to that of sedentary farmers, with the introduction of cereals in the diet, marked the beginning of the decline of human health. According to their 'unsupported' theories, Palaeolithic men were lean, strong and healthy, because they were running all day long to hunt for game or fish, which formed the main part of their diet, complemented by some berries, fruits and roots.

This concept was taken to the extreme by a group of individuals living in the US, a few of whom I have studied, who consume only raw meat, unpasteurised milk and cream: they claim to follow the 'primal diet'. Those who follow this dietary regime try to imitate their ancestor's hunter-gatherer habits, favouring the consumption of lean meats (which to be honest don't exist anymore, unless people go hunting all year around), fish, vegetables and some low-glycaemic fruits. Carbohydrates from grains and legumes are strictly prohibited.

Did any of these paleo proponents ever ask themselves how long the hunter-gatherers lived? Is there any evidence in recent history of a large group of nonagenarian or centenarians among indigenous people that follow these precepts? Native Americans, such as the famous Sioux or the Blackfeet, were hunters who ate plenty of healthy lean meat of free-ranging bison and venison, lived in pristine environments and did a great deal of physical activity every day. None of these individuals to my knowledge has ever approached 90 years of age, and the same goes for many other tribes of hunters who roamed Australia, Africa and Greenland before the colonisation of the white man took place.

On the contrary, as we have already illustrated, the Okinawans and Sardinians, who lived in the same historical period (and therefore had no access to modern medical care and technology), experienced a very high rate of healthy nonagenarian and centenarians. I will explain later why a high animal fat and protein diet, especially if enriched in four essential amino acids (methionine, valine, leucine and isoleucine), is detrimental for health and longevity.

DO ELITE ATHLETES HOLD THE KEY TO LONGEVITY?

Physicians and scientists have been debating for centuries how important fitness and exercise training are for promoting health and longevity. Accumulating evidence indicates that exercise training is essential for maximising metabolic health and wellbeing, but does not promote exceptional longevity.

Data collected from 19,012 Olympic athletes show that though on average they live three years longer than sedentary people, this is not sufficient to allow them to reach centenarian status.[37] Most of the Olympians in this large study, born between 1900 and 1904, died aged around 80, despite the fact that they led healthier lives even after the end of their competitive career. An athlete normally does not smoke, follows a controlled diet (high in calories though) and has a good, or even excellent, quality of life.

Let's take, for instance, some of the cyclists who have won the Giro d'Italia or the Tour de France. None of these has ever reached 100 years of age. The famous Gino Bartali, nicknamed 'the iron man of Tuscany', died at 85 years, Alfredo Binda at 83, Philippe Thys at 81 and Roger Lapébie at 85. Louison Bobet and Jacques Anquetil, who won three and five Tours de France, died of cancer at 58 and 53 years old, respectively. We must remember that these were special men. Nature has been particularly generous with them.

No normal person, even with the hardest training, can compete at the Giro d'Italia or the Tour de France, and least of all win those races. These are unique and rare men, who are born with hearts and lungs made of steel, and iron muscles. However, none of these exceptional human beings, who are part of an elite group of supermen from the genetic and physical point of view, has never approached the life expectancy of the centenarians living in Okinawa or Sardinia.

These observations are consistent with a fantastic set of experimental data produced by John Holloszy on the effects of endurance exercise on longevity.[38] As illustrated in figure 2 below, regular endurance exercise in the form of voluntary wheel running increases average lifespan, but not maximal lifespan in rodents.

In contrast, animals that had the same body weight as the exercising rats because of dietary restriction (they were eating 30 per cent less food) experienced a big increase in both average and maximal lifespan. This means that exercise improves health, but it does not slow the ageing process per se.

John told me, in one of our long afternoon conversations in his office, that when he designed this study, he was not interested in the effects of diet on longevity; he just wanted to prove that exercise had anti-ageing effects. He decided to study calorie restriction because he needed a weight-matched control group that had similar

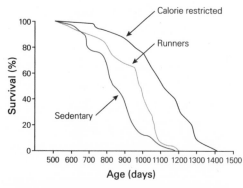

Figure 2: Calorie restriction, but not endurance exercise, increases maximal lifespan in rodents. The survival curve for sedentary control rats is significantly different from that of runners (P < 0.02), and calorie-restricted sedentary rats (P < 0.0001). The survival curve for runners is also significantly different from that of food-restricted sedentary rats (P < 0.01).[39]

weight to the exercising group. Indeed, rodents love to run on wheels, and thus, over time become super fit and lean. What is interesting about this study is that, despite the exercising rodents having much lower body fat and higher muscle mass and greater insulin sensitivity than calorie-restricted animals, they did not experience an increase in maximal longevity.

Moreover, as I will discuss later, the quantity and quality of the food that we are consuming may even interact in a detrimental way with exercise training. Data show that some elite athletes may be at higher risk of premature death, especially power athletes and overweight professional-football players. A study of 3,850 American-football athletes who died in the last century showed that offensive linemen, who are the heaviest athletes, are more than twice as likely to die before their 50th birthday as their leaner teammates.[40]

Since 1985 the average body weight in US National Football League players has increased by 10 per cent, reaching 112 kg (247 lb); and the body weight of the offensive tackle linemen has increased from 127 kg to 144 kg (280–317 lb). Overweight and obesity, due to excessive calorie and protein intake, as we will see, are major risk factors for premature death and for many of the most common chronic illnesses. Powerlifting professional athletes also have a higher mortality rate, especially those who have taken anabolic drugs.[41]

CHAPTER THREE

HEALTHSPAN AND THE MECHANISMS OF AGEING

In the last 20 years, science has made unprecedented and remarkable discoveries about the ageing pathways and processes that extend lifespan and healthspan.

It is now important to explain some of the basic mechanisms that our cells use to control the accumulation of damage, or its repair; and how these magnificent signalling pathways interconnect to slow human ageing while extending healthspan. Without understanding these basic principles, it is difficult to appreciate how human health can be manipulated in order to prevent many painful and debilitating disorders.

Healthspan is the term for the period of our life during which we are able to live without diseases, free of aches and pains, enabling us to remain independent and ultimately do what we want to do. It is a term I will use often.

WHY DO WE AGE?

Ageing is a fascinating but complex and dynamic biological process. It is characterised by progressive functional and structural deterioration of multiple cell, tissue and organ systems. As we age, the accumulation of unrepaired damage within our cells – due to the failure of the homeostatic mechanisms to completely protect or remove damage – is the key factor in the progressive decline of physical and cognitive function.[1]

Even in disease-free people, some build-up of damage with advancing age is inevitable. For instance, drying and wrinkling of the skin, thinning and greying of hair, and reductions in bone and muscle mass are universal markers of ageing.

Without looking, we can recognise with a touch of our hand the difference between the skin of a newborn and that of an old man.

Ageing is also accompanied by the replacement of normal, elastic tissue with stiffer, scar-like tissue in various organs, including the heart, arteries, lungs, and kidneys. As a consequence, cardiovascular, lung and renal function gradually decrease between the ages of 30 and 60 years, with an accelerated decline after age 70. These age-associated changes result in a reduction of physiological reserves, that are not synonymous with illness but with an increased vulnerability to challenges, that may decrease the ability to survive stressful conditions.

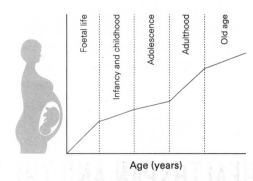

Figure 3: Accumulation of metabolic and molecular damage throughout life

It's important to understand that ageing does not itself cause chronic illnesses such as cardiovascular disease, diabetes or cancer. Instead, a persistent exposure to unhealthy lifestyles and other toxic external factors, like poor nutrition, sedentary lifestyle, psychological stress, smoking and pollution, accelerates the deterioration of organs and increases the risk of developing multiple, chronic medical conditions.

Typically, people with unhealthy lifestyles start by developing one ailment (the type varies depending on the genetic predisposition), but if they live long enough will more than likely eventually develop other chronic diseases.

DEATH IS UNAVOIDABLE, BUT A LIFE OF PROLONGED ILL-HEALTH IS NOT

Unquestionably everybody has to die, but death does not need to be painful, agonizing, or premature. Extensive evidence from experimental studies has shown that it is biologically possible to live a very long life without experiencing a cumulative increase in nasty and debilitating diseases. Twenty per cent of human centenarians do not develop any chronic illness before reaching 100.[2]

A friend of mine died at the venerable age of 107 years (one month prior to his 108th birthday) without having suffered from any major malady. Up to the age of 105 years, Arnold was still capable of driving and taking care of himself. A few months before he died, he was hospitalised with a twisted intestinal loop. While that was not the cause of his death (the problem was fixed without surgery), it was perhaps a sign that it was time for him to leave this world peacefully to begin a new journey. Like the sage Vasudeva, the ferryman of the novel *Siddhartha* by Hermann Hesse, having fully enjoyed and understood the meaning of life, Arnold began deliberately to reduce his nourishment in order to die gently in his sleep.

CAN WE PREVENT AGEING?

To date, we know of no intervention that can prevent, halt or reverse the ageing process. Nevertheless, over the past few decades we have discovered that we can slow the accumulation of damage and drastically increase healthspan. We have seen this across the animal kingdom: from worms and flies to mice; and also now in humans, as reported in a highly cited paper we have published in the journal *Science*.[3]

The most studied and reproducible intervention known to increase healthspan and lifespan is *dietary restriction* with optimal intake of vitamins and minerals. That means eating less but selecting high-quality nutritious food. Other dietary interventions that have been shown to stave off the onset of many of the diseases associated with ageing are intermittent fasting and protein and methionine-restriction (reduction of amino acids found in high concentration in animal food products), which are selective forms of dietary restriction.[4]

More recent data, collected from genetic and pharmacological studies, have confirmed that nutrition is key in slowing the accumulation of damage. Experiments in rodents, which like humans are mammals, have shown that their healthspan and lifespan can be drastically extended by inhibiting some key nutrient-sensing genes and proteins within their cells.[5] These nutrient-detectors include molecules that sense how much energy and protein are available for growth and reproduction. For example, restricting calorie or protein intake in mice or introducing mutations in nutrient-sensing pathways can extend lifespans by as much as 50 per cent.

These scientific discoveries are fantastic, because for the first time in human history we understand that ageing is not a 'wear and tear', but a highly regulated process, subject to manipulation by metabolic pathways that have been conserved during evolution. Changing a single gene within these nutrient-sensing pathways can extend lifespan dramatically, causing an animal to age normally, but just much more slowly.

IS AGEING INEXTRICABLY LINKED WITH DISEASE?

The main and striking result of these sophisticated scientific studies is that ageing and chronic diseases are **not** inextricably linked. Approximately 30 per cent of dietary-restricted rodents die at a very old age without any identifiable sign of disease.[6] Similarly, 50 per cent of mice in which we have deleted the growth hormone (GH) receptor gene, (and that as a consequence have low blood IGF-1 levels), die very old without any evidence of organ disease severe enough to be recorded as a probable cause of death.[7,8,9] They simply die of old age; probably the heart stops beating. No suffering, no pain, no medications.

Many of the diet-restricted rodents and other long-lived mutant rats or mice look like 40-year-olds when they are actually 90 or even older (in human terms). These observations are simply breathtaking!

INHIBITION OF NUTRIENT-SENSING AND INFLAMMATORY PATHWAYS PROTECTS AGAINST DAMAGE

For the scientifically minded, the best understood of these nutrient-sensing signalling pathways is the insulin/IGF-1/mTOR pathway. When food intake is reduced, levels of circulating insulin and bioavailable IGF-1 – both important growth factors – are also reduced. As a result, there is less binding to the insulin and IGF-1 receptors (present in all the cells of our body) and reduced activation of the insulin/IGF-1/mTOR signalling pathway. This leads to the activation of a key pro-longevity factor called FOXO.[10] Many remarkable things happen when activated FOXO binds to a specific site of our DNA. Among them are that it:

- activates the production of enzymes (e.g. SOD2 and catalase) that protect cells from oxidative stress
- inhibits genes and proteins that control cell proliferation. Less cell proliferation equals fewer random DNA mutations, which translates into less risk of cancer and accumulation of senescent cells. The latter are cells that have stopped dividing but remain alive in tissues where they can act like disease-causing bad apples
- triggers genes and proteins (e.g. DDB1) that increase DNA repair mechanisms, which mend the many accidental lesions that occur continually in DNA during cell division
- activates apoptosis, the cleansing suicide and renewal of cells in which DNA damage cannot be repaired, to avoid passing on the faulty DNA
- up-regulates genes and proteins that enhance autophagy, a key mechanism to remove garbage within cells, including dysfunctional and toxic proteins and organelles.

In summary, our cells become healthier, younger and more efficient in preventing and removing the accumulation of damage. See Figure 4 below.

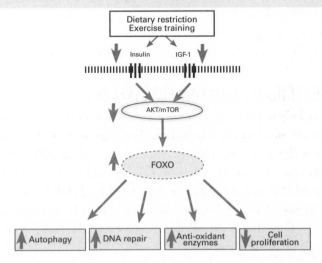

Figure 4: Effects of nutrition and exercise on cellular damage. This simplified model shows the effects of dietary restriction and endurance exercise on the insulin/IGF-1/FOXO pathway that protects against the accumulation of molecular damage.

Of course, the insulin/IGF pathway is a crucial one, but there are other signalling pathways controlled by other nutrients, for instance, the quantity and quality of protein we ingest, which interact and potentiate its anti-ageing effects. Some of these are essential to improve stress resistance or reduce inflammation that is another key factor in promoting health and longevity. All major medical conditions, including cardiovascular disease, stroke, diabetes, cancer, dementia, arthritis, and chronic liver and kidney disease, involve chronic inflammation and the activation of the immune system in the affected tissues.[11]

We will see that other lifestyle choices, including exercise, cognitive training, deep sleep and meditation, can contribute to preventing the accumulation of damage and influence the progression of multiple chronic conditions too.[12]

WHY DO PEOPLE DEVELOP CHRONIC DISEASES NOT LINKED TO AGEING ITSELF?

Modern medicine focuses on diagnosing and treating chronic diseases one at a time, mainly with drugs and surgery. We are forced to treat many of the most common chronic diseases in this way because we usually intervene after major damage has already occurred.

I use the following analogy to explain this important concept to medical students. In most cars, the timing belt, which is critical for all the internal parts of the engine to be in sync, must be replaced between 70,000 and 100,000 kilometres. If we fail to do so, the rubber belt breaks, the car stops working and we have to call a tow truck. If we are lucky, we will only need to replace a few engine valves, but in other cases the mechanic will have to partially or totally rebuild the engine. Yet simply by taking proper care of the car, we could have avoided an expensive, time-consuming operation. Unfortunately, this is how our 'sick-care' medical system works.

CHRONIC ILLNESSES HAVE COMMON CAUSES

Common, modifiable metabolic and molecular factors underlie the major chronic diseases. These factors explain the great majority of deaths for age-related illnesses at all ages, in females and males in every part of the world. As I have said, our medical system specialises in trying to fix maladies after they have occurred. The problem with this approach is that many age-associated chronic diseases begin early in life and progress over decades of unhealthy lifestyles. This triggers a wide range of physiologic, metabolic and molecular alterations that deeply influence the onset and progression of many medical conditions.[13]

The chart in figure 5 shows the interaction of many unhealthy lifestyles with chronic disease.

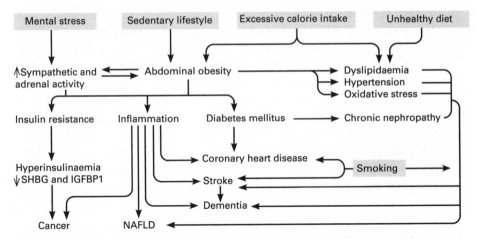

Figure 5: Unhealthy lifestyles and disease risk. The unhealthy lifestyle effectors, including excessive calorie intake, poor diets, sedentary lifestyle, mental stress, and smoking, modulate important metabolic and hormonal factors associated with the development of the most common chronic illnesses. Key: SHBG, sex hormone-binding globulin; IGFBP1, insulin-like growth factor-binding protein 1; NAFLD, nonalcoholic fatty liver disease.[14]

If we shift our focus from treatment of age-associated chronic illnesses to a general umbrella of lifestyle illnesses sharing a common metabolic and molecular cause, we can then begin to prevent the incremental build-up of molecular damage leading to these diseases.

WHY WE NEED TO FOCUS FIRST ON A BETTER LIFESTYLE

Take cardiovascular disease, for example, the leading cause of death in Western countries and now sadly also in developing ones. It takes several decades of unhealthy eating habits to develop a clinically significant build-up of a plaque in the coronary arteries, which supply oxygen and nutrients to the beating heart. Many years of high blood cholesterol and glucose, elevated blood pressure, and chronic inflammation, among other factors, are necessary before people have a heart attack or a stroke.[15]

Prescribing a statin – a cholesterol-lowering medicine – or an antihypertensive drug to a 50- or 60-year old man, who has already developed significant plaque, will reduce but not reset the risk of sudden cardiac death, heart failure or stroke. These medications can slow the progression of atherosclerotic lesions, but cannot restore the health of the arteries and heart.

Shockingly, in autopsy studies, coronary artery atherosclerotic lesions were found in three-quarters of people aged 15 to 30 years who ate a typical Western diet, and in 20 per cent of them there was a 50 per cent blockage of one or more coronary arteries. The first studies were carried out on young soldiers who died during the Korean War in 1950–53, but the results have been confirmed in road accident victims.[16]

THE FRAMINGHAM HEART STUDY

A long-term cardiovascular study of residents living in the small city of Framingham in Massachusetts, has shown that men and women with optimally low cardiovascular risk factors at 50 years of age have a very low lifetime risk of developing a heart attack and a remarkably longer survival.

- Those who had optimal levels of cholesterol, blood pressure, and glucose, a healthy body weight and were not smokers experienced a lifetime risk of cardiovascular disease of only 5 per cent.

- Having abnormal levels of one single risk factor increased the risk to 50 per cent.

- In men with two or more major risk factors the probability of developing a heart attack jumped to 69 per cent.

On average, individuals with optimally low risk factors lived more than 11 years *longer* than those with two or more abnormal risk factors.[17] Yes, 11 years! Not just a few months or a couple of years, as some detractors believe.

Unfortunately, in the Framingham study, only 4.5 per cent of women and 3.2 per cent of men had optimally low risk factors. As I will explain in this book, nutrition and exercise training have a powerful effect in optimising all these cardiometabolic risk factors.

DO YOU HAVE OPTIMAL CARDIOMETABOLIC FACTORS?

For your heart health, the optimal measurements should be:
- LDL or bad cholesterol levels of approximately 50 to 70 mg/dl (1.3-1.8 mmol/L)[18]
- fasting glucose levels less than 85 mg/dl (<4.7 mmol/L)[19]
- blood pressure below 120/80 mmHg [20]
- serum C-reactive protein (a systemic marker of inflammation) below 0.7 mg/L (6.6 nmol/L) [21]

When is the last time your doctor measured these markers?

HOW CANCER DEVELOPS

Cancer and ageing are two sides of the same coin; the metabolic and molecular mechanisms that protect against cancer are also extremely important in slowing ageing and extending healthspan and lifespan. What is underappreciated is that the metabolic alterations leading to high blood glucose, high blood pressure and low-grade chronic inflammation have a great deal in common with many other highly prevalent chronic illnesses, including cancer, the second-leading cause of death in Western countries. It is well known that overweight people have a higher risk of developing chronic illnesses. What is less known is that being overweight, especially around the abdomen, causes a long list of hormonal and immune alterations that promote tumour growth.[22]

There are exceptions, but developing a clinically detectable cancer usually takes many decades. Before a normal cell can become a malignant tumour, hundreds of mutations must accumulate in the DNA, some of which must hit genes that instruct the cell to multiply chaotically. Genes that promote uncontrolled cell proliferation must be activated, while those that trigger the suicide of irreversible mutated cells must be turned off.[23] For most tumours this process takes 30 to 40 years. This is why the risk of getting cancer increases exponentially with age.[24] The older we become, the higher the risk that we accumulate a sufficient number of DNA mutations to generate an aggressive tumour. This is why we must act to avoid the build-up of DNA replication errors.

The causes of mutations reside in our environment and include viruses, chemicals, radiation, carcinogens in food and the air, and excessive free radical levels formed during metabolic processes; for example, when our cells burn glucose and fatty acids to generate energy. Other factors such as insulin and IGF-1 promote cancer development not because they cause DNA mutations, but because they inhibit DNA repair and antioxidant cellular mechanisms, stimulate cell proliferation, and prevent the suicide of irreversible mutated cells.[25]

In the mammary gland, for example, *in situ* tumours typically take six to ten years to generate an invasive tumour, and often do not progress at all; they remain silent for decades, or may even resolve spontaneously without treatment. The same goes for lung, colon, endometrial and prostate cancer. In the prostate it is common that even an invasive tumour may remain silent for decades without symptoms and without becoming deadly.

Sometimes, however, these cancers become aggressive, and start to invade lymphatic or blood vessels, from where the malignant cells disseminate to distant organs. This is, the well-known *metastasis*, which accounts for up to 95 per cent of cancer-related deaths.[26]

We still don't know why metastasis sometimes happens and other times does not. There are more and more indications that our lifestyle affects the evolution of cancer in all its phases, with food, exercise, and mental stress being important factors.

A malignant cell, or even a tumour in the initial phase, will develop into an invasive form more easily if it finds a permissive environment, a 'fertile soil' in which the seeds (mutations) can germinate.[27] The accumulation of mutations is undoubtedly essential to cancer initiation; however, it does not appear to be sufficient for the progression of most common tumours, such as breast, colon, prostate and endometrial cancer. Although the seeds may be plentiful, they only grow if the 'soil' contains:

- available metabolic substrates (glucose and certain amino acids) to feed the hungry tumour cells

- hormones (insulin, testosterone, oestrogens, leptin), growth factors (IGF-1, TGF beta, PDFG) and inflammatory cytokines that promote cell proliferation and cancer growth

- partial suppression of immune cells that can recognise and kill tumour cells.

EXCESS BODY FAT AND CANCER RISK

If we eat more than we need, the extra calories are deposited in our fat cells, which become bigger and bigger. These large fat cells (adipocytes) produce a number of hormones, called adipokines, which cause inflammation and insulin resistance. Insulin resistance is a condition in which our cells become resistant to the signal that the hormone insulin is trying to convey, which is to move glucose from the bloodstream into our cells (to avoid high blood glucose levels and development of type 2 diabetes).

To overcome insulin resistance, the beta-cells of the pancreas produce more and more insulin. In fact, the amount of fat in our body generally correlates very well with blood insulin concentrations. The problem is that insulin is a powerful anabolic hormone that has been associated with an increased risk of developing breast, colon, pancreatic and endometrial cancers, among others.[28]

Several mechanisms are responsible for the pro-cancer effects of high insulin levels:

- High insulin levels promote cell proliferation, inhibit DNA repair and antioxidant pathways, especially in precancerous cells that express more insulin receptors than normal cells;[29]

- Hyperinsulinemia increases the bioavailability of testosterone, oestradiol and IGF-1, which are powerful growth factors that promote cancer growth as well; [30,31,32]

Recent data suggest that obesity also promotes chronic inflammation and impairs the capacity of specialised immune cells, natural killer cells and T cytotoxic lymphocytes, to recognise and kill malignant cells.[33] Finally, other factors that cannot be predicted from single-effect responses, like protective phytochemicals, toxic molecules in food and the environment, and gut microbial communities, impinge in combination on this abnormal metabolic profile to modulate tumour initiation and progression.

PART II
NOURISHING YOUR BODY

CHAPTER FOUR

THE SCIENCE OF HEALTHY NUTRITION

The power of nutrition for preventing chronic diseases and maximising health has been known since antiquity. Hippocrates of Kos (circa 460–370 BCE), the father of modern medicine, wrote in his book, *Aphorisms*:

> *When more food than is proper has been taken, it occasions disease. We must consider, also, in which cases food is to be given once or twice a day, and in greater or smaller quantities, and at intervals. Something must be conceded to habit, to season, to country and to age. ... Growing bodies have the most innate heat; they therefore require the most food, for otherwise their bodies are wasted. In old persons the heat is feeble, and therefore they require little fuel, as it were, to the flame, for it would be extinguished by much.*[1]

Sun Simiao (581–682 BCE), the most famous clinician of the Tang dynasty wrote in his treatise *Qian Jin Yao Fang* (Prescriptions Worth a Thousand in Gold for Every Emergency)[2] that both the young and the elderly should regularly consume 'natural and delicate foods like grains, legumes, vegetables and fruits'. He believed that 'vegetables should be consumed at each meal', whereas 'meat, fatty foods and refined flours should instead be limited to the minimum necessary'.

Su Shi (1037–1101 BCE), a famous physician of the Chinese Song dynasty, wrote in his treatise that to stay healthy we should eat only when hungry and stop taking food well before being completely full.[3]

The importance of the quantity and quality of the food we consume every day has finally returned to prominence in modern medicine. Solid scientific data indicate that to live a long and healthy life we need to prevent the accumulation of belly fat. How?

Well, by performing regular exercise, but most importantly by reducing the intake of foods high in empty calories, fat and animal proteins (that are rich in sulphur and branched-chain amino acids).[4]

It is of paramount importance that we also eat far more of a wide variety of minimally processed, fibre-rich foods, such as vegetables, beans, whole grains, nuts, seeds and fruit. These foods contains a unique mixture of vegetable fibres, vitamins, oligo-elements (pure trace minerals present in tiny quantities) and phytochemicals, which after being processed by our gut microbes, release a number of metabolites crucial in protection from many common diseases.[5]

In addition, the most advanced scientific research on the mechanisms of longevity suggests that for healthy people, it is important to periodically incorporate some fasting in their monthly schedule as well as to wisely distribute meals throughout the day. For instance we should ideally take in most of our calories in a limited time frame, possibly early in the day, in line with the old saying that my grandfather Natale kept repeating to me: 'Breakfast as a king, lunch as a prince and dinner as a pauper'.[6]

In the past, the main emphasis of nutrition science was the prevention of malnutrition, so establishing the recommended daily allowances for essential nutrients was the key aim. We successfully achieved this goal, as nowadays nutrient deficiencies like scurvy, pellagra and beriberi are rare in developed countries.[7]

However, other forms of malnourishment have emerged like under- and over-nutrition with foods high in 'empty' calories and low in nutrients. These are responsible for a great deal of suffering, premature death and financial cost. Examples are obesity, type 2 diabetes, hypertension, cardiovascular disease, stroke, some of the most common types of cancer, most probably dementia, and a range of allergic and autoimmune diseases.

In the following chapters, I will try to present what I believe is the best available evidence on what we should eat to maximise the probability of avoiding chronic illnesses and increase the chance of living a healthy, long life. Or, simply put, how to reach the age of 100 or more with the health of a 40-year-old.

BELLY FAT: THE ENEMY WITHIN

Around the world, scientists and physicians recognise that overweight and obese individuals are at higher risk of getting sick and ageing faster. When we habitually consume more food than what is required to move, think and maintain the basic body functions, the calorie surplus is deposited into fat cells, which become enlarged. In recent years, it has been demonstrated that these engorged fat cells are not inactive stores or passive players, but dynamic actors that produce inflammatory cytokines and a set of hormones called adipokines, which increase the risk of developing some of the most serious, debilitating and common chronic diseases.[8]

There are different ways to determine if you are overweight, obese or in the normal weight range. The simplest one is the body mass index (BMI).

DO YOU KNOW YOUR BMI?

The BMI scores give an indirect measure of body fat. As shown in the BMI chart, if your BMI is less than 18.5 kg/m^2, you are underweight. If your BMI is between 18.5 and 25, you are classified as normal weight, but if it is between 25 and 30, you are classified as overweight. If you score more than 30, you are considered to be obese.

WEIGHT lbs	90	100	110	120	130	140	150	160	170	180	190	200	210	220	230	240	250	260	270	280	290
kgs	41	45	50	54	59	64	68	73	82	86	91	95	100	104	107	109	113	118	122	127	132

Underweight · Healthy · Overweight · Obese · Extremely obese

HEIGHT ft/in	cm	90	100	110	120	130	140	150	160	170	180	190	200	210	220	230	240	250	260	270	280	290
4'8"	142.2	20	22	25	27	29	31	34	36	38	40	43	45	47	49	52	54	56	58	61	63	65
4'9"	144.7	19	22	24	26	28	30	32	35	37	39	41	43	45	48	50	52	54	56	58	61	63
4'10'	147.3	19	21	23	25	27	29	31	33	36	38	40	42	44	46	48	50	52	54	56	59	61
4'11'	149.8	18	20	22	24	26	28	30	32	34	36	38	40	42	44	46	48	51	53	55	57	59
4'12"	152.4	18	20	21	23	25	27	29	31	33	35	37	39	41	43	45	47	49	51	53	55	57
5'1"	154.9	17	19	21	23	25	26	28	30	32	34	36	38	40	42	43	45	47	49	51	53	55
5'2"	157.4	16	18	20	22	24	26	27	29	31	33	35	37	38	40	42	44	46	48	49	51	53
5'3"	160.0	16	18	19	21	23	25	27	28	30	32	34	35	37	39	41	43	44	46	48	50	51
5'4"	162.5	15	17	19	21	22	24	26	27	29	31	33	34	36	38	39	41	43	45	46	48	50
5'5"	165.1	15	17	18	20	22	23	25	27	28	30	32	33	35	37	38	40	42	43	45	47	48
5'6"	167.6	15	16	18	19	21	23	24	26	27	29	31	32	34	36	37	39	40	42	44	45	47
5'7"	170.1	14	16	17	19	20	22	24	25	27	28	30	31	33	34	36	38	39	41	42	44	45
5'8"	172.7	14	15	17	18	20	21	23	24	26	27	29	30	32	33	35	37	38	40	41	43	44
5'9"	175.2	13	15	16	18	19	21	22	24	25	27	28	30	31	33	34	35	37	38	40	41	43
5'10"	177.8	13	14	16	17	19	20	22	23	24	26	27	29	30	32	33	34	36	37	39	40	42
5'11"	180.3	13	14	15	17	18	20	21	22	24	25	27	28	29	31	32	33	35	36	38	39	40
6'0"	182.8	12	14	15	16	18	19	20	22	23	24	26	27	28	30	31	33	34	35	37	38	40
6'1"	185.4	12	13	15	16	17	18	20	21	22	24	25	26	28	29	30	32	33	34	36	37	38
6'2"	187.9	12	13	14	15	17	18	19	21	22	23	24	26	27	28	30	31	32	33	35	36	37
6'3"	190.5	11	13	14	15	16	18	19	20	21	23	24	25	26	28	29	30	31	33	34	35	36
6'4"	193.0	11	12	13	15	16	17	18	19	21	22	23	24	26	27	28	29	30	32	33	34	35
6'5"	195.5	11	12	13	14	15	17	18	19	20	21	23	24	25	26	27	28	30	31	32	33	34
6'6"	198.1	10	12	13	14	15	16	17	18	20	21	22	23	24	25	27	28	29	30	31	32	34
6'7"	200.6	10	11	12	14	15	16	17	18	19	20	21	23	24	25	26	27	28	29	30	32	33
6'8"	203.2	10	11	12	13	14	15	16	18	19	20	21	22	23	24	25	26	27	29	30	31	32
6'9"	205.7	10	11	12	13	14	15	16	17	18	19	20	21	23	24	25	26	27	28	29	30	31
6'10"	208.2	9	10	12	13	14	15	16	17	18	19	20	21	22	23	24	25	26	27	28	29	30
6'11"	210.8	9	10	11	12	13	14	15	16	17	18	19	20	21	22	23	25	26	27	28	29	30

Table 1: Body mass index calculator

To calculate your BMI you need to know your weight and your height. Divide your weight in kilos (kg) by your height in metres (m). Then divide the answer by your height again to get your BMI.

For example:

If you weigh 70 kg and you're 1.75 m tall, divide 70 by 1.75 – the answer is 40; then divide 40 by 1.75: your BMI is 22.9 kg/m^2, which is considered a normal weight for that height.

If you are using pounds and inches, either use a metric converter or apply this formula: weight (lb) x 0.45 / height (in) x 0.025 / height (in) x 0.025.

For example:

If you weigh 125 lb and you're 5'3", multiply 125 for 0.45 (the metric conversion factor), the answer is 56.25 kg; then multiply the height 63 inches by 0.025 (the metric conversion factor), the answer is 1.575 m; now divide 56.25 by 1.575 – the answer is 35.7; then divide 35.7 by 1.575: your BMI is 22.6 kg/m².

WHY IS IT IMPORTANT TO HAVE A NORMAL BMI?

As an example, the risk of developing type 2 diabetes, a silent but dangerous medical condition that damages heart, kidneys, retina and brain, rises exponentially with increasing BMI. In a study conducted at Harvard University, the risk of developing diabetes in women who are at the higher end of normal BMI (22–23.9) was 3.6 times the risk of those with BMI less than 22.[9] Gaining 2 units of BMI from 22 to 24 is not that difficult! For a woman who is 1.7 metres (5 ft 6 in) tall, that means gaining an extra 5 kg (11 lb).

However, if instead of gaining 2 units the same woman gains 9 units, and her BMI over a period of several years climbs up to 31, the risk of developing type 2 diabetes jumps an astonishing 40 times higher. For this hypothetical woman, this would mean going from 64 kg to 90 kg (141–198 lb), something unfortunately not so unusual. According to data from the 2013–2014 National Health and Nutrition Examination Survey (NHANES), approximately 40 per cent of middle-aged women in the US are obese.[10] Similar figures can be found in Australia, UK, and many other countries.[11]

Even in men a 5-unit increment in BMI (from 21 to 26) has been shown to be associated with a four times higher risk of diabetes.[12]

Because excess fat is also associated with elevated blood pressure, cholesterol, triglycerides and glucose, it is not surprising that the risk of heart attack also rises with increasing BMI.[13] Starting from a BMI of 21, the risk of heart attack increases by 10 per cent for every extra unit of BMI.[14] If a 1.8 metre (5.9 feet) tall man increases his weight from 68 kg to 100 kg (149–220 lb), this becomes a 100 per cent higher risk of heart disease.

The probability of developing a stroke, a condition with devastating consequences (e.g. paralysis of a limb, vision loss), or heart failure grows with weight gain as well.[15] For example, the risk of stroke in women with a BMI greater than 27 is 75 per cent higher than in women of the same age with a BMI of less than 21.[16]

Excess fat in overweight and obese men and women is also associated with a higher risk of developing most of the common cancers in industrialised countries.

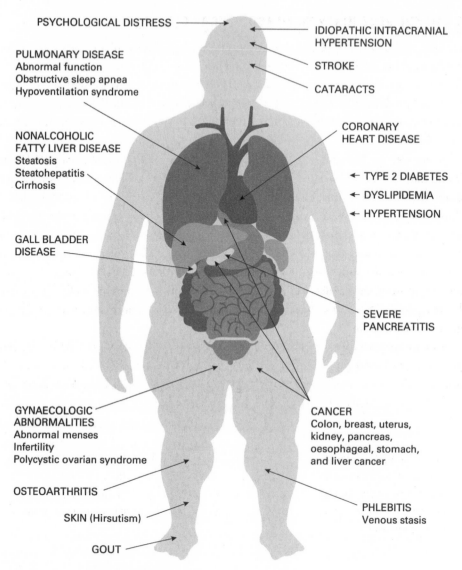

PSYCHOLOGICAL DISTRESS

IDIOPATHIC INTRACRANIAL HYPERTENSION

PULMONARY DISEASE
Abnormal function
Obstructive sleep apnea
Hypoventilation syndrome

STROKE

CATARACTS

NONALCOHOLIC FATTY LIVER DISEASE
Steatosis
Steatohepatitis
Cirrhosis

CORONARY HEART DISEASE

TYPE 2 DIABETES

DYSLIPIDEMIA

HYPERTENSION

GALL BLADDER DISEASE

SEVERE PANCREATITIS

GYNAECOLOGIC ABNORMALITIES
Abnormal menses
Infertility
Polycystic ovarian syndrome

CANCER
Colon, breast, uterus, kidney, pancreas, oesophageal, stomach, and liver cancer

OSTEOARTHRITIS

SKIN (Hirsutism)

PHLEBITIS
Venous stasis

GOUT

Figure 6: Medical complications of obesity

But that's not all. As shown in figure 6, overweight and obese people have a higher risk of developing many other illnesses, including obstructive sleep apnoea, polycystic ovarian syndrome, pancreatitis, gallstones and non-alcoholic fatty liver disease.[17] Once a rare medical disorder in the past, fatty liver disease is now the leading cause of chronic liver disease in obese patients, and may progress to cirrhosis and liver cancer.[18] Finally, carrying excess weight markedly shortens healthy life expectancy; being overweight in midlife is associated with a reduced chance of healthy survival to age 85 or older.[19]

IS BMI THE BEST INDEX TO MEASURE BODY FATNESS?

Unfortunately, even if BMI is a good start to assessing your health status, you cannot rely on it, because this is a very crude measurement of body fatness. A sedentary office clerk may display an abundance of body fat despite being in the normal BMI range, while a body builder or a heavy construction worker may be classified as overweight, despite having very low body fat and a normal metabolic health, because of substantial muscularity.[20]

Moreover, in a recent study that we conducted in collaboration with Professor Frank Hu, the Chair of the Department of Nutrition at Harvard University, we found that having a normal BMI, by itself, is not a guarantee of good health.[21] Many people in our Western societies, especially as they get older, lose weight and become lean not because of healthy eating and exercise training, but because of chronic accumulation of metabolic and inflammatory damage caused by long-term exposure to smoking, a sedentary lifestyle, and unhealthy diets. Have you ever noticed those older adults with skinny arms and legs and some belly fat. These thinner people have the same higher risk of cardiovascular and cancer mortality as obese individuals do.

In contrast, we found that slender men and women (those with a BMI between 18.5 and 22.4) who did not smoke, ate healthier diets and exercised for at least 30 minutes five days a week had a 60 per cent lower mortality risk than normal weight and overweight people with unhealthy lifestyles.

IT IS NEVER TOO LATE TO START LIVING A HEALTHIER LIFE

People who are currently overweight or obese should not despair. Our data indicate that even in overweight and obese individuals, eating healthier diets, exercising regularly and avoiding smoking can dramatically reduce their risk of chronic disease and premature death.[22]

THE IMPORTANCE OF MONITORING OUR BODY WEIGHT

An important habit we need to adopt is to monitor changes in our body weight, even if we have a normal BMI. Weight gain after age 18 is a strong predictor of morbidity and mortality, independent of current BMI.

For instance, compared with women of stable weight, the risk of developing coronary heart disease increases by 25 per cent among women who gain 5 to 8 kg (11–18 lb), and doubles in those who gain 11 to 19 kg (24–42 lb).[23] Moreover, for every 1 kg (2.2 lb) increase of weight gain after the age of 18, the odds of living a long and healthy life have been estimated to decrease by 5 per cent.[24]

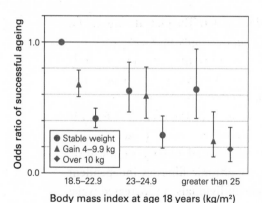

Figure 7: Weight gain in midlife related to healthy survival after 70 in women.[26]

In another study, weight gain during adulthood was associated with decreased odds of being healthy after the age of 70 (Fig. 7). Even a moderate weight gain of 4 to 10 kg (9–22 lb) was significantly associated with lower chances of healthy survival.[25] The highest risk for unhealthy survival was found among women who were overweight at age 18 and gained more than 10 kg (22 lb).

Except for a very limited number of body builders and athletes, considerable weight gain is largely due to fat accumulation. We should keep a vigilant eye on our weight, keeping it low and similar to what we had when we were practising sport in our late teens. Whenever you gain a couple of kilograms, take immediate action to bring your body weight back to the original set point. If you wait and let it spiral out of control, it will be much more difficult to reset it to normal.

Our body weight responds to a reduction of calorie intake slowly, especially in people who are very overweight, for whom reaching their new steady-state weight will take much longer than it would for those with lower initial body fat.[27] In summary, remember that preventing weight gain is more important than weight loss because once an individual becomes overweight or obese, it is harder to achieve long-term weight loss and therefore maintain an ideal weight.

WATCH YOUR WAIST, NOT JUST YOUR WEIGHT

I said earlier BMI is a crude and potentially misleading measure of body fatness. It can be used as an initial assessment, but that's all. Indeed, what is important

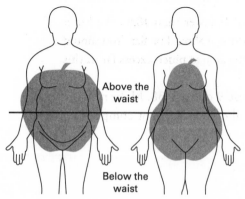

Figure 8: Apple versus pear fat distribution

is *where* fat is located. Many studies have shown that fat distribution is a much stronger predictor of metabolic health than body weight and BMI. Belly fat is the real enemy, the one that is associated with numerous detrimental metabolic conditions, including low-grade chronic inflammation.[28]

You have probably noticed that typically when men eat too much and lead a sedentary life, the calorie surplus accumulates centrally as abdominal fat. In women, instead, it gets predominantly deposited in the much 'hated' hips and thighs (gluteal–femoral adipose tissue depots). Figure 8 shows this 'apple' shape and 'pear' shape distributions of fat. The gluteal–femoral fat is metabolically less active and may be even protective, especially in the elderly.[29]

However, this sex-specific fat distribution, for reasons that are not yet fully understood, is rapidly changing, with more and more women and girls now also developing belly fat. If you do not believe me, look around you.

Multiple studies have shown that the accumulation of abdominal fat, especially the fat stored within the abdominal cavity – known as visceral fat – is the unhealthiest. Consistent evidence indicates that abdominal obesity significantly predicts the development of, and death from, many chronic illnesses independent of body weight. Indeed, even among normal-weight individuals, an increased waist circumference has been shown to be associated with a bigger risk of developing type 2 diabetes, and increased risk of death for both cardiovascular disease and cancer.[30,31]

SIMPLE WAYS TO ASSESS WHETHER YOU HAVE ABDOMINAL OBESITY

Measuring your waist circumference is an accurate marker of fat stored in the abdomen. But also ask yourself these questions:

- Has the size of your pants or skirt increased since you were in your late teens?

- How many sizes have you increased by?

- Did you need to add new holes to your belt?

If the answer to these questions is 'yes', then you have a degree of abdominal obesity.

WHAT IS A HEALTHY WAIST CIRCUMFERENCE?

Well, unlike for body weight (you do not want a BMI lower than 18.5), the lower your waist measurement, the better. Ideally, your abdomen should be flat. You should be able to see your abdominal muscle, or at least not be able to pinch excess fat. If this is not the case, check your waist measurement.

Using a flexible tape, measure as shown in figure 9 on page 38. Make sure the tape is parallel to the floor and snug around the abdomen, but not compressing the skin.

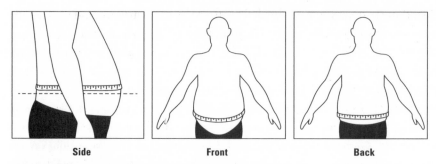

| Side | Front | Back |

Figure 9: How to position the tape to measure your waist circumference.[32]

How do your numbers stack up?

For people living in North America, the international guidelines recommend keeping waist circumference under 88 cm (34½ in) in females and 102 cm (40 in) in males. For Europeans and Asians, the criteria are much more austere. The recommended waist-size threshold for Australian and European males should be below 94 cm (37 in) and for females under 80 cm (31½ in). The cut-off for Chinese and South Asian men and women is 90 cm (35½ in) and 80 cm (31½ in) respectively.[33]

The average difference in body frame between a Vietnamese and a US woman is evident, but can we justify such a wide range of threshold for waist circumference? Probably not. Data from epidemiological studies suggest that even in the US, the ideal waistline should be much lower than the one currently recommended.

Professor Frank Hu from the Harvard School of Public Health has noted that a waist circumference of less than 71 cm (28 in) in early adulthood/midlife is associated with a very high probability of healthy survival at age 70.[34] In this study, healthy survivors were defined as women who lived beyond age 70, free from major chronic conditions, and had no major impairments of cognitive or physical function, and were in good mental shape.

In contrast, only 66 per cent of the women who at age 50 had a waistline between 76 and 80 cm (30–31½ in), and considered normal in the US, did not suffer from any illness when they reached 70 years of age. So in short, based on the available data, we should aim to keep our waist circumference as low as possible, while working hard to preserve muscle mass.

LET'S TAKE ACTION TO REDUCE OUR WAIST CIRCUMFERENCE

If you carry extra weight, especially around the belly, what should you do? What is the scientific evidence that losing weight and reducing the waistline will improve not only your silhouette and self-esteem, but metabolic health as well? How long will it take and what is the best way to achieve your goals? These are some of the questions asked by my patients every day.

The first thing to do, if you have decided to take action, is to measure and record both waistline and body weight in a personal health diary. To improve accuracy, it is better to take the measurements in the morning, when you wake up, after you have emptied your bladder, wearing only your underclothing. Then, schedule on your smartphone a reminder for remeasuring them once a month. This is already a good start!

Now you need to start to change your lifestyle. The good news is that as soon as you notice your waist shrinking, even one centimetre, you should rejoice because you have decreased the amount of harmful visceral fat trapped in the abdominal cavity. Even better, you have also increased the concentrations of a powerful anti-diabetic hormone called adiponectin, and reduced the levels of inflammatory molecules and other hormones, which increase the risk of hypertension, heart attack, stroke, cancer and, most likely, dementia. Stay on this path, reducing your waistline bit by bit, by following the advice I will give: your body will be grateful!

WHAT WILL HAPPEN WITH A REDUCTION IN WAIST CIRCUMFERENCE?

It has been shown that a reduction in waist circumference associated even with a modest 8–10 per cent weight loss greatly improves metabolic health and decreases the risk of developing multiple illnesses.[35] In a clinical trial we carried out at Washington University with 48 middle-aged overweight men and women, we found that an 8–10 per cent weight loss induced by calorie restriction or endurance exercise training over one year resulted in a striking 37–39 per cent reduction in visceral fat mass (measured by magnetic resonance imaging) (see figure 10).[36] This reduction in abdominal fat was also associated with major improvements in multiple cardiometabolic, hormonal and inflammatory factors[37,38] and cardiac function.[39]

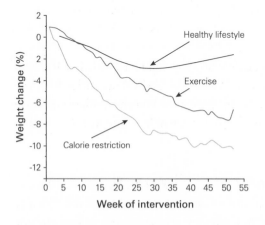

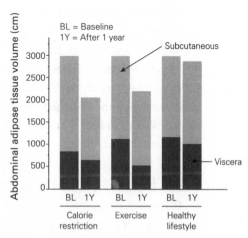

Figure 10: Body weight change throughout one year intervention. Visceral (black bars) and subcutaneous (white bars) abdominal fat by magnetic resonance imaging at baseline and after 1 year of calorie restriction, exercise training or healthy lifestyle.[40]

This amount of weight loss can even 'cure' diabetes. In the UK DiRECT trial, two thirds of patients affected by type 2 diabetes who lost at least 10 kg (22 lb) remained in remission after two years from the beginning of the dietary weight loss program.[41] Not only were their blood glucose levels normalised and all type 2 diabetes medications stopped, but their insulin levels and amount of fat in their liver and pancreas also returned to normal.

In another large trial conducted in Havana, Cuba, 90 per cent of overweight and obese patients with non-alcoholic fatty liver disease who lost more than 10 per cent of their body weight had a complete resolution of the disease, and incredibly, 45 per cent of them even had a regression of liver fibrosis.[42]

Losing 10 per cent of your body weight is not that difficult. For someone who weighs 90 kg (198 lb) that means dropping 9 kg (20 lb), which is typically associated with a substantial decrease in visceral abdominal fat.

HOW FAST SHOULD YOU LOSE WEIGHT?

An ideal and healthy plan for weight loss is to attain a slow and progressive 10 per cent drop in body weight over a six to 12-month period. In overweight and mildly obese individuals, a calorie restriction of 300–500 calories per day should result in weight reductions of about 0.25–0.5 kg (0.5–1.1 lb) per week.

However, counting calories is not easy. In the following chapters, I will provide you with some tips on how to modify your diet to achieve a healthy and successful decrease in calorie intake, without the need for weighing food and counting calories. If you can achieve this goal and maintain it for at least six months, you can consider losing further weight.

Sudden and larger drops in body weight are not associated with more favourable outcomes at the end of one year. Unless there is a medical reason to do so, I do not recommend very low-calorie diets (that is less than 800 cal/day) because there is a risk of developing serious nutritional inadequacies. Several studies have shown that rapid weight loss is almost invariably followed by regaining weight and a higher risk of serious complications, including gallstones, pancreatitis and electrolyte abnormalities.

HOW CAN YOU STOP PUTTING THE WEIGHT BACK ON?

For most people the real challenge is not shedding a few kilograms and reducing their waist circumference, but avoiding regaining the lost weight. Successful weight maintenance is defined as regaining less than 3 kg (7 lb) over two years and sustaining a decrease in waist circumference of at least 4 cm (1½ in).

> How many times have you successfully lost 10 kg (22 lb) or even 20 kg (44 lb), and then regained it with extra interest?
>
> Do you know why this happens?

One of the main reasons is the diet-induced drop in a key thyroid hormone, called triiodothyronine or T3. In several studies, my research group has shown that restricting calorie intake is always associated with a reduction in circulating T3 levels, even in young non-obese individuals.[43] The problem is that lower serum T3 causes a slowdown of your body's metabolism (resting metabolic rate), which predisposes a person to weight regain.

But there is a trick to avoid this! We have shown that similar reductions in body weight induced by endurance exercise training does not reduce T3.[44,45] This explains why a well-designed endurance and resistance exercise training program should always be prescribed as an integral component of any weight loss and maintenance program.

But that's not all, as you will see later, both the composition of your diet and the type of bacteria living in your gut may influence the metabolic response to weight loss itself.[46] From a metabolic standpoint, a calorie is not a calorie! But more on that later.

BEYOND WEIGHT LOSS: SUCCESSFUL AGEING

Our society has become obsessed with losing weight. Every few months there is a new diet craze: from low-fat to low-carb, the ketogenic diet, the 5:2 diet and so on; the weight-loss fad diets come and go on the internet, in magazines and on best-seller lists. Even among researchers there is an everlasting diet war, with different factions promoting high-protein, low-fat, paleo, vegan, keto, and a seemingly endless list of other diets. These conflicts have created public confusion and a mistrust of nutrition science.

The concept of successful ageing or healthy longevity goes well beyond weight loss alone. As we will see, people can lose weight without any metabolic benefit or, in some cases, with detrimental health consequences. So, in this book I want to divert your attention from diets to lose weight to adopting an integrated and comprehensive healthy lifestyle to maximise health and longevity. The real question we should ask is not 'How can I drop some extra kilos', but 'How can I avoid developing chronic diseases as I age, and possible live a much longer and healthier life?'

CHAPTER FIVE

LONGEVITY EFFECTS OF RESTRICTING CALORIES AND FASTING

There is now no doubt that the most powerful intervention to slow ageing and prevent the build-up of metabolic and molecular damage is calorie restriction without malnutrition.

My interest in calorie restriction started in 1990, when I read an article by Professors Roy Walford and Richard Weindruch on the amazing longevity benefits of limiting food intake in mice.[1] I wanted to understand more about this fascinating topic, but I soon realised that no one was working on this subject where I was studying, at Verona Medical School in Italy.

As soon as I finished my residency in internal medicine and started a PhD in metabolism, I wrote to Professor Weindruch, one of the world leading authorities on calorie restriction in mice, and asked about a postdoctoral position in his laboratory. He replied that his lab was working only on animal models, and suggested that I contact Professor John Holloszy, who had just been awarded a large government grant to study calorie restriction in humans. So, I did! Professor Holloszy invited me to join his lab, and this is how my scientific career was launched.

CALORIE RESTRICTION IN RODENTS: THE FOUNTAIN OF YOUTH

Since the seminal paper of Professor Charles McCay in 1935,[2] hundreds of experiments have been conducted on several animal species, which have demonstrated that a 20–40 per cent reduction in calorie intake without malnutrition (i.e. with sufficient vitamins and minerals) causes a proportionate 20–50 per cent increase in lifespan.[3]

This is equivalent to a human lifespan of 120 years and beyond.

Data from studies conducted in laboratory rodents and monkeys, found that calorie restriction increases longevity by preventing or delaying the occurrence of the vast majority of chronic degenerative diseases associated with ageing.[4] For instance, a 15–53 per cent reduction in calorie intake causes an equal linear 20–62 per cent reduction in incidence of cancer, the main cause of death in rodents.[5] The protective effect is so powerful that it is also effective on tumours that have been induced by radiation and carcinogenic chemicals.

The amazing finding is that a third of these long-lived animals do not develop any signs

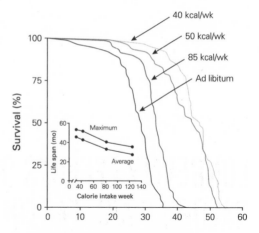

Figure 11: Calorie restriction and survival. Effects of different degree of calorie restriction on lifespan in mice. The maximal lifespan (inset) is the mean survival for the longest-lived decile of each group.[6]

of disease;[7] they die of old age without pain and suffering. Calorie restriction works not only in 'normal' disease-free animals, but also in those affected by other diseases, including progeria, a rare genetic disorder of accelerated ageing. Children born with progeria typically die in their mid-teens to early twenties. In these 'progeria' mice, calorie restriction increases lifespan three-fold and markedly retards numerous aspects of accelerated ageing, including the loss of neurons and motor function.[8]

Professor Jan Hoeijmakers from the Erasmus Medical Centre in Rotterdam, who conducted these important studies in rodents, told me about some preliminary and encouraging data in children affected by progeria. It seems they respond very well to a moderate reduction of calorie intake, with reported drastic improvements in behaviour, neurological symptoms and cognitive function.

CALORIE RESTRICTION IN MONKEYS: AGE RECORD-BREAKERS

Yeast, worms, flies and mice are very useful experimental models to study longevity, because they live much shorter lives than humans. However, the physiological differences between them and us are extensive. A better model is non-human primates, in particular rhesus monkeys, which share 93 per cent of our genetic heritage and undergo many of the same age-related adaptations in anatomy, physiology and behaviour, while exhibiting a shorter lifespan. A rhesus monkey lives on average 26 years, and has a maximum lifespan in captivity of about 40 years.[9]

In the late 1980s, two trials began in the US to determine the effect of 30 per cent calorie restriction with adequate intake of vitamins and minerals in rhesus monkeys.

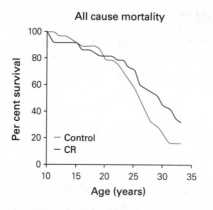
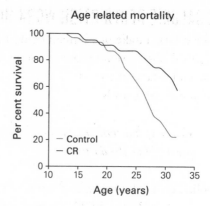

Figure 12: Effects of 30% calorie restriction in Rhesus monkeys.[10]

The results are striking. They show that moderate calorie restriction significantly extends the lifespan of monkeys, with some of the subjects breaking all known records for macaques' longevity. One-third of the calorie-restricted monkeys in the National Institute of Aging trial have lived beyond 40 years of age, which is equivalent to more than 120 years in humans.

Not only did these monkeys live much longer, but they were also much healthier. They experienced a drastic decline in the incidence of cancer and cardiovascular diseases, and were free of type 2 diabetes and even prediabetes.[11]

Most extraordinary was a monkey, named Sherman, who lived to 43 years – a longevity record for his species in captivity, and comparable to 129 years for humans.[12] Sherman lived the equivalent of seven years longer than Jeanne Louise Calment, the oldest human whose age has ever been recorded, who died at 122 years and 164 days.

While younger monkeys fed as much as they liked (or *ad-libitum* from Latin 'at one's pleasure') started to develop diseases and died, Sherman and many other calorie-restricted monkeys seemed to be immune to ageing. They looked remarkably younger – with less sagging skin and more hair that remained brown instead of grey.

In addition, these animals exhibited a slower decline of their brain and muscle mass, as well as reduced hearing loss with age.[13,14] A new study from Prof Weindruch's group shows that weakness, poor endurance, slowness and frailty were significantly lower in old calorie-restricted monkeys than in *ad-libitum* fed monkeys.[15] It disproves the scientifically unsupported claim of many physicians and scientists that calorie restriction increases the risk of muscle loss and frailty.

DOES CALORIE RESTRICTION WORK IN HUMANS?

That the calorie intake of a human could have a key role in health and longevity was an empirical observation already made in antiquity, although the ancient physicians did not understand the mechanisms. An inscription dated 3800 BCE found at the Egyptian pyramids reads:

> *Men may live with a quarter of what they eat; with the other three*
> *quarters live the doctors.*

The politician Lu Buwei, who lived in China during the last years of the Warring States period (453–221 BCE), wrote in his book that 'an indulgence in food and drink brings the ills in a swarm' and the Chinese scholar Zhang Hua of the Jin dynasty (265–420 CE) said that:

> *The less one eats, the broader his mind and the longer his life span; the*
> *more one eats the narrower his mind and the shorter his life span.*[16]

Eighteen years of clinical studies that I have conducted in my laboratory at Washington University have confirmed the importance of moderating the intake of calories in maximising health in both men and women.[17] A 20–30 per cent reduction of calorie intake, but with an optimal supply of all the necessary vitamins and minerals, radically improves multiple cardiovascular risk factors in people who were accustomed to eating typical Western diets. Blood pressure, for instance, even in those in their late 70s, is 110/70 mm of mercury: comparable to that of a child! It is simply not true that with passing years the systolic pressure will inevitably rise. It is just an unfortunate and avoidable consequence of a Western lifestyle.[18]

Similarly, it is not true that elevated cholesterol is determined primarily by genetic factors. In fact, total cholesterol in these people practising calorie restriction with optimal nutrition is very low, averaging 160 mg/dl, while the HDL-cholesterol (the 'good' cholesterol), is very high, averaging 65 mg/dl; and the latter in some of these people went from 35 mg/dl to 120 mg/dl.[19] This is fantastic, because we have found that in centenarians, a high HDL-cholesterol is one of the most reliable markers of longevity.[20] Their blood glucose is very low (average 80 mg/dl) and C-reactive protein is almost undetectable.[21]

Based on these numbers and the absence of atherosclerotic plaques in their carotid arteries, we know that the odds of these calorie-restricted practitioners having a heart attack or a stroke are virtually zero.[22] These findings have been recently confirmed by a two-year randomised clinical trial that we conducted in the US on 218 slightly overweight men and women. We found that a mild 13 per cent reduction of calorie intake markedly improved all cardiometabolic risk factors beyond normal levels even in young 20- to 50-year old individuals.[23] In addition, with a series of more sophisticated tests, we demonstrated that long-term calorie restriction prevents the age-dependent stiffening of heart and arteries.[24,25] The heart function of these individuals who decreased their average daily calorie intake to about 1800 calories is similar to that of people 15 to 20 years younger.[26]

There is no drug with similar effects across such a wide range of cardiovascular factors. We should remember that our hospitals are full of patients with vascular diseases, which are the leading cause of mortality; 35–40 per cent of deaths are due to these almost preventable illnesses.

CALORIE RESTRICTION FACTS FOR THE SCIENTIFICALLY MINDED

In humans the benefits of calorie restriction are not limited to the cardiovascular system but extend to a wide range of factors implicated in the development and progression of several common tumours and in the biology of ageing itself. For instance, we discovered that, as in long-lived calorie restricted animals, blood levels of insulin, free IGF-1, oestradiol, testosterone and T3 are low, while adiponectin and cortisol are high.[27-30] Some of these favourable adaptations have been confirmed in a series of clinical trials, including a drastic reduction in several markers of inflammation and oxidative stress.[31,32]

Finally, we have found that the improvement in these metabolic parameters are mirrored in cellular and molecular biomarkers that previous research in cells and animals has linked with slowing of ageing and prevention of cancer. These improvements include:

- an inhibition of multiple inflammatory pathways[33]
- an activation of cellular pathways that help recycle molecular debris and remove toxic misfolded proteins and malfunctioning organelles[34]
- an elevation of enzymes that protects cells against the damage of free radicals[35,36]
- an increased level of genes that repair DNA damage and chromosomal flaws[37]
- a drastic reduction in markers of cell senescence.[38]

Many factors can drive cells into senescence, including high levels of blood glucose and unrepaired DNA damage. Senescent cells, also referred to as 'zombie' cells, can accumulate in many tissues where they secrete inflammatory, protein-destroying, stem-cell-poisoning, and other cancer-promoting factors.

The incredible thing is that none of these individuals in our study, even those who were already 80 years old, take any drugs; they are all free of disease. It might surprise you that they eat huge amounts of food, and not tiny portions, as you might expect. Every day they consume many varieties of vegetables, some beans and whole grains, with the addition of nuts, seeds, fish or sometime pastured raised organic poultry. All of them have cut refined and processed foods from their diets. No sweets, sugary drinks, white bread or rice, and canned or pre-packaged foods are allowed in their diet. As we will discuss later, their high-quality diets may explain, at least in part, some of the beneficial effects on metabolic and cardiovascular health.

TOO MUCH CALORIE RESTRICTION CAN BE DANGEROUS

We need to be careful not to overdo calorie restriction; it can be dangerous, especially if you don't know what you are doing. Excessive calorie restriction can cause side effects, such as increased cold sensitivity, lower libido, menstrual irregularities and excessive loss of bone mass. It is also likely the calorie requirements needed to maximise health vary from person to person, and by factors like age, gender, levels of physical activity and genetic constitution.

In fact, recent studies have shown that in some strains of laboratory mice a calorie restriction of 40 per cent increases life expectancy in some, but in others this restriction level is too high, and 20 per cent calorie restriction is sufficient to extend lifespan.[39]

Recent experiments indicate we probably don't need to undergo a severe regimen of calorie restriction to live a long and healthy life. A combination of other less drastic interventions may lead to similar or better results.

TRICKS TO CONTROL CALORIE INTAKE
After many years of research, I came up with these easy tricks to control calorie intake:
- substitute refined and processed foods with plenty of foods rich in vegetable fibre
- stop eating before becoming full (satiated)
- once or twice a week, eat only non-starchy raw or cooked vegetables dressed with extra-virgin olive oil;
- consume most food within a restricted time frame, e.g. 8-10 hours
- eat your food slowly

WAYS TO CONTROL CALORIES, WITHOUT COUNTING

Counting calories is not easy. It requires a kitchen scale, nutritional software and, most importantly, a lot of patience and perseverance. Very few people have the knowledge, the time or discipline to perform this task day after day, meal after meal. Moreover, these nutritional software programs wrongly assume that an apple grown in New South Wales has the same nutritional value and calorie content as an apple matured in California or Spain.

We need something easier, which does not disrupt our life and take away the joy of eating and cooking a variety of foods that nourish body and mind.

THE IMPORTANCE OF REPLACING 'JUNK' WITH HEALTHY PLANT-BASED FOODS

Eating away from home in restaurants, fast-food outlets and cafeterias, and getting take-out meals has increased dramatically in many developed and developing countries. At home and away-from-home people increasingly eat highly processed and animal-derived food, which comprise a growing proportion of their overall daily calorie intake. This is the primary culprit behind the epidemic of obesity and related diseases. In contrast, many of the studies we have conducted so far show that eating plenty of food rich in vegetable fibres is the best, healthiest and easiest way to control calories, lose weight and improve metabolic health.[40]

This is a powerful tool, even for maintaining an ideal body weight as we age. Some studies have shown that just substituting refined with minimally processed plant food causes weight loss. For instance, during a five-month study, women following a fibre-rich Mediterranean diet lost 4 kg (almost 9 lb) without having to count calories.[41]

However, this was not a study where food quantities were monitored and we do not know whether the participants who lost weight ate less food as well. In order to answer this question, I designed a study where we asked people to maintain a stable body weight, while eating a diet with the same number of calories in which meat and junk food had been removed, and substituted with minimally processed plant food and fish.

For two months, our metabolic kitchen fed our research volunteers lunches and dinners of whole grains, whole-wheat bread, beans, nuts, and vegetables dressed with extra-virgin olive oil. Breakfast was composed of low-fat yogurt, oat porridge, nuts, and fruit. Fish was provided three times a week and poultry only once a week. Red meat and processed foods containing trans-fatty acids, refined carbohydrates and sugar – such as white bread, ice cream, snacks and soft drinks – were not allowed.

The fibre intake of this diet was 45 g per day, which is three times higher than the average intake of the typical Western diet. By design, in the first part of this study, we asked our participants to refrain from losing weight, because I wanted to study the metabolic adaptation to a high-quality diet (similar to the traditional Mediterranean diet, which my grandparents were consuming) in the absence of weight loss. To achieve this goal, my dieticians not only had to calculate the calorie requirement at baseline and provide an adequate and individualised number of calories for each participant, but we had to overfeed them, because most of our volunteers otherwise were losing weight quite rapidly. We calculated that, on average, we had to feed them a daily surplus of 200–300 calories in order to keep their body weight stable.

Natural fibre-rich foods, such as vegetables, whole grains and legumes induce an early feeling of satiety (because of slower gastric emptying and small bowel transit), and are also an excellent source of vitamins, phytocompounds and minerals essential to health. It's easy to slurp a dish of white rice in a few minutes, but how much brown rice can we eat before feeling satiated? The same goes for meat or cheese. One serving of 100 g (3½ oz) of Parmesan cheese contains about 384 calories (28 g fat, 0 g carbohydrates and fibre, and 33 g protein), while the same amount of cooked chickpeas contains only 164 calories (2.6 g fat, 27 g of carbohydrates, of which 7 g is fibre and 9 g protein).

In summary, it is important to clean up your diet; get rid of the processed and refined food products and begin eating real food.

LEAVE THE TABLE WHEN YOU ARE 80 PER CENT FULL

Another trick to control calorie intake (in combination with the improvement in diet quality) is to stop eating before you feel full. Many people keep eating, despite being completely satiated, because they want to empty their big plate. Instead, we should stop much earlier than that, when we start feeling gratified, but we are not satiated yet.

Li Yu (1611–1680), a doctor of the Qing dynasty, wrote:

> *Eat until you reach 70 per cent of hunger; this is the right time [to stop].*
> *It is a little too soon before that, and a little late after this point. It is*
> *like watering: water quantity must be calibrated to the size of seedlings*
> *of cereals; just what is needed to meet demand, and nothing more. Too*
> *much water will damage the plants growing. This is the right way for*
> *preserving health.*[42]

Chu Renhuo, Chinese doctor and contemporary of Li Yu, added:

> *Even when the lack of food exceeds the limit of 70 per cent for different*
> *and complicated reasons, it would be better to eat too little than to*
> *violate the rule of eating too much.*[43]

A little farther East, in Japan, traditionally home to some of the world's longest-lived human beings, a Confucian saying *'Hara hachi bun me'* educated people to eat until they are 80 per cent full. Literally, it means, 'Eat your food until you are eight out of ten parts full' or 'Consume food until your belly is 80 per cent full'. This is an easy way to obtain a roughly 20 per cent calorie restriction without counting calories.

INTERMITTENT FASTING

Typically, in human clinical studies of calorie restriction, we prescribe diets that reduce, for example by 25 per cent, the number of calories at breakfast, lunch and dinner. However, in rodents it is different. In experimental facilities, mice – which typically eat at night – are fed only once a day, in the morning. But because these mice on calorie restriction are super hungry, they eat all the food within two to four hours, which means they fast for the remaining 20 to 22 hours. Thus, the effects on health and longevity that we have noticed in all the classical animal calorie restriction study conducted so far may in part be due to intermittent fasting.

It had already been demonstrated by other researchers that intermittent fasting, or alternate-day fasting, can increase lifespan by 30 per cent in rodents, and prevent many chronic diseases, even in the absence of weight loss.[44] It is therefore possible that fasting two or three times a week could induce some beneficial health effects in humans as well.

Only recently have humans and domesticated animals had constant access to food. During their evolution, they ate only intermittently. For many organisms, lengthy periods of fasting are normal; as a result, many have evolved forms of inactivity or quiescence in response to the onset of food shortage. Interestingly, we have discovered that many of the genes that control quiescence are also important in the control of life expectancy.[45]

Fasting, moreover, has been practised for centuries in many Western and Eastern religious traditions. Philip Paracelsus, one of the most eminent physicians of the Renaissance, wrote: 'Fasting is the greatest remedy, the inner doctor'.

OUR STUDIES ON THE EFFECTS OF FASTING

In my lab in the US, we have studied the effects of intermittent fasting on human health. In these clinical randomised studies, we asked our volunteers to fast two or three times per week (the frequency depended on their baseline weight and metabolic profile), while keeping the calorie intake constant in the other four or five days. What we propose in our studies is not water-only fasting, but vegetable fasting. Participants can consume non-starchy raw and cooked vegetables, dressed with a single tablespoon of extra-virgin olive oil, lemon juice or vinegar, at lunch and dinner. We have calculated that by allowing unrestricted eating of different types of vegetables, daily calorie intake is never above 500 calories, which is equivalent to a weekly calorie restriction of about 20 to 23 per cent.

The preliminary results of this experiment have been very encouraging. The volunteers enrolled in this study lost on average 7 per cent of their baseline body weight, and some 25 kg (55 lb) in only six months, without counting calories. Be careful not to compensate in the days following those of fast though.

DIFFERENT TO THE 5:2 DIET

However it's not just about calories. Unlike the recommendations with the widely-known 5:2 diet (five days eating normally and two days restricting calories to approximately 500 calories), I believe that to maximise the results of fasting, we shouldn't eat animal protein, grains or fruit. In this way, we can powerfully shut down the insulin/IGF-1/mTOR pathway that is essential in modulating ageing and the development of cancer.[46,47]

Furthermore, with this diet it is not necessary to weigh the food and calculate calories. Vegetables generally have a very low calorie content, while each tablespoon of oil contains about 100 calories, so we shouldn't use more than two tablespoons over the course of the day.

To maximise the effects of fasting, we should also carefully select the food we consume in the non-fasting days. Preliminary data suggest that eating 'junk' negatively influences the metabolic response to fast-induced weight loss. It is not true that intermittent fasters can eat whatever they want on the non-fasting days, such as highly processed foods. What you eat on those days profoundly affects your gut microbiome and the metabolites that the bacteria produce, which have huge effects on your metabolic health and the risk of developing diseases, including cancer and many inflammatory and autoimmune disorders.

BENEFITS OF 'HEALTHY' FASTING

The benefits of this 'healthy' fasting regimen go beyond losing weight. Even lean people may benefit from fasting a few days per month. Fasting acts as a chronic mild stressor (*hormetic agent*) that provokes a survival response in the organism, helping it to endure adversity by activating longevity pathways. This explains why animals kept on a regime of intermittent fasting and reduced calories are also more resistant to a wide range of stresses (e.g. surgery, radiation, acute inflammation, exposure to heat, and oxidative stress).[48]

In fact, reducing calories results in a moderate increase in levels of blood cortisol, a stress hormone, and enhances the activity of some 'good' proteins that help the organism to remove damaged proteins and cope with a broad array of noxious agents.[49]

Fasting also increases the level of brain-derived neurotrophic factor or BDNF, a protein that promotes the growth and survival of nerve cells. Therefore, even if you are already lean, and do not need to lose weight, fasting can be used to strengthen your body and mind, or as a tool for compensating for a night of excessive eating and drinking. Performing a vegetable fast after a 'heavy' dinner can help to rebalance the metabolism and reduce the risk of weight gain.

TIME-RESTRICTED FASTING: THE 16:8 DIET

Another way to implement fasting that may better suit some people is to restrict daily food intake to between the hours of 7am and 2pm. This would result in a 16-hour fast beyond those hours. A non-starchy vegetable salad or a healthy soup might be consumed for dinner. But remember, we were not all created equal; while this might work for some, it may not for others. An intriguing thing is that experiments on animal models suggest that time-restricted feeding can produce some of the same benefits of calorie restriction, and protect animals from obesity, inflammation and diabetes. However, research on humans is still in its early stages.[51]

This concept of time-restricted feeding is not new. The sixth of the eight Buddhist Precepts requires monks to abstain from eating after lunchtime. It recommends that lay-people do the same. In accordance with the rule dictated by the Buddha, we should ingest foods only during the period from sunrise to the moment when the sun reached its zenith in the sky. Cao Tingdong (1699–1785) of China's Qing dynasty wrote in his treatise on the Gerontology Perennial Maxims:

> *Sufficient nourishment must be consumed for breakfast and lunch, and less for dinner, and at night we have to keep the stomach completely empty. Old people, in particular, should consume a very light dinner.*[52]

Simply put, they were advising us to follow a modified time-restricted fast instead of a full fast. A fascinating, but preliminary, scientific work in Israel on obese women with polycystic ovary syndrome (PCOS) supports this hypothesis. In fact, the volunteers who consumed most of their calories early in the day (980 at breakfast, 640 at lunch and 190 at dinner) lost more weight and had an improvement in blood glucose, glucose tolerance and plasma testosterone levels greater than the group who ate the same number of calories, but most in the evening (190 for breakfast, 640 for lunch and 980 at dinner).[53]

The data suggest that it would be advisable to start our day with a hearty breakfast, followed by a good lunch, whereas dinner should be early and light; for instance, just a soup or cooked and raw vegetables seasoned with a tablespoon of olive oil, lemon juice and a pinch of iodised salt.

This diet may be practised every day or intermittently – that is, every other day. Alternatively it can be practised for 30 consecutive days, once or twice a year, as in the most extreme form followed by Muslims. During the traditional Ramadan practised by religious Muslims, people consume a single, very abundant meal early in the morning, before sunrise, and then fast throughout the day. At dusk only a frugal supper, usually a few dates, is allowed. In summary, we are talking about an extreme time-restricted fast of about 22 hours.

But remember, even for the 16:8 diet the quality of food we consume is of paramount importance. In an ongoing experiment, volunteers randomised to the 16:8 diet who rushed into a fast food outlet to gorge themselves with hamburgers and French fries, just before the end of the eight-hour feeding period, experienced a huge increase in blood cholesterol levels. Fasting and time-restricted feeding are not substitutes for a healthy diet!

DANGERS OF FREQUENT EATING. DON'T SNACK. FEAST!

The way people eat has changed significantly across the globe. In particular, eating frequency has increased without any real physiological reason. People continue to snack even if they are not hungry and sit on a chair most of the day. There has been a surge not just in snacking, but also in the consumption of highly processed snack foods.

Our ancestors did not have the luxury of eating three meals a day and snacking all the time. People never opened the fridge (they did not exist until 1923) or the cupboard digging around for a sweet or salty snack. Kids were not used to asking for snacks from their parents between meals.

Based on accumulating data, I would strongly discourage nibbling many small meals throughout the day, especially late at night before bedtime. By constantly snacking, we keep stimulating the insulin/IGF-1 pathway and inhibit FOXO (see page 23), which results in the accumulation of cellular damage.[54] The take-home message is that 'being a little hungry is good'. It is a positive health sign. The feeling of hunger is caused by stimulation of certain hypothalamic neurons by a hormone produced by the stomach, called ghrelin, which has been shown to inhibit inflammation.[55]

EAT YOUR FOOD SLOWLY

Have you ever noticed how long it takes most thin individuals to consume their meals? It takes forever. The reason is that eating slowly seems to help a person to feel full faster. People who eat too fast consume too many calories before they realise they have eaten enough.

This ties in with data from a new study conducted in Japan that suggests eating at speed is associated with obesity and the future development of metabolic syndrome, a cluster of risk factors that increases the risk of developing type 2 diabetes, heart attack, stroke and some forms of cancers.[56] The study found that the incidence of metabolic syndrome among individuals who ate their meals slowly, normal and fast were 2.3, 6.5 and 11.6 per cent, respectively. The risk of metabolic syndrome in the fast-eating people was more than five times higher than in the people who ate their food slowly. Moreover, fast eating was also associated with higher triglyceride and lower HDL-cholesterol levels.[57]

A good habit is to chew everything you eat until it turns almost into a liquid. Chewing slowly helps you eat less while improving the taste and pleasure of food as well. To master the art of slow eating, first turn off the TV and concentrate on the flavour and texture of your food. Selecting high-fibre foods that take more time to chew helps to train your mind. Put down your fork while you are chewing, relax and chat with your friends or family members.

CHAPTER SIX

HEALTHY CHILDREN

The choices we make concerning health and fitness in our lifetime can reverberate over the years, with the potential to influence not only *our* children but also our *grandchildren's* wellbeing.[1,2] A growing body of scientific data indicate that the seeds of many illnesses are already planted during pregnancy or even *before*.

While every educated woman knows that smoking, drinking alcohol, and taking drugs and certain medications during pregnancy can result in long-lasting detrimental effects on her baby's health, the consequence of poor-quality unbalanced diets and obesity before conception, during pregnancy and breast-feeding is less well appreciated.

Women who have unhealthy diets at the time of conception have lower reproductive success (sub-fertility is a growing problem), and are more likely to have a complicated pregnancy and give birth to an unhealthy child.[3] Now, new data show that father's behaviour can also impinge on child's health.[4]

This is one of the reasons why the current medical approach, which consists of treating diseases only after they are clinically evident, is faulty.[5] The message is 'eat, drink and do whatever you want', and then when you become sick 'we will treat you with the most advanced and personalised drugs or surgical procedures'. This is insane!

EPIGENETICS AND FUTURE GENERATIONS: LIFE TAKES NOTES ON OUR GENES

Findings from experimental studies show that the quality and quantity of the food we eat (among many other things) can change how our genes are working. In other words, genes can be turned off – becoming dormant – or turned on – becoming active – by adjusting chemical tags on specific areas of the DNA. These are technically called 'epigenetic' modifications, that affect how cells 'read' genes, and which have been shown to play a key role in the development of diseases like obesity, diabetes, cancer or cardiovascular disease, among others.[6]

These epigenetic modifications do not change DNA sequence, with an analogy being the notes composing the musical score of a symphony. Instead they influence temporal and spatial control of gene activity, akin to how the conductor reads and interprets the notes.[7] Epigenetic regulation essentially affects which of the 20,000 genes in the DNA are read in a specific cell, and subsequently how these activated genes produce certain specific proteins that make each single cell behave and work in a definite manner.

Why is it important? Well, every single cell of our organism contains exactly the same information required to direct its function. This information is stored in the DNA, which is made up of approximately 3 billion nucleotide bases (basic blocks) and thousands of genes that provide instructions on how to make important proteins that trigger all the biological actions and functions.

However, not all the 20,000 genes are expressed (turned on) in every single cell at the same time. This is why a neuron is structurally and functionally different from a liver or skin cell. The different combinations of genes that are turned on or off is what eventually drives the differentiation of embryonic stem cells into specific differentiated cell types. This is simply amazing!

Let's take our analogy further. We need to think of epigenetic regulation of genes as the conductor's interpretation of a very long symphony. The cells are the musicians, critical units that make up the orchestra. DNA is the conductor's musical score containing all the instructions for every musician of the orchestra to perform their parts. The DNA sequence is the notes on the musical score, while the genes are particular blocks of these notes that instruct when a musician is to play or pause.

The conductor cannot delete the notes (genes) on the score, but he can make adjustments regarding tempo, phrasing, articulation, repetitions of sections, and so on, altering the musical melody for better or worse. This is why the interpretation of Mahler's Fourth Symphony by Riccardo Muti could be drastically different from the one conducted by Simon Rattle.

The problem is that epigenetic modifications also modulate our propensity to develop chronic diseases. What we have discovered in the last few years is that what we eat, how and when we exercise or sleep, our level of stress and many other things, remain imprinted not only in our memory, but also in our DNA, which accumulates several epigenetic marks, in essence influencing our future health and our genetic heritage.

BEFORE CREATION: PRECONCEPTION HEALTH FOR STRONG KIDS

What we eat and do, well before conception, exerts long-lasting health effects on the next generation and beyond. For instance, the quality and quantity of food we consume before procreation, by turning on or off key genes in reproductive cells (that is the egg and sperm cells that join to form an embryo), act as predictors of future nutritional outlook and therefore fine-tune the functioning of the body.[8]

In experimental animal models, for example, modifications in the expression of specific genes induced by calorie-restricted diets persisted for at least three generations. Offspring of the third generation of their calorie restriction great-grandparents still experienced an extension of lifespan.[9] Effects of lifestyle and nutrition of the father, and even the father's grandfather, on offspring health have been reported in humans as well, possibly mediated by modification in seminal fluid and sperm quality, its epigenetic status and DNA integrity.[10,11]

Accumulating data show that many women of reproductive age are not nutritionally ready for pregnancy, because they are deficient in one or more nutrients, including folic acid, iron, iodine and vitamin D. To show how important this can be, folic acid supplementation two or three months before conception can lower by 70 per cent the risk of delivering a baby with a neural-tube defect, and also the possibility of low birth weight, stillbirth or autism.[12-14] Replenishing the folate store also has a positive impact on mothers' health by reducing the risk of miscarriage and pre-eclampsia.[15]

An adequate dietary intake of iodine before pregnancy is equally important because even a mild deficiency has been associated with a lower intelligence quotient in the child.[16] These are just some of the most striking examples of how important the mother's preconception nutrition is on the newborn's health.

Teenage years are a particularly sensitive period of life, because many of the healthy or unhealthy behaviours – like the habit of drinking alcohol, smoking, sedentary lifestyle or consuming junk foods – originate during adolescence and extend into adulthood. These habits influence not only the teenagers' present and future metabolic health, but importantly also increase the risk of their children, grand- and great-grandchildren developing a long list of chronic illnesses. This is why it is so important to shape our health as early as possible in life.

WHY HEALTH AND LIFESTYLE IN PREGNANCY MATTER

The most crucial time of human development is the nine months that occur from conception to birth: a miraculous journey. Among millions of racing spermatozoa, only one will hit the target and successfully fertilise the female egg. The combined genetic material derived from the fusion of the maternal and paternal DNA informs the early development of the embryo.

However, the environmental forces and epigenetic modifications dictated by the mother's lifestyle play a crucial role in shaping the development of the rapidly growing organism as well. Believe it or not in only eight weeks, through rapid divisions and differentiations, a complex organism with a multi-level body plan is formed starting from a single cell, called a zygote. By week five, the embryo has already reached the size of a peppercorn, and the development of the circulatory, excretory and neurologic systems is well under way. At the end of the first semester, the foetus has developed all the internal organs, which will continue to mature through the rest of the pregnancy.

Data from multiple experimental models show that an unhealthy in-utero environment can cause epigenetic and direct toxic effects in the foetus during each one of these sensitive phases of foetal development.[17] Everybody knows that maternal smoking has major detrimental effects on intrauterine growth, and increases the risk of pregnancy loss or delivering a newborn with low birth weight. On a positive note, the implementation of legislation for banning smoking in public and private workplaces, in transport, hospitals and other healthcare facilities such as educational institutions has resulted in a 10 per cent reduction in preterm births.[18]

While alcohol and caffeine consumption during pregnancy have been associated with a similar reduction in birth weight, alcohol intake also has negative long-term consequences on the physical, behavioural and cognitive development of the newborn.[19,20] Because of its teratogenic effects, children who have been prenatally exposed to alcohol show deficiencies in associative learning, executive functioning and adaptive skills, particularly in the social domain, and emotional regulatory problems.

FOR THE SCIENTIFICALLY MINDED
Why metabolic changes in the foetus can have a lifelong impact?
It is thought that several metabolic changes in the developing foetus, caused by the mother eating a low calorie and protein diet during pregnancy, are the direct consequence of a 'survival' response that prioritises brain development over other less essential organs.[21] This results in several detrimental consequences to the child later in life, such as reduced glucose tolerance and kidney ability to remove excess sodium and toxic metabolites. This leads to a higher risk of developing obesity, type 2 diabetes, hypertension and kidney disease. These problems are greatly exacerbated by too much food and rapid catch-up growth after birth.[22-24]

Of course, a reduced insulin secretion or kidney capacity to filtrate salt and protein-derived waste would not be harmful if these individuals continued to be undernourished and remained small, trim and insulin-sensitive, and would limit salt and protein intake.

Less known are the effects of both under- and over- nourishment, especially unbalanced high-fat, low-protein diets, on birth weight and associated metabolic outcomes, including kidney and pancreatic function, and glucose metabolism.[25,26] Epidemiological data show a consistent effect on developmental programming by unhealthy early nutrition as well.[27]

Professor Susan Ozanne, Professor of Developmental Endocrinology at the University of Cambridge in the UK, has shown that a mother's diet low in protein and calories during pregnancy shortens the lifespan of mice, especially if after birth these are fed high-protein diets to accelerate their growth. In this study, however, lifespan was increased by more than 40 per cent in mice that were fed properly during pregnancy (and born with a normal birth weight), but received less protein during the weaning phase.[28,29] This experiment well illustrates the importance of the food we consume during the very early stages of our existence on our future health and potentially life expectancy.

This doesn't just apply to experimental animals. It is well known that in infants born underweight (birth weight less than 2.5 kg/5½ lb), who *quickly* regain the weight, experience an increased risk of developing obesity, diabetes, hypertension, metabolic syndrome and cardiovascular disease.[30]

We know that the Pima, Native Americans of Arizona and Mexico, who were born in environmental conditions of food scarcity and abundant physical activity, when exposed to a diet rich in calories and proteins (such as the American diet) have a much greater risk of developing diabetes, hypertension and cardiovascular diseases.

Most people don't realise that *over-nutrition* during pregnancy is just as detrimental. Excessive consumption of empty calories and animal protein during pregnancy, for example, is strongly associated with an increased risk of the offspring becoming overweight by the age of 20.[31]

It is well known that obese or type 2 diabetic pregnant women, have a much higher risk of giving birth to a large baby with a birth weight greater than 4.5 kg (10 lb), but less known is that these children will have a much higher risk of becoming obese, diabetic, cardiopathic and of developing cancer.[32]

Anyone born overweight has a higher probability of developing breast, colon, or prostate cancer.[33-35] In contrast, there is strong evidence that moderate-intensity physical activity during pregnancy can contribute to lowering the risk of excessive gestational weight gain, gestational diabetes, and symptoms of post-birth depression.[36]

HEALTHY BIRTH: HOW DELIVERY MODE AND EARLY NUTRITION CAN SHAPE THE NEWBORN'S HEALTH

During a natural birth, a wide range of bacteria, viruses and other microorganisms that dwell in the mother's birth canal and vagina will colonise the gut of the newborn for the first time. Accumulating data show that the first strains of bacteria that settle in our intestine at birth remain there for the rest of our lives, heavily influencing the development of our immune system, and the risk of developing allergic, autoimmune and inflammatory disorders.[37] Some studies suggest that even the child's cognitive brain development may be influenced by the metabolites produced by gut microbiota.[38]

It is obvious that if we are born naturally by passing through the vaginal canal, the types of bacteria that will colonise our gut will be totally different from those acquired during a caesarean delivery. The operating theatre by definition is a sterile venue, while the birth canal is host to a myriad of microorganisms, whose composition changes with diet and other behavioural habits. It is also clear that if the baby at birth immediately attaches to the mother's breast, it will be taking in a mixture of bacteria present on the breast's skin and in the mammary gland.

Lactobacillus bacteria, among the first to colonise the newborn's intestine, come from the vaginal mucosa (unless the mother has taken antibiotics just before birth).[39] Bifidobacteria, like Lactobacilli, is also very important in preventing allergic diseases; it originates in mother's milk[40] and thrives on the nutrients that are contained in it.[41] Bacteroides, crucial for the maturation of the immune system, come from the contact of the newborn with tissues surrounding the anal mucosa of women during childbirth.[42]

Of course, as we have already discussed, a mother's diet and lifestyle are crucial in affecting which bacteria reside in the gut.[43] What we eat also influences the pH of the skin and the type of bacteria that live on our bodies. Unhealthy diets rich in processed and animal foods induce an imbalance in the types of organisms present in a person's microflora, which contributes to an increased risk of developing multiple chronic diseases.[44]

In contrast, a diet rich in vegetable dietary fibre results in gut microbiota modifications which help certain immune cells, called T regulatory lymphocytes (see page 89), that are important for the prevention of many allergic and autoimmune diseases.[45] Recent data suggest that the bacteria living in our gut can even modulate our individual response to many medicinal drugs, both in terms of effectiveness and adverse effects.[46] This is important because it means that differences in drug metabolism can be explained, at least in part, by the variations in our microbiome, which depends on the food we have consumed.

HEALTHY EATING FOR BREASTFEEDING

There is no doubt that infants who are breastfed are healthier than those drinking milk formula, but the quality of a mother's diet can dramatically alter her milk's composition and its concentration of vitamins, minerals and phytochemicals.[47] For instance, data from a randomised trial have demonstrated that high fruit and vegetable consumption significantly increased total carotenoid levels in breast milk, with obvious implications for the newborn's health.[48]

But what many people do not realise is that the early exposure of the infant to various milk flavours – which are related to the type of food consumed by the mother – will also influence the infant's hedonistic response, that is, the drive to eat the same foods to obtain pleasure, for the rest of their life.[49]

BREAST MILK: PERFECT NUTRITION FOR BABIES

Breast milk has been designed by Mother Nature to provide the perfect combination of nutrients and antibodies essential for the growth and development of the newborn. Cow's milk, for example, is finely tuned to meet the nutritional requirements of the calf, which has a significantly higher growth rate than a human newborn. Table 2 illustrates that the protein content in 100 ml (3½ fl oz) of human milk is 1.3 g, which is less than half that of whole cow's milk (3.3 g). This is because the concentration of protein in milk is strictly linked to the time needed for a particular animal species to grow in size. On average a calf's weight doubles in 47 days, while for a human newborn it takes 180 days, and therefore the calf needs more proteins and minerals such as calcium to support bone growth as well.

	HUMAN MILK (100 ml/3½ fl oz)	COW'S MILK (100 ml/3½ fl oz)
Protein (g)	1.3	3.3
Casein (%)	40	82
Seroproteins (%)	60	18
Lipids (g)	3.6	3.6
Saturated (%)	47.5	60
Monounsaturated (%)	39	37
Polyunsaturated (%)	13.5	3.7
Carbohydrates (g)	7	4.8
	Lactose + Oligosaccharides	Lactose
Minerals (mg)	210	720

Table 2. Composition of human milk versus cow's milk

Cow's milk, which promotes a harmonic growth of the calf, can kill an infant due to the high concentration of proteins and minerals that damages the newborn kidney and liver. One hundred millilitres of cow's milk contains 720 mg minerals, while human milk has just 210 mg of mineral salts.

The structural composition of proteins, fats and carbohydrates is very different. Human milk contains less casein and more whey proteins, oligosaccharides and polyunsaturated fatty acids than cow's milk. Some components (sialylated oligosaccharides) of human milk can improve immune function and increase bone formation.[50]

IF POSSIBLE, BREASTFEED YOUR BABY, IT WILL IMPROVE YOUR HEALTH AS WELL

The World Health Organization recommends mothers feed their babies only breastmilk for the first six months. No water, other fluids or solid food should be added, until complementary foods are introduced at six months of age.[51] Formula milk is just food, while maternal milk contains, in the right proportions, protein, fat, lactose, glucose, fructose and galactose, iron, minerals, water, enzymes, hormones and most importantly antibodies (that formula powder does not have) that protect the newborn from infections.

The immune system at birth is not fully matured, and develops slowly during the first five years of life.[52] Breastfeeding started as soon as possible, ideally within the first hour of delivery, is associated with a much lower incidence of infections (like diarrhoea, otitis, bronchitis, pneumonia and urinary infections). In the 'Millennium project', which examined 15,890 infants, six months of exclusive breastfeeding was associated with a 50 per cent reduction in the risk of hospitalisation for diarrhoea and by 25 per cent for respiratory tract infections; this protection lasted at least up to school age.[53] The early introduction (before the fourth month) of formula milk and solid foods decreases this protection.[54]

Some studies suggest that babies who are breastfed also have better cognitive development and are psychologically healthier, probably thanks also to a stronger maternal-infant bond that develops because of the maternal-infant skin-to-skin contact.[55,56] When the newborn attaches to the breast, a symbiotic relationship is created. The close contact with the mother's body provides the newborn with all the biological and emotional information (heart, respiratory and circadian rhythms) that are necessary to maintain physiological harmony. Newborns use their mother to help regulate their own metabolic systems and to keep their body at 'tempo'. Most importantly, breast milk does not need to be prepared; it is pure and is consumed by the baby at the right temperature and quantity, whenever needed.

But that's not all. Breastfed children also experience a reduced likelihood of developing allergic diseases (e.g. asthma, atopic dermatitis) and autoimmune diseases (type 1 diabetes mellitus).[57] The risk of developing obesity and type 2 diabetes is also lower.[58,59]

In two randomised clinical trials of formula-fed infants, those who were fed a higher-protein content formula at birth had a much higher BMI and body fat later in childhood (five to eight years of age) than those consuming the standard or lower-protein formula.[60,61] The higher protein intake caused an increase in blood concentrations of branched-chain amino acids, which translated into insulin resistance and increased insulin levels.[62]

BREASTFEEDING PROMOTES MOTHER'S HEALTH

The great thing about breastfeeding is that it protects both the child and the mother.[63,64]

Some of the immediate benefits of initiating breastfeeding within one hour of delivery are:

- reduced bleeding after childbirth
- a faster shrinking of the volume of the uterus
- a faster return to pre-pregnancy body weight.

The long-term benefits of breastfeeding are:

- reduced risk of developing type 2 diabetes. Women who breastfed their infants experienced a 20–30 per cent lower risk for each year of breastfeeding.[65]
- a lower risk of developing breast and ovarian cancer; reduced by 4–8 per cent for every five to 12 months of breastfeeding.[66,67]

BALANCING NUTRITION IN OUR GROWING CHILDREN THROUGH PUBERTY

We know that underfeeding our growing children results in stunted growth, however overfeeding them, especially with ultra-processed energy-dense foods and excessive animal products results in other detrimental consequences. One is overweight and obesity, the other is a rapid and excessive growth that leads to high stature and early puberty. Indeed, average adult height, which has increased markedly in many countries during recent generations, is positively associated with an elevated risk of colon, prostate and breast cancer, as shown in figure 11.[68-70]

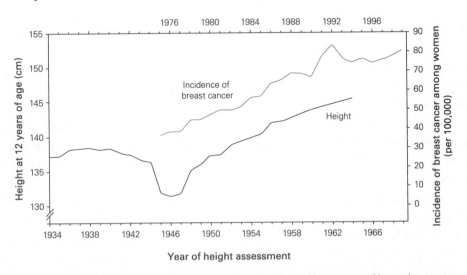

Figure 11: Relationship between girls height at 12 years old and incidence of breast cancer 30 years later among Japanese women 40 to 44 years of age.[71]

Over-nutrition during child development, which is correlated with girls' height and weight, is also correlated with age at first menstruation.[72] An early menarche is a well-established risk factor for the development of breast cancer, and in many developed countries it is now happening in girls aged around 10 to 12 years, four or five years earlier than for our grandmothers. It is estimated that for each year earlier that menarche occurs in a girl, the probability of her developing breast cancer increases by 5 per cent.[73]

Not only early menarche, but also rapid growth in the period of the greatest development of the mammary gland (between eight and 14 years of age), is a powerful risk factor for breast cancer. This is because, even if DNA mutations accumulate across the entire lifespan, the most rapid build-up occurs between the first menstruation and the first pregnancy, a period in which breast cells, especially stem cells, undergo rapid proliferation and differentiation in order to develop into fully developed mammary glands that produce milk. During this crucial time the risk is higher because any mutated cell grows at a faster pace and is rapidly multiplying.[74,75]

More cell proliferation translates into more random DNA mutations (see page 23). Indeed, after the first breastfeeding period, when the mammary gland is fully differentiated, the breast cells seems to be more cancer-resistant.[76] This is the reason why women who do not have children, or procreate later in life and do not breastfeed have a much higher risk of developing breast cancer.[77]

Therefore, limiting nutrition and providing a wide range of nutritious food to maintain a healthy normal weight during early childhood and puberty not only prevents obesity, type 2 diabetes and cardiovascular disease, but also prevents accelerated growth in children and reduces the risk of cancer in adulthood.[78]

CHAPTER SEVEN
DIET QUALITY MATTERS

When I started to work in this field almost 20 years ago, the belief was that only the reduction of calories, regardless of nutritional quality, was responsible for the anti-ageing effects of calorie restriction. I still remember my discussions with Professors Edward Masoro and Richard Weindruch, two giants of calorie restriction research in rodents, who were adamant that the nutrients of a diet were irrelevant. They both stated with force that: 'Only calories were important!'

Now we know that this is not true. The types of foods our meals comprise are key, and the macronutrient composition as well.[1] It is not true that 'a calorie is a calorie', at least from a metabolic point of view. When we practise calorie restriction or time-restricted feeding, eating just half a hamburger, half a bag of French fries and half a glass of sweetened soda is not a viable option if we are interested in healthy longevity, and not merely in shedding some extra kilos.

The hypothesis that only calorie restriction was effective in extending lifespan was primarily based on a flawed interpretation of experimental data showing that 40 per cent calorie restriction, but not 40 per cent protein restriction, increased lifespan in rats.[2] However, the protein-restricted rats were not food restricted, because their growth rate was normal, a point overlooked by the authors of the study. A subsequent series of studies in many experimental animal models has clearly demonstrated that a reduction in specific nutrients, in particular dietary protein, can preserve health and extend lifespan (even if at lesser extent), independently of calorie intake.[3]

Determining the best overall intake and dietary ratios of protein, carbohydrate and fat is important, because, as I will explain, eating too much protein is not good for our health.[4] However, the effects of reduced consumption of a specific macronutrient will depend partly upon the composition of the rest of the diet and the quality source of the macronutrients. If we reduce our protein intake, we must either increase the consumption of carbohydrates or fat, or both. But which type of carbohydrates? Should we eat refined flour, sugar and high-fructose corn syrup or complex wholegrain carbohydrates and legumes? Should we consume animal fat and margarine or monounsaturated-rich extra virgin olive oil, avocado and nuts?

HOW MUCH PROTEIN SHOULD WE EAT?

High-protein diets and supplements are very trendy nowadays. People are obsessed with proteins and believe that eating plenty of them will be instrumental in losing weight, gaining muscle mass and staying healthy. The global protein supplements market size is expected to reach US$21.5 billion by 2025, according to a new report by Grand View Research, Inc.

Because of this new fad (that has been smartly advertised), almost every person I know favours foods rich in animal protein and tries to avoid any type of carbohydrate. For these people, a typical breakfast might consist of milk or yoghurt, omelette with various vegetables (fried in butter or vegetable oil) or scrambled eggs and bacon; for lunch grilled chicken or salmon with vegetables; and for dinner a steak, pork chops or a cheeseburger (no bun), served with vegetables and salsa sauce. Snacking on protein-packed bars and drinks in the morning, afternoon and at bedtime is also part of this daily picture.

At many restaurants, a typical menu consists of beef, lamb, chicken or fish as the main courses, accompanied by the usual few strips of carrots and broccoli in quantities that merely add some colour. At the gym, people are advised by their personal trainers to consume lots of meat, egg whites, high-protein bars, shakes and supplements.

The fad started in 1972 when Dr Robert Atkins published his first book 'Dr Atkins' Diet Revolution', which sold tens of millions of copies. His 2002 follow-up book, 'New Diet Revolution', made high-protein diets and fortified food products even more trendy. Since then, many other popular books on the benefits of low-carb diets for weight loss have been published, such as the Dukan diet, the South Beach diet, the Paleo and the Ketogenic cookbook, among many others. Because of this and other campaigns, high-protein foods have acquired an aura of health and goodness.

But where are the scientific data supporting the claimed, magical effects of low-carb diets? Are these diets really healthy or potentially dangerous for your health?

Supporters believe that high-protein diets and fortified products reduce hunger, increase the capacity of the body to burn fat, and make people lose more body weight than other diets while minimising the loss of lean body mass. However, the evidence for these statements is very weak at best.[5]

Multiple observational studies, including the EPIC study (one of the largest cohort studies in the world, with more than half a million participants recruited across 10

European countries and followed for almost 15 years), have found that high-protein intake is associated with an increased risk of gaining weight and becoming obese.[6] In addition, the results from the most recent randomised clinical trials revealed that high-protein intake does not result in long-term greater weight loss than standard-protein intake and has only a very small effect in preserving lean body mass (about 700 g after 10 per cent weight loss).[7]

Some small studies have found that in the short-term (first three months), dieters on the low-carb diets experience greater weight loss than those on a low-fat diet, presumably because short-term adherence to a low-carb diet is easier. Most people love meat and cheese, and they can get away with eliminating starchy foods for some time.

However, a large multicentre clinical trial found no differences in weight, fat or bone mass between people consuming a low-carbohydrate diet (20 g of carb per day) or a calorie-restricted low-fat diet (1200 to 1800 kcal/d; ≤30 per cent calories from fat) at six, 12 or 24 months.[8] Moreover, the participants who consumed the low-carb diet reported more adverse symptoms, such as bad breath, hair loss, constipation and dry mouth. A more recent large randomised clinical trial published in JAMA (*Journal of the American Medical Association*) shows there is no significant difference in weight change over a 12-month period between a healthy low-fat diet versus a healthier version of the low-carbohydrate diet.[9]

DOES EATING MORE PROTEIN INCREASE MUSCLE MASS?

The claims that high-protein diets or protein-fortified foods are important for building muscle mass and reducing muscle wasting during weight loss or ageing is also another scientifically unsupported myth. Yes, it is true that consuming a high-protein diet can reduce muscle loss during weight loss, but the effect is very small and, most importantly, can have serious detrimental effects on metabolic health.

Data from a comprehensive systematic review show that eating a high-protein diet can preserve at the most 400 to 800 g (14–28 oz) of lean body mass in people who have lost 5–10 per cent body weight with a calorie restriction diet.[10] A well-conducted clinical trial by my colleague Bettina Mittendorfer from Washington University showed that protein supplementation during 10 per cent weight loss in obese postmenopausal women resulted in a mere 200 grams (7 oz) (bilateral) sparing of thigh muscle mass without any change in muscle strength.[11]

Moreover, accumulating data show that high protein intake has no proven beneficial effect on muscle mass in individuals who consume weight-maintaining or high-calorie diets. Data from the Framingham Third Generation Study show that muscle mass of arms and legs did not differ between people who consumed 1.1g of protein per kg of body weight per day and those eating 1.8 g per kilogram of bodyweight per day.[12]

This finding is consistent with the results from multiple randomised clinical trials demonstrating that:

- daily supplementation with 56 g of protein for 6 months did not increase lean mass in overweight or obese men and women[13]

- daily supplementation with 30 g of protein for 24 months did not help maintain muscle mass in older women[14]

- daily supplementation with 22 g protein per day for three months or 40g for six months did not increase the exercise-training induced increase in the size of skeletal muscle, even in healthy young adults[15–17]

- consuming a high-protein diet (25 per cent of energy from protein) did not induce more gain in lean body mass than a diet containing 15 per cent of energy from protein.[18]

WHAT IS A HEALTHY PROTEIN INTAKE?

Proteins are essential nutrients. We need them to maintain health. But how much? According to the Institute of Medicine, a non-profit organisation affiliated to the National Academies of Science in the United States, the estimated average protein requirement (EAR) for adults is 0.6 g per kilogram of body weight a day. It has proposed that the recommended daily intake (RDI) for protein needed to meet the requirements of 97.5 per cent of the population is 0.8 g per kilogram of body weight a day.[19] The FAO/WHO/UNU and European Food Safety Authority Population Reference Intake (PRI), which is considered adequate for all adults, is 0.83 g per kilogram of bodyweight a day.[20]

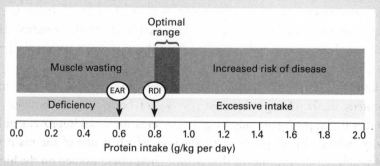

Figure 12: Optimal protein intake[21]

What this means is that if your body weight is 70 kg (154 pounds), you should consume about 58 g (2 oz) of protein per day in terms of the PRI. By the way, this value is more or less what the centenarians of Okinawa had been consuming for centuries. This means that too many people in Western countries, and now even in many developing countries, eat much more than they need – on average 1.3 g of protein per kg of bodyweight every day. In a 70-kg man that means 90 g (3.17 oz) per day.

These and many other studies clearly show that protein supplementation is essentially ineffective for increasing muscle mass[22-26] and strongly suggest that the marked effect of weight-bearing exercise alone is mostly responsible for maintaining and increasing muscle mass when consuming an adequate intake of protein.

Well-conducted clinical studies show that the synthesis of new skeletal muscle protein reaches a plateau when we consume about 30 g of protein at each meal.[27,28] All the excess is oxidised and at the same time activates the pro-ageing IGF/mTOR pathway.[29] Eating more protein than what is needed, therefore, will not increase muscle mass, but will accelerate ageing and increase the risk of developing many chronic diseases.

HIGH-PROTEIN DIETS PROMOTE DISEASE AND AGEING

A growing body of data demonstrates that high protein intake in humans is unhealthy, correlating with an increased risk of diabetes and cardiovascular disease.[30-34] The risk of developing type 2 diabetes has been estimated to increase by 20–40 per cent for every 10 g of protein consumed in excess of 64 g (2.25 oz) per day.[35-37]

In contrast, reducing protein intake seems to be beneficial for metabolic health.[38] Our group, in collaboration with Dudley Lamming of the University of Wisconsin, has found that a moderate reduction in protein intake (close to the intake consumed by the centenarians of Okinawa) improves metabolic health in both humans and mice. Humans fed isocaloric 7–9 per cent protein diets, lost 2.6 kg (5.7 lb) in only four weeks and experienced a significant decrease in fasting blood glucose levels.[39] We also observed a doubling of the levels of an important pro-longevity hormone, called FGF21,[40] in subjects fed this lower protein diet. In the parallel study, the mice fed the 7 per cent protein diet gained less weight than mice on the standard 21 per cent protein control diet over the course of two months.[41] This was despite the low-protein diet mice consuming more food.

In another clinical trial, Bettina Mittendorfer showed that in obese individuals high protein intake (1.3 g of protein per kg of body weight), but not a normal protein diet (0.8 g per kg of body weight), prevents the usual improvement in insulin sensitivity induced by 10 per cent weight loss, which is one of the main metabolic goals of weight loss.[42] This means that despite these obese women on the high-protein diet having lost 10 per cent of their body weight (and a considerable amounts of visceral and liver fat), they were still insulin resistant and therefore at increased risk of developing type 2 diabetes. As explained, insulin resistance and compensatory high levels of insulin trigger the activation of the insulin/IGF pathway that promotes accelerated ageing and cancer (see page 23).

Some epidemiological studies even suggest that high protein intake may increase overall mortality. In one study of 6381 adults from the National Health and Nutrition Examination Survey, men and women aged 50 to 65 who consumed a high-protein diet had a 75 per cent increase in overall mortality and a four-fold increase in cancer and diabetes mortality during the 18-year follow-up.[43] Studies in multiple experimental animal models support these data.

Among the three macronutrients, protein has been found to be the most likely to influence ageing and mortality. Across many species of animals, the greatest longevity is generated by diets that are lower in protein and higher in carbohydrates, where the optimum ratio of protein to carbohydrates is about 1:10, with the protein content of the diet as low as 10 per cent or less.[44]

In mice, the median lifespan progressively increased up to 30 per cent as the dietary protein-to-carbohydrate ratio was decreased.[45] Interestingly, the longest-living population in the world, the people of the Japanese island of Okinawa, have traditionally eaten a diet where the protein intake is 9 per cent.

These experimental animal and human studies are very important because they demolish two misconceptions:

1. A calorie is simply a calorie.

2. High-protein diets are good for health and important to avoid obesity, build muscle and live a long and healthy life.

The data available are clear: we must avoid consuming too much protein on a daily basis, especially animal protein (rich in branched-chain and sulphur amino acids), because it increases our risk of getting fat, developing diabetes, cardiovascular diseases and cancer and, most likely, dying prematurely.

THE QUALITY OF PROTEIN IS MORE IMPORTANT THAN QUANTITY

Many thousands of different proteins exist, each one formed by long and convoluted strings of peptides. The building blocks of proteins are amino acids. There are 20 different types of amino acids; nine of them (leucine, isoleucine, methionine, phenylalanine, valine, threonine, tryptophan, lysine and histidine) are essential, which means they cannot be made by our bodies, and therefore must be supplied with diet.

ANIMAL PROTEIN

Meat, eggs and cheese do contain all the required amino acids. However, when we eat animal products we are also consuming:

*   excessive amounts of saturated fat, which drives hypercholesterolemia[46]

- choline and l-carnitine, which when fermented by gut bacteria produce a substance (called TMAO) that accelerates the formation of coronary atherosclerotic plaques[47]

- excess iron, which drives oxidation and colon cancer[48]

- high levels of methionine and branched-chain amino acids, which by activating the IGF/mTOR pathway can promote insulin resistance, type 2 diabetes, cancer and accelerated ageing.[49]

Consistently, data from randomised controlled trials demonstrate that consuming high-protein diets (comprising dairy and meat products and whey protein supplements) causes a drastic reduction in insulin sensitivity and an associated increase in blood insulin levels.[50,51] In an another trial of patients with type 2 diabetes, high consumption of chicken, fish, eggs, low-fat milk and cheeses prevented the expected improvements in glucose metabolism and insulin sensitivity induced by a two-month weight loss intervention.[52]

These data support findings from epidemiological studies, where the association between total protein consumption and type 2 diabetes was largely explained by animal protein intake, whereas there was no association, or even an inverse association between plant protein consumption and type 2 diabetes.[53,54]

Is it true that only animal foods contain the right and complete proportion of all the essential and non-essential amino acids, and that without consuming an adequate amount of animal protein daily we cannot build muscle mass and function well?

Have you ever noticed the impressive muscle mass of a Shire horse, or a Holstein bull? They are herbivores; they eat only grass, hay and some whole grains such as oats. Typically, most adult horses require only 8–10 per cent protein in their diet. The same is true for African elephants, which can weigh up to 10.4 tons and are the largest and heaviest animals on earth, and for the silverback male gorillas, which can weigh up to 260 kg (580 lb).

This is because plant foods contain all the essential amino acids, even if in different proportions. Legumes, for instance, are high in lysine, but low in tryptophan and methionine. In contrast, whole grains are low in lysine but high in tryptophan and methionine. A meal of brown rice and lentils or durum wheat pasta with chickpeas, therefore, provides a complete protein – no different from the protein found in eggs or meat. That is why it's important to combine whole grains and legumes some time during the day.

PLANT PROTEIN

Why the metabolic effects of plant proteins differ from those of animal proteins is unclear. It may be due, at least in part, to the differences in their amino acid profile.

In a recent study, we found that feeding mice a diet specifically with less branched-chain amino acids (found in dairy products, meat, chicken, fish and eggs) is sufficient to reduce body weight (and fat) and blood glucose levels.[55] Dietary branched-chain amino acids have also been shown to play a crucial role in promoting insulin resistance and cancer development, and in humans, predict cancer mortality risk.[56,57] Consistently, in another study we found substituting plant for animal proteins markedly inhibited prostate and breast cancer growth in human xenograft animal models of cancer.[58] In these xenograft models, human tumour cells are transplanted into immunocompromised mice that do not reject human cells.

It is also possible that the neutral or protective effect of plant protein consumption on type 2 diabetes and cancer risk may be due to increased consumption of beneficial bioactive substances that are associated with dietary plant proteins. Finally, epidemiological data suggest that substituting plant protein for animal protein is also associated with lower mortality.[59]

In particular, the risk of death from all causes among participants of Harvard's Physician and Nurse Health Studies was 34 per cent lower when 3 per cent of energy from plant protein was substituted for an equivalent amount of protein from processed red meat, 12 per cent lower for unprocessed red meat, and 19 per cent lower for egg.[60]

These epidemiological data are in line with those of animal studies showing that in rodents restriction of methionine, a key essential amino acid found in high concentrations in meat and dairy, extends average and maximal lifespan.[61] Restricting methionine to about 65–80 per cent of standard intake increased the lifespan of rats and mice by up to 30 per cent and reduced their glucose, IGF-1 and insulin levels.[62] Plant-based proteins are lower in methionine than animal proteins, which may explain, at least in part, their health and anti-ageing benefits, which have been documented in some human populations eating predominantly plant-based diets.

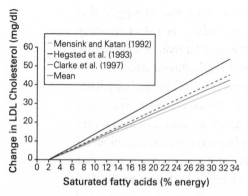

Figure 13: Relationship between dietary saturated fat intake and blood LDL-cholesterol levels.[63]

FAT: IS DIETARY FAT OUR REAL ENEMY?

The nutritional gridlock so many Americans, European and Australians are now in is largely a result of a misinterpretation of dietary recommendations that created phobias of fat and then carbohydrate. It began at the end of World War II, when US and North European newspapers began reporting on a drastic increase in deaths from heart attack in relatively young and apparently healthy men.

Several observational studies were put in place (including the famous Seven Countries study), which showed a direct correlation between dietary animal fat intake, in particular saturated fat, and blood cholesterol levels, a major risk factor for heart disease. For every 1 per cent increase in calories from saturated fat, blood LDL-cholesterol rises by 2 per cent.[64]

Because of these findings, doctors and nutritionists started to recommend their patients substitute food rich in animal fat with alternatives rich in carbohydrates and vegetable fat, such as exchanging butter with the newly developed margarines prepared with trans fatty acids. We now know margarines are worse than butter and cream in increasing blood cholesterol, inflammation and the risk of heart attack.[65]

The result of this over-simplistic approach was the explosion of an unprecedented epidemic of obesity and related chronic diseases. The real problem was that dietary fat was not substituted with healthy sources of carbs, but with highly processed foods such as white bread, polished rice, sugar, all kind of sweets, fruit juice, sweetened yogurts, and plenty of soft drinks.

Then, because of the obesity crisis, in the early 2000s a new fad began focusing on reducing carbs and consuming high-protein diets and, more recently, high-fat diets (the ketogenic diet). The enemy, the 'bad guy', is now carbohydrate. But the words 'carbohydrate' or 'fat' are generic and potentially misleading. It is, instead, essential to distinguish between healthy fats and bad fats, and healthy carbs and bad carbs.

NOT ALL FAT IS CREATED EQUAL

Vast differences exist in the composition of fats from plant and animal origin. In the case of animal fats, what the animal eats also influences the final fatty acid composition. Saturated fats, for example, found in meats and dairy products, raise blood levels of cholesterol. But extra-virgin olive oil, avocado, nuts and fish, which contain primarily monounsaturated and polyunsaturated fatty acids, do not increase cholesterol and protect the heart.

Data from the Nurses' Health Study and other observational studies suggest that fats from olive oil and other monounsaturated fats can even reduce the risk of coronary heart disease.[66] Substituting monounsaturated fat for saturated fat reduces low-density lipoprotein (LDL)-cholesterol without affecting the good HDL-cholesterol.[67]

Another set of data suggest that monounsaturated fats, unlike carbohydrate, reduce blood sugar and triglycerides in adult onset diabetes.[68] Even the word 'monounsaturated' fat does not mean much, unless we know the source of it. A recent study found that monounsaturated fatty acids from plant origins, such as olive oil and avocado, are associated with lower cardiovascular and cancer death rate, but monounsaturated fatty acids from animal sources are related to higher mortality.[69]

What about polyunsaturated fat intake? Should we increase the consumption of oils rich in these fats, such as corn or sunflower oil? Multiple animal studies show that high intake of oils rich in omega-6 polyunsaturated fat promotes inflammation, coronary thrombosis and cancer.[70,71] These results have not been confirmed yet in human studies, but I recommend limiting the consumption of vegetable oils rich in polyunsaturated fatty acids (PUFA); also, they quickly become rancid if left at room temperature and are often extracted with chemical solvents.[72] I advise using cold-pressed extra-virgin olive oil, in moderation, as the main condiment for our food, because it is an excellent source of vitamin E and other precious phytochemicals.[73]

CARBS: HEALTHY VERSUS UNHEALTHY CARBOHYDRATES

There are many legends about the consumption of carbohydrates, the main one being that they make you fat and must be avoided as much as possible. But this belief is based on false premises, as well as a misunderstanding of the scientific literature.

Foods rich in carbohydrates are cereals (wheat, rice, maize, barley, millet, oats, rye, triticale and sorghum), starchy vegetables (potatoes, corn, rice), fruits, beans, sweets, soft drinks, honey and, of course, brown and white table sugars. Sugars are simple and starches are complex carbohydrates, but ultimately all of them are broken down into glucose and absorbed into our blood. This occurs faster for free sugars (e.g. table sugar and corn syrup, which are added to soft drinks and jams, biscuits and sweets) and a bit slower for starch found primarily in potatoes, rice, corn and all other cereals.

The problem is that starchy foods from highly processed grains, such as white bread and white rice, which have been stripped of their fibre, behave just like simple sugar. They are quickly digested and absorbed, causing steep spikes of blood glucose, which in turn trigger big rises of insulin. The high amount of insulin released by the pancreas to lower blood glucose can overshoot the mark and result in rapid and sharp declines in blood glucose, which in turn induces appetite, creating a vicious circle of hunger, fat deposition and obesity.

The food matrix and the fibre properties found in whole foods are mostly lost when whole grains are milled into refined flours[74,75] or when fruit or vegetables, such as apples, oranges or carrots, are juiced.[76] And adding fibre supplements does not reintroduce the lost structural food matrix properties found in unprocessed plant foods.

In unrefined or minimally refined whole grains, the fibre-rich cell wall restricts the rate at which starch and sugars are digested and absorbed in our small intestine. Slow-releasing carbohydrate foods have multiple beneficial health effects.

Carbohydrates that slowly release glucose and have a low glycaemic index* induce satiety and decrease hunger, therefore reducing the risk of obesity.[77] Both low-glycaemic foods and whole grains offer protection from the risk of developing type 2 diabetes,

---

* The glycaemic index (GI) measures how fast and how much a certain food increases blood glucose concentration. Foods with higher GI values raise blood sugar more rapidly and intensely than those with lower GI values do. Examples of high GI foods are: potatoes, white rice, white bread, cookies, cakes, candies and sweet drinks; those with lower GI, include whole grains, nuts, legumes, fruits, non-starchy vegetables.

coronary heart disease and colorectal cancer. For example, regular consumption of whole grains induces a 20–40 per cent reduction in the risk of cardiovascular disease and a 20–30 per cent decrease in the risk of diabetes.[78-80]

As always things are a bit more complicated than we would like them to be, because the rate of glucose absorption and its concentration in our blood is influenced by many other factors, such as:

- the total carbohydrate content of the food, also called glucose load
- the fat and protein content of the added meal components
- the type of food processing
- the volume and frequency of our meals
- the timing since our last bout of physical exercise
- our body weight and metabolic health.

These factors modify the levels of circulating insulin in our blood and the clearance of glucose from blood into our muscles, liver and fat cells. For example, white bread and carrots have similar glycaemic index values, but carrots have much lower carbohydrates. But you would not eliminate carrots from your diet, because (despite their high glycaemic index) they provide only a small percentage of the total carbohydrate load and, more importantly, lots of healthy vitamins and other phytochemicals.

In contrast, foods like baked potatoes and French fries, white bread (especially the sugar-enriched buns used for burgers), white rice, rice cakes, cornflakes, pretzels and instant oatmeal should be eliminated or drastically reduced from our diet because they possess both a very high glycaemic index and a very high glucose load. At the other end of the spectrum, whole grains (brown rice, farro, barley), legumes (chickpeas, lentils, fava beans, black beans), and some fruits (berries, apples, prunes) have a smaller effect on blood glucose. Most green vegetables (lettuce, cabbage, broccoli, spinach, arugula, chard, kale) have so little an effect as to be almost undetectable.

How we process and cook our carbohydrates is also very important. For instance, food should not be overcooked, as this changes the starch's structure, and modifies how fast carbohydrates are digested and absorbed. For example, when rice – especially white rice – is overcooked in water, the starch granules get disrupted and gelatinised into a form easily available to pancreatic amylases, the enzymes that break up starch into simple sugar units.[81]

Spaghetti cooked 'al dente' behaves differently because of the dense food matrix of the durum wheat flour, which is digested more slowly than white rice and induces a much lower glycaemic spike.[82,83] A trick to help lower the absorption of carbs is to add extra-virgin olive oil to our meal, because this is known to slow the absorption of carbohydrates into our intestine.[84]

FIBRE

Beneficial effects of dietary fibre

A heathy diet should contain lots of dietary fibre. For instance, people consuming a traditional Mediterranean diet consume at least 45 g (1.6 oz) of dietary fibre per day, particularly insoluble fibre. This is more than triple what is in the usual Western diet (on average 14 g/day). A cup of cooked brown rice, for example, contains 3 g of fibre, while a cup of white rice has only 1g. In 100 g (3½ oz) of cooked lentils there is 8 g of fibre, while 100 g (3½ oz) of beef has no fibre at all. To illustrate further, table 3 shows the major differences in dietary fibre and other key nutrients in different processed and unprocessed foods.

	Brown, rice cooked	White, rice cooked	Lentils cooked	Almonds unroasted	Beef cooked
Dietary Fibre, g	2	0	8	12	0
Calories, kcal	110	130	129	578	288
Fat, g	1	0	2	51	20
Protein, g	3	3	9	21	26
Carbohydrates, g	23	28	20	20	0
Vitamin A, µg	0	0	18	0	1
Vitamin B12, µg	0	0	0	0	2
Folate, µg	4	3	176	8	7
Magnesium, mg	43	12	35	25	22

Table 3. Fibre and total nutrition content of 100 g (3½ oz) of different foods

If we eat 2 cups of organic brown rice, 1 cup of lentils, 20 almonds, 1 cup of green cabbage, 1 cup of spinach, 2 medium carrots, 1 apple, 1 orange, 2 tablespoons of olive oil, the juice of 1 lemon and 1 tablespoon of flax seeds in one day, we will obtain 73 g of fibre in only 1886 kcal, 76 g of proteins, 64 g of fat (with only 4 per cent saturated fat) and more than 100 per cent of the recommended daily intake for each nutrient with the exception of vitamins D and B12.

Data from a large European epidemiological study suggest that people who consume only 14 g of fibre per day have a 30 per cent higher risk of mortality than those consuming 30 or more grams per day.[85] Other epidemiological studies suggest that individuals who consume at least 25–29 g of fibre per day have a reduced risk of dying of diabetes, heart attack, and colorectal and breast cancer.[86] In these studies, for each increase of 10 g of fibre per day there was a 10 per cent reduction in mortality risk;[87] and consuming 35 g of fibre per day reduced the risk of colon cancer by 40 per cent compared to those who consumed only 15 g a day.[88] Data from clinical trials have demonstrated that people who consume more fibre have significantly lower body weight, systolic blood pressure and total cholesterol.[89]

The healthiest fibres seem to be those from whole grains, cereals and non-starchy vegetables. In the prospective NIH-AARP Diet and Health Study, which followed 367,442 men and women for 14 years, the individuals with the highest intake of wholegrain fibre had a 19 per cent lower risk of mortality from all causes and 15–34 per cent lower risk of mortality from specific diseases, such cancer or respiratory infections.[90]

The ways in which higher dietary fibre intake protects against several metabolic, inflammatory and autoimmune disorders and cancer are multiple:

1. Dietary fibre increases stool weight and bulk. Larger, softer stools dilute colonic content of potential carcinogens and move through the intestine faster so that the colon mucosa is exposed to food-derived carcinogens for less time.[91]

2. Dietary soluble fibre reduces the pH of our gut,[92] and increases bile acid excretion.[93] This is beneficial as bile acids can be converted into cancer-causing molecules.

3. Foods high in fibre are typically lower in fat, which may also help protect against colon cancer by reducing bile acid production.

4. Insoluble fibre alters the colonic flora[94] and serves as a substrate for the generation of short-chain fatty acids that are the preferred substrate for the lining cell of our colon mucosa and the local immune cells.[95]

However, don't take the short cut of using fibre supplements. Data from a three-year randomised clinical trial show that individuals taking 3.5 g of fibre supplements (ispaghula husk) had a significant increase in the risk of small and larger tumour recurrence, especially in the presence of high calcium intake.[96] There are a number of possible explanations for these unexpected results, but they emphasise the complexity of interactions among nutritional factors and strongly suggest caution before taking supplements.

POTENTIAL HEALTH RISKS OF VEGETARIAN AND VEGAN DIETS

Well-balanced and planned vegetarian diets offer many positive nutritional benefits, including lower consumption of saturated fat, cholesterol and animal protein, and higher levels of complex carbohydrates, soluble and insoluble fibre, mono- and poly-unsaturated fatty acids, magnesium, boron, carotenoids, folic acid, vitamin C, vitamin E and many other phytocompounds.

However, some vegetarians, especially those who avoid all animal products for ethical reasons, are at greater risk of developing certain vitamin-deficiency illnesses.[97] Vitamin B12 is an essential vitamin, produced by certain strains of soil bacteria that animals ingest when grazing grass. During digestion large amounts of vitamin B12 are formed and incorporated in the animal's meat, milk and eggs. Fish and shellfish also contain considerable amount of vitamin B12; for instance 100 g (3½ oz) of clams contain up to 49 µg of vitamin B12. We humans are unable to produce it, and because we wash vegetables before eating – to reduce the risk of contracting parasites – we must consume foods of animal origin in order to obtain this substance essential for the proper functioning of our cells.

An alternative nowadays for vegetarians is to consume foods supplemented with vitamin B12, including B12-fortified nutritional yeast, which has a nutty, cheesy flavour and can be used as a cheese substitute. Many of these enriched foods can be found on the market, and orthodox vegans need to consume them, or alternatively take vitamin B12 tablets. Note that vitamin B12 in spirulina or other algae is not bioavailable and may even inhibit B12 metabolism.[98] Lacto-ovovegetarians should be able to obtain the recommended allowance of vitamin B12 by regularly eating eggs and cheese.

Be careful, because vegan diets rich in folic acid can mask anaemia induced by vitamin B12 deficiency for long periods. Some studies suggest that chronic vitamin B12 deficiency could also accelerate cognitive decline. Therefore, vegans should regularly check their blood levels of vitamin B12.[99]

Other potential deficiencies that vegetarians may develop are those from iron, zinc, calcium and occasionally riboflavin.[100] These deficiencies are especially important in vegan children, pregnant women and those who experience heavy periods. Many plant foods contain iron and zinc, but they are less absorbable than those from meat, because of substances that inhibit absorption, such as fibre, phytate and calcium.

One way to increase iron and zinc absorption is to add vitamin C. Even in non-vegetarians it is always a good idea to use lemon juice to cook and season vegetables, legumes and grains, because it helps to increase the absorption of iron and other minerals.[101,102] Organic acids present in fruits and some vegetables increase absorption of iron as well.[103]

Another helpful trick is to sprout or ferment beans, cereals and seeds, because this destroys phytates.[104] Slow-fermented bread (where sourdough is used as a starter) can also reduce phytate levels and increase the absorption of both iron and zinc.[105] Conversely, we should avoid consuming tea, coffee and cocoa during meals because they reduce the absorption of these and other minerals.[106]

Calcium deficiency might be another potential problem if vegans do not eat plenty of calcium-rich vegetables and other foods. Many plant foods contain calcium, and in some of these, calcium bioavailability is very high. For instance, 40–60 per cent of the calcium contained in cabbage, broccoli or broccoli sprouts is absorbed (because these vegetables are low in oxalates), against only 31–32 per cent of the calcium in cow's milk.[107] Legumes, soy products (especially tofu made with calcium sulphate) and figs provide further dietary calcium.[108]

However, certain vegetables rich in oxalate, such as spinach, chards and beets, hinder calcium absorption. Diets high in salt increase calcium loss from bones, while vitamin D facilitates its absorption. In lacto-ovo vegetarians, there is no problem with the calcium balance, but in strict vegans deficiency may arise.[109]

In a study I conducted in St Louis, we found that people following a raw food vegan diet had significantly low bone mass at clinically important skeletal regions, but without evidence of increased bone turnover or impaired vitamin D status.[110]

Finally and most importantly, vegetarians should pay close attention to the composition of their diet and the quality of the foods they eat. For example, data from a recent epidemiological study suggest that men and women consuming plant-based diets rich in healthier plant foods (whole grains, fruits, vegetables, nuts, legumes, oils, tea, coffee) have a 25 per cent lower risk of coronary heart disease. In contrast people eating plant-based diets that emphasise less-healthy foods (juices, sweetened beverages, refined grains, potatoes, fried goods and sweets) had a 32 per cent higher risk of coronary heart disease.[111] Similar results have been found for type 2 diabetes.[112]

Consistently, in some clinical studies that I conducted at Washington University, we observed that many 'ethical' lacto-ovo vegetarians and vegans consume excessive amounts of refined and processed high-glycaemic foods, rich in empty calories, trans-fatty acids and salt. In these studies, we found many of them were overweight (mean BMI 27.8 with excessive abdominal fat accumulation), had low blood HDL-cholesterol, high blood LDL-cholesterol and abnormal inflammatory markers. Some had frank hypertension or abnormal blood glucose levels.

Like many people in North America, they often consumed pre-packaged foods such as 'vegan' pizzas, vegetarian lasagne, ice cream and desserts that were full of preservatives, refined carbohydrates, simple sugars and trans-fatty acids.[113] Trans-fats are worse than animal-derived saturated fatty acids in promoting formation of atherosclerotic plaques. Some 'ethical vegetarians' also consumed lots of sugary drinks, candy, white bread and rice, and vegetable oils rich in polyunsaturated fats; whereas the lacto-ovo-vegetarians often ate excessive amounts of cheese and eggs.

To summarise, being a vegetarian in itself does not mean much. Vegetarians can decide not to consume meat, but instead overindulge in sweets, cakes and many other energy-dense foods loaded with trans-fatty acids, vegetable oil and salt.

PART III

FROM THE MEDITERRANEAN TO THE MODERN HEALTHY LONGEVITY DIET

CHAPTER EIGHT

THE MEDITERRANEAN DIET: WHERE TASTE MEETS HEALTH

My grandmother Faustina was born in Mandatoriccio, a charming small village facing the Mediterranean Sea on the east coast of Calabria. She used to tell me stories about her family and their diet before the 1950s.

Unfortunately, after the end of World War II, their dietary habits began to change because of growing economic wealth and the unhealthy influence of the American diet. Consumption of greater quantities of meat, dairy and white bread were considered a symbol of success and wealth.

Before the war, homemade bread and pasta were their staple foods, prepared weekly with freshly ground local durum wheat. This flour, which contained all the wheat germ and a high percentage of the bran (some of the coarse bran was fed to the pigs), was used to make a delicious bread, leavened very slowly using a sourdough starter containing a unique culture of lactobacillus bacteria living in symbiotic combination with yeasts. The dough was alive and ready to use, because every woman shared their starter sourdough, taking it from one home to the next and nurturing it with love. The nutritional qualities of the flavourful, crisp-crusted sourdough bread were exceptional, quite unlike the plain white bread of today, made out of refined flour and baker's yeast.

I still have wonderful childhood memories of my grandfather Natale and I sharing my grandmother's homemade bread. As a treat, Grandma would put out a small plate with some amazing homemade pickled eggplant or sun-dried tomatoes preserved in extra-virgin olive oil with wild fennel, garlic and some hot pepper to eat with her delicious bread. It was a feast! Sometimes, she would use the same dough to prepare a magnificent thin-crusted pizza topped with fresh tomato and mozzarella or tomato sauce, basil and anchovies.

Another wonderful snack that I loved was wholegrain friselle bread with tomato. Friselle is a kind of bagel-shaped crispbread made of durum wheat and barley. (In the old days, friselle was a common food for sailors to take with them on their journeys. The hard, dry crispbreads would be softened in seawater before they were eaten.)

My grandmother served friselle with a topping of diced ripe tomatoes, garlic, some leaves of basil, oregano, a pinch of sea salt and a dash of excellent extra-virgin olive oil. The secret to maximise the sensory experience was to let the friselle absorb the juice of the tomatoes along with the oil and garlic. Sometimes she would add artichokes, capers, anchovies or sardella (a relish made of tiny fish fermented in salt with plenty of dried chilli powder).

The same freshly ground wholegrain durum wheat flour was used to prepare tagliatelle or fusilli (made by wrapping the pasta dough around a knitting needle). Grandma used to serve this homemade pasta with a spicy sauce of chickpeas, lentils or fava beans. Vegetables, both raw and cooked, were (and in my house still are) an essential part of the cuisine.

No main meal was complete without lots of *verdure* or greens. I still remember the colourful and tasty mixed salads Grandma Faustina would prepare with different types of lettuce, wild herbs, dandelions, plantain, watercress, mallow or purslane onions, sliced carrot or pumpkin, capers, olives and, of course, a dressing of olive oil and lemon juice. Chard, spinach or escarole was cooked, and then slightly stir-fried in olive oil, with garlic, red pepper and some wild fennel seeds. All these salads were accompanied by a variety of small dishes: home-cured fresh fish (such as anchovies, sardines or bottarga), preserved eggplant, dried tomatoes, mushrooms, zucchini or olives. These preserves captured the taste of the vegetables at the peak of their flavour, with that heightened taste that produce acquires when it reaches full ripeness.

At my grandfather's home a glass of red wine was consumed regularly but only with meals. Dessert was usually the seasonal fruits or, during the winter, sun-dried peaches, nectarines, grapes or figs with nuts. A slice of bread with jam made from fully ripe figs (which does not require sugar) was also common for breakfast.

On special occasions such as weddings, birthdays or Christmas, Grandma Faustina would prepare some delicious yet simple sweets using honey, mosto cotto or miele di fichi as the main sweeteners. Mosto cotto is made from the juice of wine grapes cooked down to a dark syrup; miele di fichi or fig honey is made by draining the syrup of cooked figs through a cloth.

It is not surprising that this traditional Mediterranean diet consistently comes out on top as the best for our health.

THE 'DISCOVERY' OF THE MEDITERRANEAN DIET

Some people say that Ancel Keys (1904–2004), a professor at the University of Minnesota, 'discovered' the Mediterranean diet. This is far from true, people living in some of the beautiful countries facing the Mediterranean Sea had been eating and sharing this diet for hundreds of years. Ancel Keys was just the first researcher to study its cardiometabolic effects.

Professor Keys met Gino Bergami, the Director of the Institute Filippo Botazzi of Naples, at an international meeting in Rome in 1951.[1] During a coffee break, Prof Keys was complaining about the extremely high rate of heart disease deaths among business executives in the US. Dr Bergami told Professor Keys that in Naples, coronary heart disease was not a problem, and invited him to visit his hospital in Naples.

At the beginning of 1952, Professor Keys went to Naples to look into Dr Bergami's claims. With the help of Flaminio Fidanza, a young local assistant professor, he started to analyse the blood of the people living in Naples and found that their blood cholesterol level was very low (160 mg/dl [4.1 mmol/L]). During all the months he spent there, no patient was admitted to the 60-bed clinic at Naples University Hospital having suffered a heart attack. However, in the private clinics, where the wealthy Neapolitans were treated, the number of heart attacks was high, as were their blood cholesterol levels.

At that time, as Keys describes in an article he wrote about his work there, the average Neapolitan man and woman consumed very little meat (only every week or two), extra-virgin olive oil was used as a dressing; butter and cream were not part of their diet and milk was only used in small amounts in coffee (caffé macchiato) or for infants. Lunch comprised half a loaf of homemade bread crammed with boiled lettuce or spinach; pasta was eaten every day.[2] According to his dietary survey, about a quarter of the calories in the diet came from extra-virgin olive oil and wine.

In another article, Professor Keys further described the diet of the people living in this beautiful region of southern Italy:

> *Meat, fish, milk, cheese, and eggs were definitely luxuries for all the men, the great bulk of the diet being bread, pasta (macaroni, spaghetti, etc.) and local vegetables. Sugar and potatoes were eaten only in very small amounts, and butter was never used. Fruits and very small amounts of cheese were quite regularly consumed.[3]*

This traditional Mediterranean diet was consumed in many of the southern regions of Italy, including Puglia, Sicily, Sardinia and Calabria.

HEALTH EFFECTS OF THE MEDITERRANEAN DIET: HOW SOLID IS THE SCIENTIFIC EVIDENCE?

After the surprising observations made in Naples, Professor Keys was more intrigued than ever. He realised that this was the tip of the iceberg. In mid-1952 he accepted an invitation to travel to Spain from Dr Carlos Jiménez Díaz, a professor of medicine in Madrid. Keys found that the people living in the Vallecas and Cuatro Caminos, the workers' districts of Madrid, had a much lower incidence of heart attacks than inhabitants of the wealthy district of Salamanca. The dietary surveys showed that the working-class inhabitants did not consume milk or butter and rarely meat – and had much lower blood cholesterol levels – while the tables of the wealthy people from Salamanca were loaded with rich foods and all sorts of red and processed meat.

In 1955, Keys went to Cagliari in Sardinia and Bologna in Emilia Romagna. He found that people from Cagliari were eating the same diet as Neapolitans and that they too experienced an extremely low rate of heart attacks. He recorded that the blood cholesterol level of Sardinian men was very low, despite the fact they ate lots of eggs (more than the average man ate in his home town of Minnesota), but their consumption of meat and dairy products was extremely low.

In Bologna things were quite different. Italians call this area of Italy 'Emilia la grassa' (Emilia, the fat land), because Bolognese cuisine is very rich in animal products: salami, raw and cooked ham, mortadella, lard, butter, cheese, and the world-famous Parmigiano Reggiano. Here, cholesterol levels were much higher than in Sardinian men, and the Department of Medicine of the University of Bologna had a good share of patients with coronary heart disease.[4] Similar studies were carried out by Dr. Noboru Kimura in Fukuoka prefecture in Japan and by Dr Martti Karvonen in North Karelia in Finland.

To cut a long story short, in 1970, after 15 years of observational studies of more than 12,000 men living in Italy, Greece, Yugoslavia, Finland, Holland, Japan and the US, the results of the 'Seven Countries Study' conducted by Professor Keys and colleagues were published. This study strongly suggested that there was a high association between the amount of dietary saturated fat intake, blood cholesterol levels and the risk of death from cardiovascular diseases.[5]

Of the people living in these seven countries, Finland, Holland and the US had the highest animal food consumption, the highest saturated fat intake, the highest blood cholesterol levels and the highest percentage of cardiovascular deaths. In contrast, the Mediterranean countries and Japan were at the opposite end of the spectrum.

One of the most important discoveries of the Seven Countries Study was that both the inhabitants of Crete in Greece and North Karelia in Finland obtained more than 40 per cent of their calories from fat. However, the percentage of deaths from heart attack was much higher in Finland than in Crete – the average middle-aged Finnish man was consuming butter, milk and cheese as the main source of fat, while for men in Crete it was fish, nuts and extra-virgin olive oil. According to Professor Keys' notes, a favourite after-sauna snack of Finnish lumberjacks was 'a slab of full-fat cheese the size of a slice of bread on which was smeared a thick layer of butter'.[6]

In recent years, new population-based epidemiological studies in the US and Europe suggest that the Mediterranean diet might also have a protective effect against diabetes, hypertension, several type of cancers, allergic conditions, and, as most recently reported, against Alzheimer's diseases and Parkinson's disease.[7] However, epidemiological studies are by nature observational and do not imply a cause-effect relationship.

A series of randomised clinical trials have since confirmed a strong protective effect against heart disease. The first to demonstrate the beneficial effect of a Mediterranean-style diet was the Lyon Diet Heart Study.[8] In this trial, 605 men and women who had already had heart attacks were randomised to either the diet recommended by the American Heart Association or a Mediterranean-like diet, supplemented with a margarine rich in alpha-linolenic (plant-based omega-3, polyunsaturated, fatty acids).

Patients randomised to the Mediterranean-type diet consumed more bread, vegetables, fruit and fish, and less red meat (that was replaced with poultry), while butter and cream were exchanged for the margarine rich in alpha-linolenic acid. Interestingly, after only two years, the study had to be terminated because people eating the Mediterranean-like diet experienced an amazing 70 per cent reduction in mortality. This was due to a 73 per cent reduction in coronary heart disease death and major reductions in non-fatal complications. The diet had a striking protective effect against the recurrence of heart disease.

In another trial, patients at high risk or with existing coronary heart disease who were randomised to an 'Indo-Mediterranean diet', rich in whole grains, fruits, vegetables, walnuts, almonds, mustard or soybean oil, experienced a significant 50 per cent reduction in the rate of non-fatal heart attacks and a 60 per cent reduction in the rate of sudden cardiac death.[9]

More recently, the five-year PRIDIMED trial has demonstrated that in men and women at high cardiometabolic risk, but with no evident cardiovascular disorders at baseline, consuming a Mediterranean diet supplemented with extra-virgin olive oil or nuts is associated with a significantly lower number of cardiovascular events, in particular fewer strokes.[10] Secondary analysis of this trial suggests that individuals randomised to the Mediterranean diet may also experience a reduced risk of developing type 2 diabetes, other heart-associated disease (peripheral artery disease, atrial fibrillation) and breast cancer.[11-13]

MECHANISMS BEHIND THE BENEFITS OF THE MEDITERRANEAN DIET

Several factors have been hypothesised to explain the benefits of consuming a traditional Mediterranean diet. The three most important are:

1. lowering of cholesterol

2. reducing oxidative and inflammatory damage

3. modifying the composition and function of the gut microbiome.

Lowering of cholesterol

The traditional Mediterranean diet of my grandmother Faustina was rich in high-fibre vegetables and low in animal fat, and this combination explains most of its positive effects on cholesterol. A lower intake of saturated fat translates into lower blood cholesterol. Because of the very low consumption of meat, milk and butter, the intake of saturated fat is very low: less than 8 per cent of energy. Replacing 5 per cent of calories from saturated fats with similar quantities from polyunsaturated vegetable fat, monounsaturated vegetable fat, or carbohydrates from minimally processed whole grains is associated with a 25 per cent, 15 per cent and 9 per cent lower risk of coronary heart disease, respectively.[14] Alternatively, substituting saturated fats with refined carbohydrates increases the risk of a heart attack.[15]

FOOD RICH IN SATURATED FAT

Examples of foods rich in saturated fats are:

- dairy products, including butter, cream, whole milk and cheese
- meat, especially fatty cuts of beef, pork and lamb
- lard and processed meats such as sausages and salami
- chicken skin.

Saturated fats are also frequently found in processed and packaged foods including:

- biscuits, pastries, cakes, and desserts
- fatty snacks like potato crisps and deep-fried foods like French fries cooked in palm oil.

In the Mediterranean diet, extra-virgin olive oil, nuts and seeds provide most of the fat, in particular plenty of monounsaturated and polyunsaturated fatty acids. Fish and walnuts, for instance, are a good source of polyunsaturated omega-3 fatty acids, while almonds, hazelnuts and pine nuts provide omega-6 fatty acids and plant sterols, which seem to play an important role in reducing LDL-cholesterol levels and heart disease risk.[16]

A trial conducted in Canada found that eating a range of cholesterol-lowering foods, such as nuts, soy protein, oats, barley and psyllium, can lower LDL-cholesterol by 13 per cent;[17] and data from epidemiological studies suggest that consuming five servings of nuts per week is associated with a 40–60 per cent reduction in the risk of heart attack.[18] Moreover, growing data suggest the naturally occurring trans-fatty acids found in milk and red meat have similar adverse effects on blood lipids.[19]

Another factor responsible for the lower levels of cholesterol in people consuming a Mediterranean diet is the high intake of fibre. A typical Mediterranean diet provides 30–45 g of fibre per day which comes from eating lots of whole grains, legumes, vegetables, nuts and dried fruits.

Data from several trials indicate that high consumption of water-soluble fibre can lower cholesterol quite substantially because it blocks the (re)absorption of cholesterol and bile acids in the small intestine. For each additional gram of water-soluble fibre it is estimated that LDL-cholesterol drops by approximately 1.12 mg/L.[20] In addition, low-glycaemic foods rich in dietary fibre have been shown to reduce circulating insulin and increase the levels of short-chain fatty acids produced by fibre fermentation, which have both been demonstrated to inhibit the production of cholesterol by the liver.[21]

REDUCED OXIDATIVE AND INFLAMMATORY DAMAGE

Mediterranean diet staples, such as vegetables, beans, unrefined whole grains, nuts, seeds, fruits and extra-virgin olive oil, are loaded with antioxidant vitamins and minerals (vitamin C, vitamin E, beta-carotene, selenium, folate), and a wide range of phytochemicals. For example, we have calculated that people consuming a healthy Mediterranean diet on a normal day ingest about 400 mg of vitamin C, 17 mg of vitamin E, 6000 mg of beta-carotene equivalents (derived from provitamin A carotenoids) and 120 mg of selenium. These are powerful antioxidants that have been shown to be extremely important in protecting cells and tissue against oxidative damage.

Oxidative stress plays a main role in the onset and progression of many chronic diseases, including cancer and dementia. Results from large epidemiological studies suggest there is a protective effect of the Mediterranean diet and its dietary antioxidants against heart disease not only induced by an unhealthy lifestyle but also by long-term exposure to air pollutants.[22,23] Not eating enough antioxidant-rich food contributes to the development of plaque in arteries (atherosclerosis) by oxidising the lipids contained in LDL-cholesterol particles. Oxidised LDL particles bind to specific receptors on endothelial and immune cells, boosting the growth of atherosclerotic plaques.[24] Results from a recent trial of the Mediterranean diet showed a significant reduction in circulating oxidised LDL and inflammatory markers.[25,26]

Multiple nutrients from the many diverse foods are responsible for the anti-inflammatory effects of the Mediterranean diet.[27] They synergise with the high-fibre and low-energy density of minimally processed plant foods in lowering inflammation. Fish consumption, which is rich in omega-3 fatty acids, contributes to reducing inflammation by activating some anti-inflammatory pathways.[28,29] Several phytochemicals (such as ferulic acid and olechantal) found in whole grains and extra-virgin olive oil may also play a role in inhibiting inflammation.[30]

GUT HEALTH

Did you know that trillions of microorganisms live in our gut, including bacteria, viruses, prokaryotes (unicellular organisms that lack a distinct nucleus) and yeasts? Some can be our best friends, but others may become our worst enemies, contributing to the development of many chronic ailments. What we eat can determine which ones will thrive or die. If we eat meat, for example, we boost the growth of bacteria that break down peptides, whereas consuming vegetables favours those synthetising proteins.

My research group, together with Professor Jeffrey Gordon, one of the world's leading experts in microbiota biology, has demonstrated that, of all the nutrients, protein and insoluble fibre are the most important influences on the type of bacteria in our intestine.[31] What is interesting is that each family of bacteria produces specific metabolites with important biological functions.

A Mediterranean diet high in dietary insoluble fibre has been shown to increase the production of certain bacteria (called Bacteroidetes and Firmicutes), which produce high levels of short-chain fatty acids (such as butyrate and propionate).[32,33] These metabolites, by binding to specific receptors, inhibit inflammation[34,35] and increase the levels of certain immune cells, called regulatory T cells, which protect us from the development of allergic and autoimmune disorders.[36,37] The drastic drop in consumption of fibre-rich vegetables, legumes and whole grains in Western diets may be responsible, at least in part, for the remarkable increase in asthma, type 1 diabetes, and multiple sclerosis.

Data from a recent study showed that the amount of dietary fibre and protein is also the strongest determinant for the development and progression of inflammatory bowel disease (IBD). Among all the types of vegetable fibre tested, psyllium, pectin and cellulose fibre reduced the severity of colitis, whereas methylcellulose and protein, especially casein from milk, worsened the colitis.[38]

The harmful inflammatory effect of excessive protein is supported by epidemiological data suggesting an increased rate of ulcerative colitis relapses in people consuming excessive amounts of meat and other animal proteins.[39] The beneficial effects of vegetable fibre are supported by other epidemiological studies showing a 53 per cent reduced risk of Crohn's disease with higher consumption of vegetables and fruit,[40] and a greater risk of Crohn's recurrence in those who avoid eating fibre-rich foods.[41] A small randomised clinical trial of patients with ulcerative colitis in remission showed that psyllium fibre supplementation caused a substantial improvement in gastrointestinal symptoms.[42]

Finally, the digestion of animal proteins by certain gut bacteria can also influence the risk of heart disease. For instance, animal and human studies have clearly shown that when gut bacteria digest dietary choline and L-carnitine – abundant in red meat, eggs and cheese – they produce a metabolite called trimethylamine N-oxide (TMAO), which increases the risk of developing cardiovascular disease by 20 per cent, independently of traditional cardiometabolic risk factors.[43] We estimated that the intake of choline and L-carnitine is more than 50 per cent lower in the traditional Mediterranean diet than in a typical Western diet.

Even if some bacteria respond to dietary changes within a couple of days, there is growing evidence that you need to stick to the changes for a long time to substantially modify the composition of the microbial community in your gut. We have shown that long-term consumption of a calorie restricted, plant-rich diet results in a richer and more diverse microbiota.[44]

In contrast, exposure for multiple generations to a Western diet causes specific microbiota and bacterial lineages to become extinct.[45] This could have serious detrimental effects on the immune system and brain development of your children and your long-term health.[46]

CHAPTER NINE

MOVE TO THE MODERN HEALTHY LONGEVITY DIET

It is very difficult to define what a healthy and balanced 'Mediterranean diet' is, because no single one exists. Twenty-three countries border the Mediterranean Sea, and their inhabitants' dietary habits, the ingredients and types of dishes they make and eat, and their lifestyles and cultures vary considerably.

Also today's Mediterranean diet has transformed radically, and has little to do with the quality and quantity of the traditional Mediterranean diet of my grandmother Faustina. Pizza made with white refined flour covered with mozzarella cheese, ham or prosciutto, big portions of white bread and pasta with meat sauce, and many other products labelled as Mediterranean foods were not consumed when Professor Ancel Keys visited Italy in 1952.

We must also bear in mind that many other things have changed since my grandparents were born. Most people in industrialised countries live a sedentary life; they do not need to perform hard manual work anymore. After tractors rolled onto farms in the early 20th century, manual labour declined steeply, and consequently so did the calorie requirements.

If we were to consume the same amount of olive oil, pasta and bread that my grandparents were eating, we would become obese and unhealthy in no time. A single tablespoon of olive oil contains about 120 calories, so if we were to eat 10 tablespoons of it every day, that extra 1200 calories would cancel out the positive effects of the vitamins and phytocompounds contained in this precious and healthy condiment.

The Mediterranean diet has some great aspects that we can all learn from, but there are other elements to take into account for healthy longevity. The knowledge we have acquired over the past couple of decades about the metabolic and molecular mechanisms that regulate ageing is allowing us to more accurately choose what to eat, how much of it and when, to meet our nutrient needs.[1]

There is no doubt in my mind that consuming the appropriate amounts of calories and proteins is the most important factor in promoting health and longevity, but the quality of these calories and proteins is also key. Reducing calories by eating smaller portions of unhealthy foods won't extend lifespan and will just lead to malnutrition. If you force an obese person to eat only bread and water, in the short-term they may experience some weight loss-induced benefits, but they eventually will develop major nutrient and vitamin deficiencies that will cause life-threatening illnesses and dramatically shorten their lifespan.

NO MAGIC INGREDIENT OR SUPERFOOD EXISTS

People are fascinated by the promise of a silver bullet to improve health and cure all sorts of infirmities. Some people concentrate their attention on selected superfoods – such as extra-virgin olive oil, broccoli, kale, almonds, goji berries, chia seeds, green tea; the more exotic, the better – while others consume supplements or single isolated compounds (e.g. resveratrol, quercetin) hoping for dramatic health benefits.

The truth is that no magic ingredient or superfood exists. Everything in nature has been optimised for maximal efficiency in the right combination and proportion. Different foods, as we will see, need to be consumed in the right amount in order to balance out the consumption of calories and protein with our energy expenditure, while providing all the essential nutrients, fibres and phytochemicals.

Our diets need to provide not just the right amount of calories and proteins, but all the essential nutrients as well. To achieve 100 per cent of the recommended daily intake for each essential vitamin and mineral and stay within your target calorie and protein intake, it is essential to eliminate processed and refined food from your diet and choose a combination of nutritious foods.

For example, preliminary data suggest a synergistic interaction between certain bioactive phytochemicals in food and a moderate reduction of calorie intake, since both promote a reduction in oxidative stress.[2] In contrast, excessive calorie intake may mute the antioxidant and anti-inflammatory effect of certain foods.[3] We also need to learn to maximise the extraction of essential nutrients while transforming them into deeply satisfying meals. We don't have to sacrifice flavour to eat healthy food!

So, based on the knowledge gained so far, how can we start to design our healthy diet?

THE IMPORTANCE OF HEALTHY FOOD DIVERSITY

Eating healthily, first and foremost, means diversifying. It is a natural law. We know, for instance, that monoculture farming leads to the development of plant pathogens and diseases. In contrast, plant diversity is essential for healthy ecosystems. If you observe the composition of a forest, you will see that ferns, moss, lichen, wildflowers and many small plants live on the forest floor, while a variety of shrubs fill in the understorey, and tall trees occupy the higher level. All these different plants live together and help each other in a perfectly self-sustained cycle.

Similarly, a healthy diet should be as diverse as possible. Vegetables contain compounds that can target sick cells and keep normal cells happy. Eating a wide variety of vegetables allows different unique bioactive molecules to interact, playing different roles in helping us to fend off disease.

Different foods can also have synergistic interactions.[4] For example, combining foods like garlic (rich in S-allylcysteine) with tomatoes (rich in lycopene) can inhibit the progression of stomach cancer at much lower intakes than if these foods are eaten individually.[5] Likewise, consuming soybeans (genistein-rich foods), with apples or capers (quercetin-rich foods), can block prostate and ovarian cancer cell growth at a much lower level than when consumed in isolation.[6] Preliminary data suggest that quercetin and fisetin (also found in apples) may even be able to kill abnormal senescent cells in our body.[7]

Diversity, however, doesn't mean eating a little bit of everything (including little bits of junk food), but selecting the healthiest foods and eating them in the right proportions. The saying 'everything in moderation' may not be the best dietary rule of thumb. In fact, in several studies conducted in the US and other Western countries dietary diversity was associated with suboptimal eating patterns, greater energy intake and increased weight gain.[8]

Individuals who ate a wide variety of foods were also more likely to consume higher amounts of processed foods, refined grains and sugar-sweetened beverages. As we will see, eating a selected number of minimally processed highly nutritious foods is the key for the prevention of a wide range of chronic illnesses.

THE MODERN HEALTHY LONGEVITY FOOD PYRAMID EXPLAINED

The foundation of a modern healthy diet includes a wide variety of colourful vegetables, beans, minimally processed whole grains, nuts, seeds and fruits. These plant-based foods should be consumed every day and form the largest portion of our calories.

Extra-virgin cold-pressed olive oil and avocado fruits can be used daily as condiments together with a range of spices, lemon juice and very small amounts of iodised salt.[9]

Fish, shellfish and molluscs can be consumed two to three times per week.

Small portions of cheese and a few eggs can be consumed one to two times per week.

Meat and sweets should be eaten only occasionally.

Spring water and herbal teas are the best drinks to stay hydrated. All sugary beverages, such as soft drinks and fruit juices, and highly processed foods, should be avoided.

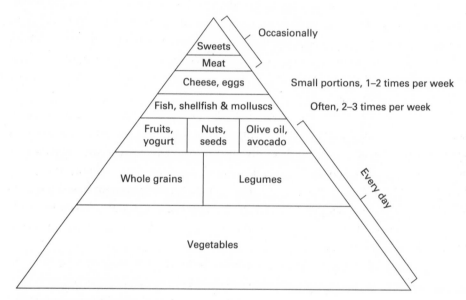

Figure 14: The modern food pyramid

VEGETABLES: THE STAPLE FOOD OF THE MODERN DIET

Starting at the bottom of the pyramid, vegetables are essential for our health; they nourish our organs, tissues and cells. The word 'vegetable' derives from the Latin word 'vegetabilis', which means growing or flourishing, and is still used to describe all edible plant foods, including vegetables, grains, legumes, nuts and fruit. Of these plant foods, leafy green and yellow-orange vegetables are those with the lowest calorie density and glycaemic load, but with the highest concentration of healthy vitamins, minerals and oligo-elements (i.e. pure trace minerals, present in minuscule quantities, but essential for metabolic health).[10]

These leafy green, purple, yellow and orange coloured vegetables are the most botanically diverse, and are packed with thousands of biologically active phytochemicals, which contribute significant variety and complexity to human diet and health.[11] Polyphenols, for instance, are phytochemicals produced by plants to protect themselves from environmental stresses, such as UV light, drought, lack of certain nutrients and predation. Interestingly, accumulating data suggest that these molecules may also improve stress resistance in plant eaters, including humans. This phenomenon is called 'xenohormesis'.[12,13]

What do we know about the health benefits of vegetables?

Data from large cohort studies suggest a high vegetable intake, especially raw vegetables, is associated with a lower risk of death from ischemic heart diseases, stroke, chronic respiratory disease, liver disease and some types of cancer.[14-16] In particular, higher consumption of green leafy vegetables, beta-carotene- and vitamin C-rich fruit and vegetables, and citrus fruit is associated with a lower risk of heart disease.[17] A high intake of vegetables seems to contribute to the reduction of blood pressure, a major cardiometabolic risk factor; the active ingredients responsible for this effect are most likely potassium and magnesium.[18]

Because body fat, smoking and other lifestyle factors are powerful variables, data about cancer are less certain. In many studies fruits and vegetables are analysed together, which may obscure potentially protective effects of certain vegetables or fruit families on some cancers.[19] Also in many Western countries, about 30 per cent of fruit is consumed as fruit juice, and high-glycaemic index potato-based products (like baked white potatoes, potato chips, etc.) constitute 27 per cent of total vegetable intake. Generally dark green vegetables and cabbage contribute to less than 1 per cent of total vegetables consumed.

Nonetheless, data from a pooled analysis, including 993,466 women from 20 studies, suggest the more vegetables eaten the better outcomes for breast cancer (especially oestrogen-receptor-negative breast cancer), bowel and kidney cancers.[20,21] Higher intake of vegetables, especially fresh vegetables, has seen a reduced risk of developing lung, throat and oesophageal cancers.[22-25] Some carotenoids, such as lutein and zeaxanthin, contained in green leafy vegetables, have also been related to a decreased risk of developing cancer and cataracts.[26]

Weight control

Because of their high fibre and water content and low glycaemic load, non-starchy vegetables are essential for maintaining a healthy body weight. Indeed, scientific data show that the higher the intake of vegetables, the stronger the reduction in body weight.[27,28]

Counting calories is difficult and boring. One strategy I use is to start my meals with a variety of non-starchy organic raw and cooked vegetables, like leafy greens, carrots, peppers, pumpkin, avocado, onion that help to fill me up while providing lots of vitamins, minerals and phytochemicals.

Vegetable consumption and gut health

Recent data also indicate that the variety of plants we consume is the single most important contributor to gut microbiome biodiversity, which I have earlier noted is enormously important to good health.

In the past decade the incidence and prevalence of type 1 diabetes, for example, has increased approximately 2–3 per cent per year, especially among children younger than 15 years. A similar increase has been noted for allergic (asthma, atopic eczema) and other autoimmune disorders (multiple sclerosis, inflammatory bowel diseases). Clearly, this striking surge cannot be explained by genetic modifications; genes do not change that fast. Data suggest that it is the changing diet of infants and therefore decreased gut-microbiome diversity that may play an important role.[29] The burden of chronic disease in old age is also associated with lower microbiota biodiversity, probably due to immune alterations and increased inflammation.[30]

'Eating the rainbow': consume the widest possible range of vegetables

For many people, eating vegetables means consuming potatoes, tomatoes, lettuce, carrots and maybe one or two stems of broccoli. Typically this is what we are served at restaurants too. However, if we take into account the different types of leaves, stems and roots, there are more than 40 botanical families of vegetables, each one containing *hundreds* of varieties.

Accumulating data suggest it's ideal to eat as many as we can. Results from epidemiological studies suggest that increasing the variety of vegetables in our diet offers extra protective effects against type 2 diabetes[31] and cancer.[32-35]

The exact mechanisms through which biodiversity boosts health is not clear. However, it is well known that different types of vegetables contain different concentrations of vitamins, minerals, oligo-elements and some unique phytochemicals, which synergistically stimulate or inhibit specific key pathways. A recent study has shown that eating a greater variety of vegetables, more than 13 categories per month, is associated with lower systemic inflammation as well.[36]

Ideally, every single one of our meals should contain a variety of raw and cooked vegetables; so experiment and use a diverse array of vegetables. Science tells us that the higher the biodiversity of vegetables we consume, the greater the health benefits. So eat the rainbow.

Large dark-green leafy vegetables

Include large dark green leafy vegetables in your diet because they are nutritional powerhouses rich in chlorophyll, folic acid, carotenoids and vitamin K, and are essential to neutralise excess acidity caused by the animal food-rich Western diet. In a small randomised clinical trial, supplementation with folic acid caused a three-fold reduction in the recurrence of precancerous colon lesions, called adenomas.[37] Dark-green leafy vegetables also contain lutein and zeaxanthin, which are important for protecting eye tissues.[38]

There are many varieties of dark green leaves that can be eaten raw or lightly steamed. Avoid overcooking them by boiling, as this will strip them of essential vitamins and minerals. My favourites are silver beet, spinach, beet greens and mustard greens. Did you know 100 g (3½ oz) of cooked silver beet contains 312 per cent of the recommended daily allowance (RDA) for vitamin K (which plays a key role in blood clotting, as well as bone health), 38 per cent of the RDA for vitamin A and 22 per cent of the RDA for vitamin C?

There are also many different varieties of tender green-purple vegetables suitable for raw salads, such as lettuce, endive, chicory, garden cress, and dandelion greens. Common varieties of chicory include radicchio, puntarelle and endive, while common lettuce includes loose-leaf, romaine, iceberg and butter.

I like to prepare colourful, healthy raw salads dressed with extra-virgin olive oil, lemon juice or balsamic vinegar, with a sprinkling of finely sliced onion, chopped nuts, olives and a pinch of salt.

TIP: From time to time, the stems and leaves of purslane can be added to salads because of their interesting slightly sour and salty taste, and purslane's relatively high concentration of vegetable omega-3 fatty acids. 50 g of fresh purslane contain approximately 200 mg of alpha-linolenic acid, a healthy essential fatty acid.[39]

Cruciferous vegetables

Part of the family Brassicaceae, cruciferous vegetables include cabbage, broccoli, cauliflower, Brussels sprouts, kale, savoy cabbage, collard greens, watercress, arugula (rocket), bok choy, turnip greens, kohlrabi and gai lan. These interesting and healthy vegetables contain high levels of vitamin C and some unique phytochemicals, such as isothiocyanates, indol-3-carbinol and sulforophane, which seem to play a role in cancer prevention and longevity.[40]

Many of the precious compounds in these vegetables are heat-sensitive and are rapidly destroyed by cooking. The best way to eat broccoli, for instance, is raw or steamed for just two to three minutes. The same applies to other cruciferous veggies, including kale, cauliflower and cabbage.[41]

It is better to consume these cruciferous veggies in combination with some mustard, because it contains an enzyme called myrosinase, which helps convert the dorment phytochemical glucoraphanin into the powerful cancer-suppressor molecule isothiocyanate. One of my favourite salads is finely sliced cabbage dressed with extra-virgin olive oil, lots of lemon juice, a pinch of marine salt, and a honey mustard dressing on the side.

TIP: Add some capers to your salads. They are one of the richest sources of the flavonoid quercetin, which has antioxidant and potential anti-inflammatory and anti-cancer properties.[42] In several animal models, quercetin has also been shown to lower blood pressure and other metabolic syndrome factors.[43,44]

FOR THE SCIENTIFICALLY MINDED

Powerful anti-cancer effects of cruciferous vegetables

Epidemiological studies show eating cruciferous vegetables is linked with a reduced risk of several cancers, including prostate, bladder and lung.[45] Sulforophane of broccoli, for example, has been shown to trigger detoxifying enzymes that play a role in protecting against colon and skin cancer,[46] and in the prevention of type 2 diabetes[47] and autism.[48]

Isothiocyanates and indoles, which are formed when we chew raw cruciferous vegetables, have been shown to reduce the incidence of tumours in experimental animals exposed to carcinogens.[49,50]

A recent paper in the prestigious journal *Science* shows that indole-3-carbinol is a powerful inhibitor of a cancer-promoting enzyme called WWP1. This enzyme blocks the activity of one of the most potent tumour suppressors called PTEN. Basically, indole-3-carbinol activates a complex chemical response that sets free PTEN to do its job, which is preventing the growth of tumours.[51] PTEN is also involved in longevity. Indeed, mice that are engineered to produce surplus PTEN not only are healthier and protected from cancer, but also live much longer.[52]

Pumpkin, carrots and sweet potatoes

Eat carrots, pumpkins and sweet potatoes often. They are loaded with different carotenoids – responsible for their orange colour and for the production of vitamin A. This vitamin plays a key role in eye and immune-function health, and in prenatal and postnatal development. Several studies have shown that plasma beta-carotene levels are three times higher when we eat carrots and spinach that have been steamed (but not boiled) and pureed, than when these vegetables are consumed raw.[53]

Carrots, like celery and parsley, are members of the Apiaceae or Umbelliferae family, and all contain the compound polyacetylene, which displays some preventative effects against thrombosis (blood clots) and cancer.[54]

Sweet potatoes contain the highest concentration of beta-carotene (31 mg in 100 g (3½ oz) of cooked product), but pumpkin also provide generous amounts of alpha-carotene, zeaxanthin and lutein, making it a superior source of antioxidants.

Pumpkin's delicious, sweet flavour makes it a versatile ingredient for many recipes. Sometimes I cut thin slices and eat them raw. Raw pumpkin can also be added to a morning smoothie with fruits, avocado, nuts and dates or raisins. It can be roasted or baked, or used to prepare nutritious winter soups. Cooked pumpkin can be pureed with chickpeas, tahini, garlic and lemon juice for a colourful hummus.

> TIP: In order to optimise carotenoid absorption and conversion to vitamin A, fat (for instance extra-virgin olive oil) needs to be eaten at the same meal as carrots, pumpkin or sweet potato.[55]

Tomatoes

Red tomatoes and in smaller amounts, watermelon, contain lycopene, a strong antioxidant, which has been shown to be important in the prevention of certain cancers, including prostate, digestive tract and cervical.[56]

Preliminary data from a small randomised clinical trial of lycopene supplementation before radical prostatectomy suggest a reduction in prostate cancer growth.[57] This anti-cancer effect might be mediated, at least in part, through a direct effect of lycopene in reducing IGF-I bioavailability.[58] Eating cooked tomato puree results in a greater elevation in lycopene than consuming raw tomato juice.[59]

Allium genus

Onion, garlic and leeks are members of the *Allium* genus and are loaded with unique volatile organo-sulphur compounds, which give these vegetables their characteristic aroma and flavour.[60] When garlic is cut or crushed, the compound alliin is exposed to alliinase, an enzyme that is essential to produce allicin. Heating destroys garlic's active allyl sulphur compound formation.[61]

Cell culture and some animal studies suggest that allicin may lower the risk of heart disease by lowering blood pressure and cholesterol levels. Allicin can also be transformed into several bioactive compounds. Data from animal studies suggest that supplementation with one of garlic's bioactive compounds, (gamma-glutamyl-Se-methylselenocysteine), protects against the development of breast cancer.[62] Diallyl sulphide, one of the main bioactive compounds of garlic, when given to mice, inhibits the incidence of bowel cancer by 74 per cent.[63]

Human studies show that regular garlic-powder intake has a protective effect against hypertension and the age-dependent stiffening of arteries.[64] Several case-controlled studies suggest garlic consumption is associated with a reduced risk of developing some common cancers, including gastric, colon, prostate and endometrial.[65,66]

Onion, *Allium cepa*, is one of the richest sources of dietary flavonoids (fructo-oligosaccharides and thiosulfinates). Flavonoids, in particular, have shown to be important in the prevention of cardiovascular diseases and cancer, especially gastric cancer.[67]

There are many different types of onions, in shape, colour of the outer scales (red, pink, yellow, white), spiciness (from sweet to very pungent) and storage life. Red onions, my favourite, contain the highest levels of flavonols, while yellow onions contain only half as much.

Interestingly, the Italian sweet red onion, Tropea, a staple in the diet of centenarians in Mediterranean countries, contains high concentrations of taxifolin, a compound that has been shown to be a powerful inhibitor of many types of cultured cancer cells.[68]

Other vegetables that I love to eat are asparagus, artichokes, garden peas, cucumbers and radishes. They call contain bioactive compounds.

WHITE POTATOES ARE STARCH BOMBS

White potatoes don't behave like most other vegetables – they are starch bombs. Several studies suggest that people who consume seven or more servings per week of baked, boiled, mashed and especially fried potatoes have a higher risk of developing type 2 diabetes compared to those who consume less than one serving per week.[69] Similar results have been observed for the risk of developing high blood pressure and obesity.[70]

In Australia and the US, potatoes are the most consumed vegetable, with Americans each consuming on average 52kg (114 lb) of potatoes every year, of which two-thirds are French fries and potato chips. Fried potatoes are the worst. We found that people who eat fried potatoes two to three times per week have an increased mortality risk.[71]

WILD EDIBLE WEEDS: A WELL OF NUTRIENTS

Did you know that several wild common weeds are edible and more nutritious than any vegetables you can buy in a store? Because they have not been bred commercially, they possess higher concentrations of vitamins, oligo-elements and phytochemicals.[72,73]

Typical vegetables are bred in protected fields to optimise yield, for bigger and less bitter leaves. In contrast, edible wild vegetables have been naturally selected to resist adverse conditions, including cold, aridity, wild animals and insects. This is why they are loaded with phytochemicals.

These weeds are healthier, and produce a stronger, more alive taste. Take for example, wild dandelion, plantain, borage, clover, purslane, wild brassica, mallow, Japanese knotweed, nettles, chickweed, sheep's sorrel and ground ivy: all these can be added to our salads to enhance taste and nutrient content. Wild dandelions, which are an excellent source of vitamin A, vitamin K, calcium and iron, can be eaten raw in a salad, and the leaves can also be cooked and eaten like spinach.

NOTE: You must be very careful to forage for edible weeds safely – you need to be absolutely certain that the weeds you are picking are what you think they are and also that they are growing in healthy unpolluted soils. It is essential to know beyond any reasonable doubt that what you are consuming is edible; there are very toxic plants, some of which are poisonous. Look out for edible weed foraging courses so you can learn about the plants that can be safely foraged.

HERBS AND SPICES: MAXIMISING FLAVOUR

Since antiquity, culinary herbs and spices have been used to provide a wonderful range of flavours, aromas and colour to our food, as well as being used as preservatives because of their well-known antimicrobial and antiviral properties. However, one of the main reasons to learn how to incorporate flavourful fresh, dried or powdered herbs and spices in your recipes is to reduce the consumption of less healthy ingredients such as salt, sugar, butter and vegetable oils.

Chilli pepper, basil, parsley, coriander (cilantro), dill, rosemary, sage, thyme, oregano, turmeric, black pepper, cumin, caraway and many other herbal seasonings can be used to transform a so-so recipe into a memorable culinary masterpiece that is delicious and enhances your health.

Culinary herbs and spices contain high concentrations of unique phytochemicals that clearly alter metabolic and cellular processes with potentially positive clinical effects. I use the word 'potential' because it is very difficult to demonstrate in human randomised clinical trials the independent effect of one or more of these herbs and spices in preventing cancer or cardiovascular disease.

However, according to the Phenol-Explorer database, the richest sources of polyphenols are spices and herbs (see table 4). Cloves, peppermint and star anise comprise the highest concentrations of phenolic compounds (eugenol in cloves, eriocitrin in peppermint and anethole in star anise), followed by oregano, sage and rosemary.[74] Herbs of the Lamiaceae family – peppermint, sage, rosemary, spearmint, thyme – contain the highest amounts of a powerful antioxidant compound, hydroxycinnamic acid.

Here is a list of the spices and herbs that I use when I cook.

Chilli pepper or cayenne (*Capsicum* species)

I often use this to add a spicy, hot taste to many of my favourite dishes. The bioactive compounds that give chilli pepper its pungent intensity are capsaicin and capsaicinoids, which not only have potent analgesic (pain relief) effects,[75] but might also play a role in the prevention of obesity and its related complications by activating two important molecular pathways called TRPV1 and AMPK.[76]

Data from animal studies indicate that dietary capsaicin inhibits inflammation in fat and liver cells, and improves glucose control.[77] In a very small randomised clinical trial, diet supplementation with capsinoids was associated with abdominal fat loss in mildly obese people.[78] In another human study, daily ingestion of capsinoids for six weeks increased energy expenditure by enhancing the heat producing activity of brown adipose tissue.[79]

Sweet peppers contain a series of less pungent compounds, called capsinoids, which share a similar structure and function to the hot pepper capsaicinoids.[80]

Turmeric (*Curcuma longa*)

This is another of my kitchen staples. It can be used fresh (grated) or as a dried powder to give curries or vegetables dishes a distinctive sun-yellow colour and a slightly bitter, peppery, earthy taste. But most importantly, this precious rhizome will provide high concentrations of a phytochemical called curcumin.

Several studies show a potential anti-inflammatory, antioxidant and anti-cancer effect. Curcumin's ability to affect the activity of our genes and to induce the programmed death (apoptosis) of cancer cells in preclinical models is likely to be of particular relevance to colon cancer prevention.[81,82]

Research on rodents shows that curcumin has inhibitory effects against colon, skin and oral cancer.[83] In a pilot study, six months of treatment with curcumin and quercetin resulted in a significant reduction of colon polyp number and size.[84,85] Finally, some very preliminary data suggest that curcumin might also play a role in the prevention of dementia, because it seems to inhibit the formation of amyloid plaques.[86]

> TIP: Unfortunately curcumin is poorly absorbed by the human body when consumed on its own.[87] A trick to improve its absorption is to combine turmeric with black pepper; the latter contains a compound called piperine which can double blood curcumin levels.[88]

Cumin (*Cuminum cyminum*)

This has been used for centuries throughout the world for its rich, spicy pungent flavour and its purported medicinal effects. What we typically consume are the dried yellow-brown seeds of the herb *Cuminum cyminum*, a member of the Umbelliferae family, which also includes caraway, dill and parsley. Cumin seeds can be used as whole seeds, or even better, as a powder in combination with other spices, the most famous being garam masala and dukkah.

When I have time, I gently toast the whole seeds and freshly grind them to produce a flavour-rich powder. While enriching my food with its nutty taste, the freshly ground cumin also provides plenty of valuable polyphenols, among which the most prominent are quercetin, elagic, syringic and p-coumaric acid. Ongoing but very preliminary studies suggest some of these compounds might play a role in the prevention of cancer and diabetes.[89]

Cinnamon (*Cinnamomum verum*)
Ground cinnamon adds a sweet, warm flavour to tea or to gently poached fruit such as apples, pears or prunes. I also use it to give a bit of zing to my lentil soup. Bear in mind that ground cinnamon loses it fragrance very quickly, so buy only what you need or, alternatively, freshly grind cinnamon sticks, which have a shelf life of up to three years. Consuming cinnamon has potential anti-diabetic effects. Some of its extracts (hydroxycinnamaldehyde) not only possess strong antioxidant and anti-inflammatory properties,[90] but also seem to improve symptoms associated with metabolic syndrome in rodents and humans.[91] Preliminary data suggest long-term supplementation with cinnamon extract can lower blood glucose levels[92,93] and reverse insulin resistance induced by eating fructose-rich food products.[94] Cinnamon also has a mild blood cholesterol-lowering effect in both animals and humans.[95]

Ginger (*Zingibar officinale*)
This is another one of my favourite spices. Ginger is a rhizome with a pungent taste that I use finely chopped in many hot bean, lentil and vegetable dishes. I also love to prepare thinly sliced ginger pickled with white vinegar and salt that I enjoy consuming with my sushi. A small piece of fresh ginger added to my morning smoothie is delicious. And its spicy-hot flavour goes very well with fruit, in particular mango, bananas and peaches.

The dominant active molecule of ginger is gingerol, which is converted into zingerone when cooked. Very preliminary animal studies suggest that ginger might play a role in the prevention of cancer and dementia,[96,97] but these effects have not been studied in humans. Studies in healthy men and women have shown ginger speeds up gastric emptying, promotes satiety and increases the heat-producing (thermic) effect of food,[98,99] all factors that can help in the prevention of obesity.

Several clinical trials indicate that ginger may reduce nausea and vomiting during chemotherapy,[100] but it should be used with caution before surgery, as several studies have shown a potential blood-thinning effect.[101]

Food	Polyphenols	Antioxidants
Cloves	15188	16047
Peppermint, fried	11960	980
Star anise	5460	1810
Cocoa powder	3448	1104
Mexican oregano, dried	2319	—
Celery seed	2094	—
Dark chocolate	1664	1860
Flaxseed meal	1528	—
Chestnut	1215	2757
Sage, dried	12073	2920
Rosemary, dried	1018	2519
Spearmeint, dried	956	6575
Thyme, dried	878	821
Blueberry, lowbush	836	471
Capers	654	3600
Black olive	569	117
Blueberry, highbush	560	205
Hazelnut	495	687
Pecan nut	493	1816
Soy flour	466	—
Plum	377	411
Green olive	346	161
Sweet basil, dried	322	4317
Curry powder	285	1075
Sweet cherry	274	144
Globe artichokes	260	1142
Blackberry	260	570
Roasted soybean	246	—
Milk chocolate	236	854
Strawberry	235	268
Red chicory	235	129
Red raspberry	215	980
Coffee, filter	214	267
Ginger, dried	202	473
Wholegrain hard wheat flour	201	186
Prune	194	1195
Almond	187	191
Black grape	169	205
Red onion	168	91
Thyme, fresh	163	1173
Spinach	119	248

Table 4: Polyphenol and antioxidant content of some of the richest foods (mg per 100 g (3½ oz)).[102]

Other precious spices

There are many other precious spices that are part of my pantry. These include oregano, coriander, black pepper, fennel, dill, clove, star anise, caraway, fenugreek, nutmeg and bay leaf. Each one of these contains a unique set of bioactive compounds that can activate or inhibit a number of enzymes or receptors with significant disease-preventative actions.[103] However, more studies are needed to confirm these effects.

Culinary herbs

There are also several culinary herbs that are important to learn to use and incorporate in your recipes.

In my apartment I always grow rosemary, sage and basil. Growing plants that I can harvest, eat or decoct for teas is one of my greatest pleasures. Even if you don't have a garden, herbs are quite happy growing in pots, especially if they are kept close to a window that gets plenty of light throughout the day.

The herbs that I most often use are parsley and basil, as well as marjoram, lemongrass, peppermint, spearmint, rosemary, sage, tarragon and, when possible, saffron. Here are descriptions of some of these vital herbs.

Parsley (*Petroselinum crispum*)

Parsley is one of my favourites. Because of its fresh, peppery and grassy flavour, it complements most other ingredients. I use finely chopped parsley leaves and garlic to prepare a superb fresh tomato sauce or a delicious dip called salsa verde. Preparing salsa verde is easy and it takes less than five minutes. You simply chop up parsley, capers, anchovies, garlic and some stale wholegrain bread. Parsley can also be used as a garnish on almost any dish. Chopped parsley is the main ingredient in the Mediterranean salad tabouli and essential in falafel.

Parsley contains high levels of the flavone apigenin, which has been shown to inhibit the proliferation of tumour cells, at least in experiments conducted in cell culture systems.[104] Other foods that are particularly rich in apegenin are onions, oranges, chamomile and wheat sprouts.

Basil (*Ocimum basilicum*)

I love fresh basil leaves for their fragrance and slightly sweet, but savoury and minty taste. The secret to good cooking is using fresh ingredients as much as possible. This is particularly true for basil; the difference in flavour between fresh and dried basil is enormous. This is one reason I always grow several basil plants at home.

Using fresh-cut, organic basil to prepare a delicious homemade pesto sauce is easy and rewarding to add to your pasta. During the hot summer months, I use basil, oregano, red onion and extra-virgin olive oil to make a colourful and refreshing tomato salad. The anise- and clove-like flavour and aroma of basil is primarily due to estragole, linalool and eugenol, but most of its antioxidant activity is mediated by the interaction between rosmarinic acid and tocopherol.[105]

Rosemary (*Rosmarinus officinalis*)

Rosemary is an aromatic evergreen plant native to the Mediterranean countries, a prominent member of the mint family Lamiaceae. This spikey, distinctively scented herb contains many interesting phytochemicals; in particular, it is rich in rosmarinic acid and carnosic acid, compounds with potential antioxidant, central nervous system and liver-protective properties.[106,107] I really like rosemary, it is one of my favourite herbal teas.

Sage (*Salvia officinalis*)

Sage has become another staple in my tea cabinet. In the 'The Salernitan Rule of Health', the textbook of the most famous Medieval School of Medicine in Europe, it is written 'How can a man die when sage grows in his garden?'. Indeed, sage is considered to be one of the richest sources of potent antioxidants and an impressive range of biologically active compounds. Animal studies and some very preliminary human trials suggest a potential cognitive-enhancing and protective effect of sage.[108]

WHOLE GRAINS AND LEGUMES: COMBINING ENERGY, FIBRE AND PROTEINS

Wheat, barley and legumes rather than meat were the staple food of gladiators in Ancient Rome, as a study on their bones by the Department of Forensic Medicine at the Medical University of Vienna has demonstrated.[109] Beans and minimally processed whole grains were also the staple foods of populations rich in healthy nonagenarians and centenarians. As the food pyramid shows, grains and beans should be consumed daily. Unlike refined carbohydrates, the consumption of minimally processed whole grains and beans are essential for optimal health.[110]

Consuming legumes and unrefined grains has been shown to reduce glucose levels after the meal at which they are consumed and also at subsequent meals. This effect is lost if we instead use highly milled grain flours or overcook legumes and grains at high temperatures. If we eat brown rice and lentils at lunch our glycaemia at dinner will be lower. Or even better, if we consume, for example, a quinoa and garbanzo bean salad for dinner, our night-long blood glucose will be reduced.[111] This subsequent meal effect is very important not only for healthy individuals, but particularly for people with prediabetes and diabetes.

A combination of legumes and whole grains also provides all the essential amino acids, important to form all proteins in our body, without atherogenic fatty acids promoting plaque builds up inside the arteries. Indeed, unlike animal products and vegetable oils, they do not contain any saturated or trans-fatty acids, or other unhealthy ingredients.

However they do contain many calories; this is why we need to consume the right amount of them, based on our physiological needs. If we perform lots of manual work, or exercise hard, we need to eat higher amounts of whole grains and legumes to provide the essential amino acids and energy required to replenish our glycogen (liver and muscle concentrated glucose) stores in the liver and skeletal muscle. If we are sedentary, we need to eat less. But the higher the consumption of minimally processed whole grains and beans, the higher the intake of a variety of protective vitamins, minerals, phytochemicals and dietary fibres as well.[112]

PRACTICAL IDEAS FOR INCREASING THE CONSUMPTION OF WHOLE GRAINS AND LEGUMES

- Always have a variety of whole grains and legumes in your cupboard. Unlike many other food products, they will last for several months as long as they are stored at room temperature and in dark conditions.
- When you go to the kitchen to cook, put a pot of water on the stove and add a cup or two of legumes (like dried beans, lentils or chickpeas). Within an hour or two of simmering, they will be ready to cool and store in the fridge ready to use. Cook brown, rice, farro or barley ahead of use too.
- Use cooked brown rice or legumes as a side dish for your lunch, or to add to a vegetable soup for dinner. A legume salad with lots of fresh vegetables is a healthy option for lunch or as a side dish for dinner.
- Once you become comfortable cooking grains and legumes, try preparing two different kinds at one time, so you always have them in the fridge ready to use.

Whole grains: a gift of nature

Whole grains contain the integral bran, germ and endosperm. In contrast, refined grains have been milled and most of the bran and germ have been taken out to improve their shelf-life. Examples of *refined* grain products are white rice, white flour, white bread and de-germed cornmeal. However, the germ and the bran are rich in important bioactive compounds, essential for our health. For instance, the aleuron layer of wheat bran contains a number of phyto protectants (e.g. ferulic acid, alkylresorcinols, apigenin, lignans and phytic acid), which have been shown to have antioxidative and anticarcinogenic activities in rodent animal models of colon and skin cancer.[113-115]

The germ of whole grains contains a polyamine, called spermidine, that Professor Frank Madeo of the University of Graz has demonstrated can extend lifespan in animal models. Spermidine helped increase the removal of damaged cells and reduced inflammation.[116]

Data from large human epidemiological studies suggest eating whole grains has a protective effect against obesity, type 2 diabetes, cardiovascular disease and cancer.[117-120] In the NIH-AARP Diet and Health Study, individuals with the highest intakes of whole grains had a 17 per cent lower risk of mortality from all causes.[121]

Data from studies with a total of 286,125 participants suggest that consuming two servings per day of whole grains is associated with a 21 per cent reduction in risk of type 2 diabetes, even after adjustment for BMI and other factors.[122] In another meta-analysis, men and women consuming three to five servings of whole grains (approximately 40–80 g) every day had a 21 per cent lower risk of cardiovascular disease compared to those who never or rarely consume whole grains.[123]

Intake of whole grains has also been reported to be associated with a lower risk of developing hypertension,[124] and colon[125] and breast cancer.[126] In particular, higher brown rice consumption has been associated with lower premenopausal breast cancer risk. In contrast, in the same study white bread consumption was associated with a higher risk of breast cancer.[127]

Grains are not all created equal

Today's most-consumed cereals are refined wheat, rice and corn. However, there are a wide variety of fibre-rich whole grains that we can use, including different varieties of wheat and rice, along with barley, millet, oats, rye and quinoa. Next time you are thinking of using white rice or pasta, cook one of these nutritious, high-fibre grains instead. Each one has its own nutritional properties and individual taste.

Here are some important characteristics and nutritional values of the main whole grain cereals:

Wheat (*Triticum aestivum*)

This is one of the oldest cereal grains. There are two basic varieties of wheat: 'hard' or durum, and 'soft' wheat, plus other subspecies such as spelt (*Triticum spelta*), known as farro in Italy.

Durum wheat has more protein than soft wheat and is used to make pasta. Personally, I prefer to use durum for making my homemade pasta and sourdough bread. Durum wheat is the ideal grain for baking bread, because it contains high levels of an elastic protein called gluten. Two or three slices of my marvellous homemade nutrient-rich and tasty whole-wheat bread for lunch is a genuine lifesaver. I have it with chopped fresh vegetables and some spicy dahl.

There are other ways to make good use of this nutritious cereal. One is to concentrate the gluten protein into a meat-like substitute called *seitan*. Another way is to eat it as couscous, a staple food of many countries facing the Mediterranean Sea, especially in North Africa and Sicily. Couscous is made from semolina, the coarse grind of high-protein durum wheat. Whole-wheat couscous is more nutritious that the regular variety.

Of course, the nutrient and protein content of wheat varies depending on the variety and soil quality. The protein content of wheat is higher, on average, than that of other grains (14 g in 100 g/3½ oz), but it is relatively low in two essential amino acids, lysine and threonine. This is why it is best to combine it with legumes.

One hundred grams (3½ oz) of whole durum wheat contains high concentrations of niacin (7 mg, 42 per cent RDA), thiamine (0.4 mg, 38 per cent RDA), vitamin B6 (0.4 mg, 32 per cent RDA), manganese (3 mg, 139 per cent RDA), phosphorus (508 mg, 73 per cent RDA), magnesium (144 mg, 34 per cent RDA), zinc (4 mg, 38 per cent RDA), copper (1 mg, 68 per cent RDA) and iron (4 mg, 44 per cent RDA). Whole wheat is also an excellent source of selenium (89 mcg in 100g (3½ oz), 163 per cent RDA).[128] The germ fraction of wheat contains healthy fatty acids and spermidine.

When buying flours, get them fresh and store them in the fridge if possible, to prevent rancidity due to oxidation of the precious fatty acids contained in the germ.

Rice (*Oryza sativa*)

This is the second most consumed cereal in the world and a staple food in Asia. Many varieties of rice exist. The most healthy and common are:

- long-grained brown rice (seeds are longer and thinner, but less glutinous and expand more)
- short round-grained brown rice (contains more dextrin, more glutinous and expands less)
- basmati brown rice.

Unlike refined white rice, wholegrain brown rice retains higher concentrations of nutrients with protective attributes. The side hulls, brans and germ of brown rice are rich in minerals, vitamins and phytochemicals. One hundred grams (3½ oz) of brown rice contains high concentrations of manganese (4 mg, 163 per cent RDA), phosphorus (333 mg, 48 per cent RDA) and selenium (23 mcg, 43 per cent RDA). It is also a good source of vitamin B6 (1 mg, 39 per cent RDA), niacin (5 mg, 32 per cent RDA), pantothenic acid (1 mg, 30 per cent RDA), and vitamin E (1 mg, 5 per cent RDA).

Brown rice is also an excellent source of fibre. Refining removes approximately 80 per cent of thiamine and other B vitamins, such as pyridoxine, B6, and riboflavin, B2, and two-thirds of the niacin, B3, and some of the minerals; spermidine and essential fatty acids are lost as well.

I always buy organic brown rice because it contains lower levels of harmful pesticides and chemicals. High-quality brown rice usually requires 40 to 50 minutes of cooking. Besides just boiling it and combining it with a hundred different types of vegetable dishes, legumes, tofu or fish, my family enjoys a dish of cream of brown rice. Organic brown rice cakes are a very healthy snack for our kids. They are a low-sodium, low-cholesterol, high-fibre snack that can be eaten plain, but children also like them with tahini or almond butter.

Barley (*Hordeum vulgare*)

This is one of the most ancient cultivated grains, and it is very rich in dietary fibre made up of cellulose, amylose, pentosans, and beta-glucan. The latter is found in appreciable amounts only in barley and oats, and is probably an important contributing factor in lowering glucose, insulin and cholesterol levels.[129-131] This is one of the reasons why I try to incorporate this nutty and slightly chewy grain into all sorts of dishes, from soups to breads, and as a substitute for brown rice when I prepare risotto, paella and pilaf.

Toasting barley before it is cooked gives it a delicious nutty flavour that I use with pistachios, raisins, tahini and a range of roasted vegetables to make a gloriously rich dish that never fails to satisfy. Barley can also be used to prepare a variety of non-alcoholic drinks, such as barley water, barley tea, and a roasted barley drink similar to coffee.

As with other cereals it's best to buy the natural unrefined grain. I use only hulled barley and not pearled barley. Pearl barley, which is more commonly found in stores, has been polished or 'pearled' to remove most of the outer bran layer and germ along with the hull. Hulled barley is a healthier choice, but will increase the cooking time quite considerably. The intact hulled kernels of barley are very rich in fibre, riboflavin (0.3 mg, 20 per cent RDA), thiamine (1 mg, 54 per cent RDA), and trace elements such as iron (4 mg, 45 per cent RDA), copper (0.5 mg, 55 per cent RDA), and zinc (3 mg, 25 per cent RDA).

In some barley cultivars, chromium levels are ten times higher than those of brewer's yeast (generally regarded as the richest natural source of chromium). Other components that have been associated with its health benefits include tocotrienols, lignans, phytoestrogen and a number of phenolic compounds.

Millet (*Pennisetum millet*)

This is another interesting grain that should only be eaten from time by time, because some studies suggest that a compound called C-glycosylflavone, which is primarily contained in the outer millet's bran fraction, may inhibit the activity of an enzyme that is crucial for the production of thyroid hormones. Especially in areas of iodine deficiency, its ingestion may contribute to the genesis of goitre.[132]

Apart from this, the tiny millet kernels with their mild, slightly nutty taste (pan-roasting enhances the nutty flavour) are quite versatile. I use them with beans to make crispy bean patties and serve them with a spicy avocado sauce, or I make millet fritters with chickpea flour as the binder. Millet swells a lot when boiled and becomes a great alternative to oatmeal for breakfast. It can be added directly to soups or pre-cooked to sprinkle over salads. Lightly toasting the millet kernels before cooking adds extra flavour.

Millet is gluten-free and therefore can be consumed by coeliac patients. It is a hearty healthy cereal, with a higher fibre content than rice, and is rich in manganese, copper, magnesium, iron, niacin and thiamine. Easily digested, it is a very nutritious food: half a cup of millet contains 380 kcal and 11 g of protein with a higher content of essential amino acids (leucine, isoleucine and lysine) than wheat, rye and corn.[133] Millet is also an excellent source of selenium, which is essential to protect cells from oxidative damage.[134]

Corn (*Zea mays L.*)

Even if corn is not as nutritious as other cereals, my family love to consume this sweet and very tasty grain. We simply boil or slightly roast the corn cobs and eat the kernels right off the cob. Certain varieties of dried corn kernels can be made into popcorn, which makes a healthy snack for kids.

Organic yellow corn flour (or maize) can be made into a thick porridge (polenta in Italy, mămăligă in Romania or mush in the US) or used to prepare delicious flat breads, tortillas and thin, crisp corn chips. I love using organic corn tortillas as a small scoop to eat one of my favourite dips, guacamole. It is super easy to prepare, just mix the flesh of three ripe avocadoes with chopped onion, sweet pepper and coriander (cilantro), add salt and lots of lime or lemon juice, which will help to balance the richness of the avocado.

> TIP: Note that the bioavailability of niacin in corn is very low, and it also has a very low content of two essential amino acids, lysine and tryptophan. Combining corn with beans will re-establish an amino acid balance and a complete range of amino acids for normal protein synthesis.

Oat (*Avena sativa*)

This cereal grain is commonly bought as rolled oats and used for making porridge. Oat flour is also used in baked goods or as an ingredient in multi-grain muesli. Like barley, oat kernels can be soaked and boiled to use as a drink.

Oat is a good source of proteins and it is the only cereal grain containing the globulin protein, called avenalins. Globulins are water-soluble and therefore cannot be transformed into bread but can be made into milk. Oat kernels have the highest protein concentration (15 per cent) among all the cereals and their protein score is pretty high.[135]

One cup (156 g/5½ oz) of oat kernels contains high concentrations of thiamine (1.2 mg, 95 per cent RDA), manganese (6 mg, 246 per cent RDA), phosphorus (739 mg, 100 per cent RDA), magnesium (231 mg, 55 per cent RDA), zinc (5 mg, 44 per cent

RDA), copper (1 mg, 59 per cent RDA) and iron (7 mg, 82 per cent RDA). Oat bran, oatmeal and oat flour contain a high concentration of a specific insoluble fibre (beta-glucan), a no starch polysaccharide, that has a small but significant cholesterol-lowering effect by reducing cholesterol's intestinal absorption.[136]

TIP: Germinating grains can increase the bioavailability of certain vitamins and phytochemicals, such as folate, tocopherols and tocotrienols.

Rye (*Secale cereale*)

I love the taste of rye when I bake bread. Usually, I use one-third rye flour combined with two-third durum wheat flour. This nutrient-rich flour adds a strong acidic flavour to my bread. Making sourdough bread increases the bioavailability of some important vitamins and phytochemicals, such as folate, tocopherols and tocotrienols.

Rye is an extremely good source of fibre and some minerals. On average one cup (170 g/16 oz) of wholemeal rye flour contains 25 g of fibre, 5 mg of manganese (198 per cent RDA), 60 mcg of selenium (109 per cent RDA), 1 mg of copper (85 per cent RDA), 6 mg of zinc (58 per cent RDA), 5 mg of iron (57 per cent RDA), 2 mg of pantothenic acid (50 per cent RDA) and 7 mg of niacin (45 per cent RDA). The outer bran of rye contains three to four times more phenolic compounds and one and a half to two times more sterols, folates, tocopherols and lignans than wholemeal rye.

Buckwheat (*Polygonum fagopyrum L.*)

Sometimes, I like to add a small amount of buckwheat flour to my sourdough bread. Buckwheat is commonly referred to as a cereal, though its seeds are achenes: small, dry, one-seeded fruits that do not open to release the seed. Like sunflower seeds, they have a hard exterior shell and soft inner core.

Buckwheat flour is much darker than wheat flour. In Italy and Japan, the flour is also made into short stripes of pasta (called pizzocheri) and noodles (soba). Buckwheat is the only grain containing rutin, a bioactive compound, with potential protective effects against diabetes.[137] It is also a good source of proteins, quercetin, fibre, vitamins and some precious minerals. On average one cup (170 g/6 oz) of buckwheat contains 17 g of fibre, 12 mg of niacin (75 per cent RDA), 1 mg of riboflavin (56 per cent RDA), 393 mg of magnesium (93 per cent RDA), 2 mg of copper (208 per cent RDA) and 2 mg of manganese (96 per cent RDA).

Like rice and corn, it does not contain gluten, and can be consumed by people with coeliac diseases.

Legumes: love them and they will love you back

I love legumes, an excellent source of healthy proteins and vitamins. Legumes, also known as beans or pulses, have been a staple food for many populations around the world, especially those in the Mediterranean countries with many nonagenarians and centenarians.[138] Chickpeas, lentils, fava beans, soybeans or black beans, prepared in healthy, tasty recipes, were consumed every single day.

With the Westernisation of food consumption patterns, they have unfortunately become a forgotten dish.[139] When I advise my patients to increase their consumption of legumes, they either ask, 'What is a legume?' or 'How do I eat them?' For some strange reason legumes became stigmatised as food for the poor, and people began to eat meat and dairy products instead. This is very unfortunate, because they are such an excellent source of healthy protein, carbohydrates and fibre, and they are loaded with myriad vitamins and bioactive molecules. They also provide B vitamins, iron, copper, magnesium, manganese, zinc and phosphorous. Most people are surprised when they learn just how nutritious they are.

Most beans, apart from soya, are naturally low in fat, and practically free of saturated fatty acids and cholesterol. One serving of legumes, approximately half a cup, provides on average 120 calories, 20 g of complex carbohydrate, 6–10 g of fibre and 8 g of protein. Let's keep in mind, however, that proteins in beans, with the exception of soybeans, are incomplete. They are poor in some sulphur amino acids, methionine and cysteine in particular, which are found in high concentrations in whole grains. But bean and grain combos provide all nine essential amino acids in a balanced and healthy proportion.

Legumes are especially advisable for overweight and obese people, particularly individuals at high risk of diabetes. This is because they contain complex carbohydrates and higher quantities of amylose than most other cereals or tubers, which are slowly digested and have a low glycaemic index.[140] Indeed, legumes do not raise blood glucose and insulin levels as much as other foods with a similar calorie content.

In a three-month clinical trial, patients with type 2 diabetes who increased their legume intake by at least one cup per day experienced a much greater reduction in blood sugar, cholesterol and blood pressure than those who consumed whole-wheat products.[141] In another trial, where legumes replaced red meat, they significantly decreased fasting blood glucose and insulin, triglyceride and LDL-cholesterol.[142]

The cholesterol-lowering effect of bean consumption has been confirmed in many other clinical trials.[143] On average the mean reduction in total cholesterol for people treated with a legume diet was 11.8 mg/dl. The high intake of fibre and phytosterols from legumes (but also from nuts, seeds, whole grains, vegetables and fruits) may play a significant role in lowering plasma cholesterol levels by competing with intestinal cholesterol absorption.[144]

A diet rich in legumes may also help with weight control and reducing blood pressure.[145] Obese patients who participated in a weight-loss program that included legumes and wholegrains benefited with significantly reduced waist circumferences and improved blood pressure and triglycerides levels.[146]

Other small trials have shown legumes lower blood pressure, independent of weight loss, in people with and without hypertension.[147] By making people feel fuller, the high content of indigestible fibres may promote weight loss.

The fibres also provide a perfect substrate for probiotic bacteria. Some intestinal bacteria that thrive on bean fibre produce a wide range of metabolites that can lower systemic inflammation. In a small randomised cross-over trial, replacing two servings of red meat with legumes significantly reduced C-reactive protein and two key pro-inflammatory cytokines (IL-6 and TNF-alpha) in overweight diabetic patients, independent of weight change.[148]

Dietary potassium is another factor that lowers blood pressure. A meta-analysis of several trials found that for each 2 g per day increase in potassium excretion there is a reduction in systolic and diastolic blood pressure.[149] Foods rich in potassium are fruits, vegetables and beans. For instance, half a cup of cooked white beans contains 595 mg of potassium, while one medium sweet potato contains 542 mg and a quarter of a cup of canned tomato paste contains 700 mg.

Legumes are also one of the best sources of folate, a water-soluble B vitamin essential for creating new red blood cells and for preventing some birth defects such as neural tube defects, which affect more than 300,000 newborns each year worldwide. Folate may also help in preventing cancer. This vitamin cannot be stored in our body, which is why we need to consume plenty of folate-rich foods every day, such as legumes, leafy green vegetables, fresh fruits and yeast. Liver is also an excellent source, if you like it. I don't!

In addition, other bioactive compounds (formononetin, biochanin A, coumestans) in legumes may contribute to their cancer-protective effects. In particular, two phytoestrogens – genistein and daidzein – mimic oestrogen in the body. They can bind to a person's oestrogenic receptors and thus play a role in blocking cancer cell proliferation.[150]

> TIP: It is true that legumes more than other foods tend to make us produce some extra gas (flatulence), which in some people may cause bloating. Producing gas is a sign that our gut and our microbiome are healthy and working well. Gas itself from the fermentation of the beans' fibre won't cause any injury, but there are steps that we can take to minimise this problem. Introduce legumes into your diet gradually, and at the beginning remove the skins (rich in fibre) by passing them through a sieve.

Simple tricks for storing and using different legumes in your kitchen

There are many myths about how difficult it is to cook legumes. The reality is that beans are very easy to use, once you master some easy skills. First of all, storing a supply of precooked legumes for the entire week in the refrigerator means you can use them in almost any dish you make. Try to prepare two different kinds at the same time and change the variety you make every week. For instance one week cook green lentils and lima beans, the following week boil fava beans and kidney beans, and then chickpeas and borlotti beans.

A legume salad or soup can be made with any combination of cooked legumes, together with fresh or steamed vegetables. You can also serve your favourite grain – brown rice, quinoa or barley for example – with some chickpeas or lima beans and a range of colourful roasted vegetables, which will not only improve the nutritional value but most important will enhance the taste.

COOKING TIPS ON HOW TO USE BEANS

- Large beans such as chickpeas, fava beans and borlotti should be soaked for 24 hours in cold water before cooking. Lentils require much less time.
- Beans are like sponges; they absorb lots of water during cooking. Add at least three cups of water for each cup of legumes.
- During cooking, skim off the foam that rises to the top and discard it.
- Only add salt at the end of the cooking process.
- If you plan to store beans in the fridge, drain off all the water and add some salt to increase their shelf-life.
- Legume salads taste much better if you marinate the legumes with the other ingredients for at least 30 minutes before serving.
- Adding lemon juice to a legume salad or soup improves the taste and the availability of minerals and vitamins.

Lentils (*Lens culinaris*)

Lentils are one of my favourite legumes, because of their characteristic earthy flavour and beautiful lens shape. There are a wide variety of lentils of different sizes and colour, ranging from green to brown, black, orange and red. Red lentils contain a third of the dietary fibre of green lentils (11 per cent rather than 31 per cent) and break down more during cooking, ending up almost in a soft puree.

Lentils have a relatively short-cooking time, typically 15–20 minutes, especially if the husk has been removed, such as in red lentils. If you use a high-pressure cooker, green lentils cook in ten minutes and six minutes for red or yellow lentils. Cooked lentils can be stored in the refrigerator up to five days and can be used in a wide variety of highly nutritious soups, spicy colourful dahl and pasta sauces. Additionally, you can sprout lentils to add to salads and other dishes. In South India slightly fermented lentils and rice are used to prepare the batter of the masala dosa, which is one of my favourite Indian dishes, and is filled with onion and potato and served with a spicy-hot green coconut chutney on the side.

After soybeans, lentils are the legume with the highest protein content, on average 27 per cent.[151] One cup of green boiled lentils (198 g) provides 230 calories, 16 g of dietary fibre, and only 1 g of fat. They are an excellent source of iron (7 mg, 82 per cent RDA), zinc (3 mg, 31 per cent RDA) and selenium (6 mcg, 10 per cent RDA). Lentils are also very rich in folate (358 mcg, 90 per cent RDA), thiamine (1 mg, 30 per cent RDA) and vitamin B5 (1 mg, 25 per cent RDA). They also possess one of the highest concentrations of phenolic compounds and antioxidants.[152] Epidemiological data suggest that the consumption of these small legumes is associated with a lower risk of developing cancer and cardiovascular disease.[153]

Chickpeas or garbanzo beans (*Cicer arietinum*)

Chickpeas are yellow-brown, pea-like beans with a nutty flavour and buttery texture. They provide a concentrated source of protein, dietary fibre, vitamins, minerals and low-glycaemic starches. One cup of boiled chickpeas contains 270 calories, 12 g of dietary fibre, 15 g of protein and 4 g of fat (mainly mono- and poly-unsaturated). They are a rich source of copper (1 mg, 64 per cent RDA), iron (5 mg, 59 per cent RDA), manganese (2 mg, 73 per cent RDA), calcium (80 mg, 8 per cent RDA) and zinc (3 mg, 23 per cent RDA). Chickpeas also provide plenty of folate (282 mcg, 40 per cent RDA), which is essential for our health.

Chickpeas need to be soaked in water for at least 24 hours, and can then take up to an hour to cook until they are tender. They can be served in salads, soups or sauces, and to garnish pasta dishes. Chickpea flour is used in Italy's Tuscany and Liguria regions to prepare the famous crunchy farinata, a baked chickpea pancake.

In the Middle East, mashed chickpeas seasoned with tahini (sesame cream), chopped garlic, lemon juice and extra-virgin olive oil are blended together to make *hummus*, a super-healthy dip. Uncooked chickpeas are also used to make *falafel*, crispy patties that are served with fresh vegetables and tahini sauce.

Fava beans (*Vicia fava*)

I love fava beans (or broad beans) with their nutty, slightly sweet creamy taste. They are perfect for salads, soups, pastas, dips and so much more. Fava beans were widely cultivated in the ancient Mesopotamian civilisation and were considered a delicious treat by the Greeks and Romans. They are healthy high-fibre and cholesterol-free legumes that deserve a regular place in our cuisine.

Fresh fava beans can be harvested in late spring while they are still very young and tender, and the entire pod can be cooked. Lightly sautéed fresh baby fava beans served with olive oil, salt, garlic and pinch of lemon zest create a perfect sauce for a delicious pasta dish. Alternatively, you can remove the beans from their pods and steam or boil them. If you have never eaten them fresh, you should, they are really delicious and complement many dishes.

Because they have a very short season in spring, if you want to enjoy them year-round you can either freeze the podded beans or use the classic dried broad beans. Dried beans are cheaper than canned beans, and they do not contain additives like sodium, sugar or potentially toxic BPA released by the can's lining.

Soak dried fava beans in water for eight to ten hours, then remove the outer skin and cook in a large saucepan of water until tender. Fava beans are delicious in a soup or as an addition to other dishes. They can also be pureed with olive oil to create a smooth dip. Toasted and salted fava beans are a popular snack in many Asian and South American countries. A plate of mashed, cooked fava beans mixed with olive oil, salt and cumin, known as *ful medames*, is a traditional breakfast dish of Egypt.

> NOTE: People diagnosed with fauvism, a rare hereditary deficiency of the enzyme glucose-6-phosphate dehydrogenase (G6PD), should not consume fava beans, because they can trigger an haemolysis of red blood cells.[154] If you ever experience discomfort after eating fava beans, you should be tested for this genetic deficiency.

Soybeans (*Glycine max*)

I rarely consume cooked whole mature soybeans, but tofu and edamame are staple foods in my diet. Tofu, also known as soy cheese, is a protein-rich food prepared by coagulating soymilk with lemon juice or calcium sulphate. One hundred grams (3½ oz) of tofu contains 10 g of proteins packed in only 91 calories. Notably, the quality of soy protein is much higher than that of all the other beans and very similar to animal protein.[155] Zen Buddhist monks use tofu as their main substitute for meat and fish.

I love to grill thin slices of tofu and dress them with olive oil and a few drops of tamari (soy sauce). They taste so good and are very easy to prepare. Because tofu has such a subtle flavour, small cubes of tofu can be added to most soups and sauces.

> TIP: Add the tofu for the last 10–15 minutes of the preparation to allow it to absorb the flavours.

There are many other ways to consume soybeans. One is to eat the sweet immature soybeans, called edamame. The still tender and green pods are typically picked a month before they fully ripen, and frozen to use later. The pods are boiled in salted water and eaten while still warm as a very healthy snack. One cup of edamame, approximately 150 g (5 oz), provides 18 g of protein and 20 per cent of an adult's iron needs, 16 per cent of vitamin C, 10 per cent of calcium, 52 per cent of vitamin K and 121 per cent of the daily recommended amount of folate.

Another way to consume soybeans is fermented bean paste such as miso, natto, tempeh and tamari. Miso is a salty thick fermented paste of soybeans and cereals such as rice or barley, which is used to make a delicious Japanese style-soup.

Consumption of soy products in general appears to modestly lower blood pressure and improve the health of our arteries.[156] Several studies have shown that diets low in saturated fat and cholesterol and high in soy protein can reduce LDL cholesterol levels, especially when soy protein replaces foods that contain animal fats. Soy isoflavones have been associated with a reduced risk for osteoporosis and cancer, and a lower frequency and severity of hot flushes in postmenopausal women.[157-159] One hundred grams (3½ oz) of tofu contains approximately 25 mg of isoflavones.

Cannellini, kidney, pinto and a host of other incredible legumes
There are plenty of other beans we can eat, including cannellini beans, navy beans, kidney beans, borlotti beans, pinto beans, northern beans, black beans, black-eyed peas and adzuki beans. Experiment and try lots of different types of legumes because they all contain their own special phytochemicals and oligo-elements. Some of their health benefits have not even been studied yet.

LEGUMES LOWER CARDIOVASCULAR AND CANCER RISK
Epidemiological studies suggest that people who often consume legumes, say two to four times per week, have a reduced risk of death, in particular for cardiovascular disease.[160] Eating beans is associated with a reduced risk of developing a heart attack, probably because beans are instrumental in lowering blood pressure and the levels of plasma cholesterol and glucose, C-reactive protein.[161-164] Regular bean consumption has been associated with a reduced risk of colon, breast and lung cancer.[165-168] Analysis of the Harvard Nurses' Health Study suggests that women who consume two or more servings of legumes per week might have a 24 per cent lower risk of developing breast cancer.[169,170]

THE WONDERS OF NUTS AND SEEDS

Nuts and seeds are nutritional powerhouses that most of us forget to consume regularly. Ideally, we should be eating some every day. They are a great natural source of essential amino acids and fatty acids (mostly healthy monounsaturated and polyunsaturated fats), and dietary fibre as well. They also provide a wide variety of essential vitamins (B group vitamins, folic acid, vitamin E); important minerals such as potassium, magnesium, calcium, iron and zinc (including the antioxidant minerals selenium, manganese and copper); plus other key phytochemicals such as flavonoids, resveratrol and plant sterols.

A handful of raw nuts or toasted seeds are a very healthy snack, especially for our kids. When I travel on an airplane, I always take a small bag of organic almonds, pecans or cashews. Because of their subtle sweet and savoury taste, they combine well, and add taste and texture, to all kind of salads, sauces, dips or smoothies.

Nuts in general, and in particular almonds, are better digested and absorbed when soaked in water overnight: soaking reduces the levels of an anti-nutrient, called phytic acid.[171] Be aware that many commercial nuts and seeds have added salt, vegetable oil and sugar, all of which have detrimental effects on blood pressure and body weight, and can increase the risk of diabetes.

Try to buy raw nuts still in their shells so you know they have not been treated. Unshelled nuts and all seeds should be kept refrigerated, because they easily become rancid due to the large content of highly oxidisable polyunsaturated fatty acids.

A growing body of epidemiological studies suggests that people who consume at least five servings of nuts per week experience a 40–60 per cent lower risk of developing heart disease.[172]

Here are six reasons why nuts may protect our cardiovascular system:

1. Nuts (with the exception of macadamias) are low in saturated fats, and rich in the cardio-protective monounsaturated and polyunsaturated fats.

2. They are rich in soluble fibre that reduces the absorption of cholesterol in our intestine.

3. All nuts, particularly almonds and walnuts, are the main dietary source of the powerful antioxidant vitamin E and of antioxidant minerals, such as selenium, copper and manganese.

4. Raw nuts are naturally low in sodium and high in potassium and magnesium, factors that have an important effect in lowering blood pressure. The exceptions are processed, roasted and salted nuts.

5. Many nuts, but in particular pine nuts, are very rich in arginine, an amino acid that is converted to an anti-atherogenic molecule called nitric oxide.

6. Walnuts are a source of omega-3 alpha-linolenic acid, which lowers triglycerides levels, inflammation and protects against several irregular heartbeat conditions.

Data from clinical trials show that consuming 30 to 50 g of nuts per day significantly reduces triglycerides and fasting glucose, and also ameliorates circulating lipid levels, particularly among those with higher cholesterol.[173,174] The results of a six-month randomised clinical trial showed that eating a range of cholesterol-lowering foods, including almonds, led to a 15 per cent reduction of blood cholesterol.[175]

Which nuts are best for health?

Mother Nature has supplied us with a great variety of beautiful and tasty nuts, each one with a particular chemical composition as shown in table 5 below.

Nut	Energy (kj)	SFA (g)	MUFA (g)	PUFA (g)	a-linolenic (g)	Fibre (g)	Protein (g)	Arginine (mcg)	Folate (mcg)
Almond	2418	3.88	32.15	12.21	0	8.8	21.26	2.47	29
Brazil	2743	15.13	24.54	20.57	0.06	8.5	14.32	2.15	22
Cashew	2314	7.78	23.79	7.84	0.16	5.9	18.22	2.12	25
Hazelnut	2629	4.46	45.65	7.92	0.09	10.4	14.95	2.21	113
Macadamia	3004	12.06	58.87	1.5	0.2	6.0	7.91	1.4	11
Pecan	2889	6.18	40.8	5.6	1	8.4	9.17	1.18	22
Peanut	2220	6.83	24.42	15.55	0.01	8.5	25.8	3.1	240
Pistachio	2332	5.44	23.31	13.45	0.26	9.0	20.61	2.03	51
Walnut	2738	6.12	8.93	47.17	9	6.4	15.23	2.28	98

Table 5: Nutrient composition of nuts per 100 g (3½ oz)[176]

Almonds (*Prunus dulcis*)

Almonds are a very rich source of the powerful antioxidant, vitamin E. A small handful of almonds (approximately 30 g) provides 37 per cent of the RDA for vitamin E and 20 per cent of the RDA for magnesium, which plays a role in lowering blood pressure. They are also a good source of protein and calcium. I use chopped almonds to garnish salads; they add warmth and a depth of crunchy flavour. Homemade almond milk, made from spring water and raw almonds, is a terrific substitute for dairy milk in smoothies.

Walnuts (*Juglans regia*)

Known for their distinctive brain-like shape, walnuts are an excellent source of omega-3 alpha-linolenic acid, besides being a rich source of vitamin E and other polyphenols that may contribute to the prevention of oxidation of bad

LDL-cholesterol particles.[177] One hundred grams (3½ oz) of walnuts provide 9 g of alpha-linolenic acid that in our body is converted into docosahexaenoic acid (DHA) and ecoisopentanoic acid (EPA).[178] These two omega-3 fatty acids, also typical of healthy fish, have cardio-protective properties, because they reduce inflammation and platelet aggregation.[179,180]

Hazelnuts (*Corylus avellana*) and pine nuts (*Pinus pinea*)

Both are an excellent source of vitamin E. Hazelnuts are richer in fibre, folate and potassium. Hazelnuts are also one of the richest sources of proanthocyanidins,[181] which seem to play a role in lowering lipid free radicals.[182]

Pine nuts contain high levels of arginine, an amino acid needed for the production of nitric oxide, which is essential for lowering blood pressure and preventing the aggregation of platelets.

Brazil nuts (*Bertholletia excelsa*)

The fruits of a South American tree, brazil nuts are one of my favourite nuts. They are the richest source of selenium: six nuts supply approximately 780 per cent of the RDA for selenium, a powerful antioxidant mineral that helps to prevent tissue damage caused by free radicals. They are also a good source of fibre. Two or three times a week, I add a couple of these nuts, together with a couple of teaspoons of organic unsweet dark cocoa powder, to my morning fruit smoothies.

> TIP: A paper published in *Nature* shows that eating plain, dark chocolate, which is rich in epicatechin, causes an increase in plasma antioxidant capacity; an effect that is markedly reduced when the chocolate is consumed with milk or if milk is incorporated as in milk chocolate.[183]

Pistachios (*Pistacia vera*)

A good source of protein and potassium, pistachios contain higher carotenoids and chlorophylls than other tree nuts; they also have appreciable amounts of the polyphenol stilbenes, which seems to possess anti-cancer, anti-inflammatory and antioxidant activities.[184] A small clinical study showed that the addition of pistachios to high-glycaemic foods, such as white bread, lowers the glycaemic response.[185]

Cashews (*Anacardium occidentale*)

A good source of iron (non-heme), cashews contain more magnesium than almonds – 246 mg per 100 g (3½ oz) versus 220 mg – but much less vitamin E.

Macadamia (*Macadamia integrifolia*)

Among all the nuts, these are perhaps the least healthy as they contain relatively high levels of saturated fat (10 g per 100 g or 3½ oz).

Chestnuts (*Castanea sativa*)

The chestnut is considered to be a tree nut, however chestnuts differ quite considerably to most nuts because they are very low in fat and high in low glycaemic index carbohydrates. They are also a good source of fibre and vitamin C.

> TIP: Boiling chestnuts destroys part of their vitamin C; it's better to eat them roasted or raw.

COUNTING YOUR NUTS

A healthy handful of nuts each day promotes your health.
A 30 g (1 oz) serve of nuts is equivalent to approximately:

- 20 almonds
- 9 walnuts
- 15 pecans
- 20 hazelnuts
- 30 pistachios
- 15 cashews
- 2 tablespoons of pine nuts

Peanuts (*Arachis hypogaea*)

These are actually legumes, and they are rich in folate, which plays a key role in DNA synthesis and repair, and in brain development.[186]

Depending on the soil, climate and weather in which they grow, different nut crops may be relatively richer or poorer in particular amino acids, fatty acids, minerals and phytochemicals. It is the same for many other vegetable foods.

> TIP: Remember, a rule of thumb is to eat a diet as rich as possible in diversity. Having the same food every day isn't going to be as healthy as eating a rich diversity of foods, because we may miss some important nutrients or consume too much of some others. No single food can supply all the nutrients one needs, so 'healthy' food diversity is necessary to promote health. Moreover, dietary diversity makes meals more interesting and less repetitive.

The health benefits of seeds and how to enjoy them

Small but packed with a wealth of nutrients, edible seeds eaten as part of a healthy diet can contribute to a reduced risk of developing cardiovascular disease. They are very rich in monounsaturated and polyunsaturated fats, antioxidant vitamins (vitamins E, A and B) and minerals such as magnesium and phosphorus that play a key role in maintaining low blood pressure.

Many seeds are also a good source of proteins (proportionally many more than in cereals), zinc, iron, calcium and copper. Their oils contain generous amounts of phenolic compounds that protect the seed, and also our cells, from oxidation.

Edible seeds come in all sorts of different colours, forms and sizes.

Sesame seeds (*Sesamum indicum*)

Sesame seeds are also called the 'seeds of longevity'; they are considered to be the oldest oilseed crop known to humanity. These very small white seeds grow on plants that can survive in harsh climatic conditions (drought and high heat) and need little farming support. These tiny, super tasty seeds can be used whole in salads or ground into a cream called tahini, which you can buy by the jar in many stores.

I typically use organic tahini on bread or to prepare baba ghanoush and hummus, my favourite dips. Hummus is made of cooked, mashed chickpeas blended with tahini, olive oil, lemon juice, salt and garlic.

Unhulled sesame seeds are more nutrient-rich; black seeds have a toasty and smoky flavour. Slightly toasted they provide a formidable snack for our growing kids.

Sesame seeds contain several specific antioxidant compounds. Sesamin, one of the most abundant lignans, is associated with reduced serum levels of cholesterol in rodents and humans.[187]

Flaxseeds (*Linum usitatissimum*)

Also called linseeds, flaxseeds are the fruits of a plant cultivated in some of the cooler regions of the world. They are also an important source of antioxidant lignans (up to 13 mg per gram) and heart-friendly omega-3 alpha-linolenic acid. After oily fish, flax seeds are the main source of omega-3 fatty acids in our diet. Interestingly, it takes less than two weeks for the flax seed omega-3 alpha-linolenic acid to be incorporated in significant amounts in the membranes of our cells.[188]

Data from several randomized clinical trials indicate that consuming whole flaxseed results in a small but significant reduction in total and LDL-cholesterol.[189] As with other seeds, because of the high polyunsaturated fat content, it's best to keep the flaxseeds and their oil in the refrigerator to avoid oxidation.

TIP: Omega-3 fatty acid bioavailability in flaxseeds is greater when the seeds are ground. Grinding flaxseeds in a mortar or a powerful blender also improves the bioavailability of certain enterolignans. Dietary plant lignans are converted by the gut microbiota in the upper part of the large bowel to enterolignans. Experimental data suggest that high concentrations of enterolignans in blood are associated with a lower risk of heart disease and cancer.[190]

Pumpkin seeds (*Cucurbita pepo*)

The flat and asymmetrically oval pumpkin seed consists of 30 per cent proteins. These vibrant green slightly sweet, chewy seeds make a great snack when lightly toasted, but they are also delicious when used as a garnish on salads, soups and bread. They can also be used instead of pine nuts to make a pesto sauce.

Sunflower kernels (*Helianthus annuus*)

These are another types of seeds that I consume regularly. They are the fruit of the beautiful plant *Helianthus annuus*, whose big yellow flowers look like the sun. These nutty-tasting seeds are rich in vitamin E and zinc and can be used to prepare a fabulous creamy spread, which is an excellent replacement for peanut butter.

Chia seeds (*Salvia hispanica*)

Chia seeds have recently become popular as a healthy food. They can be easily added to a morning fruit smoothie or to a bean soup for extra texture and nutrition. Recent studies have shown them to be one of the richest plant sources of omega-3 fatty acids. One tablespoon of chia seeds (14 g) contains approximately 70 calories, 6 g of fibre, 3.5 g of unsaturated fat and 2 g of complete protein, containing all the essential amino acids. They are also a rich source of calcium, phosphorus, zinc and copper. Several studies suggest a potential protective effect of chia seeds in reducing cholesterol and body weight. These results have not been confirmed in human clinical trials.[191,192]

Other seeds

There are many other interesting seeds that we can use to diversify our diet, for instance alfalfa, nigella and mustard seeds. There are also other ways to use seeds like sprouting.

SPROUT SECRETS

Green sprouts have been consumed in many cultures for much of recorded history. The culinary benefit of including sprouts in our diet is that they are very low in calories and rich in vitamins, but most importantly they do not need to be cooked. There are many types of sprouts, the most common being: alfalfa, radish, fenugreek, clover, sunflower, mustard, dill, garlic and pumpkin, as well as various legumes and grains, such as mung, kidney, pinto, navy and soybeans, and wheat berries.

An interesting one is broccoli sprouts. They contain extremely high concentrations of a cancer-fighting bioactive compound called glucoraphanin.[193] Three-day-old sprouts of broccoli and cauliflower contain 10 to 100 times higher levels of glucoraphanin than the corresponding unsprouted plants do.[194] Accumulating animal data suggest that glucoraphanin is highly effective in reducing the incidence and development of breast cancer.[195]

How to grow sprouts

The sprouting process is not difficult. Soak beans, seeds or grains for 8 to 24 hours, drain the water and then spread them in a single layer on a large tray covered with a clean damp kitchen towel. They are ready when tiny sprouts appear. It is better to consume them immediately, but if stored in the fridge they should be eaten within three or maximum four days. Always keep the sprouts refrigerated.

Be careful, because fresh sprouts, if not properly prepared, might be a vehicle for harmful bacteria. Do not consume sprouts that have turned brown or changed colour.

If you decide to sprout seeds at home, buy only seeds suitable for home sprouting, because they are subjected to strict controls. And always wash your hands carefully before handling the seeds and use equipment like spoons that have been cleaned thoroughly, preferably boiled in hot water.

FRUIT IS THE BEST DESSERT TO NOURISH THE SKIN

It's becoming increasingly clear that what we eat affects the vitality and health of our skin, and how quickly it ages. Cherries, blueberries, blackcurrants, strawberries, apples and pears are low-glycaemic fruits rich in vitamins and phytochemicals that possess skin-protecting properties. Together with other foods (see page 126), they are instrumental in keeping our skin glowing, smooth and clear. Eating fruits daily that are rich in carotenoids, lutein and zeaxanthin improves skin tone and luminance, and protects against UV-induced redness and photo ageing.[196]

Fruits rich in carotenoids are papaya, watermelon, cantaloupe, mangos and oranges, while excellent sources of lutein and zeaxanthin are kiwi fruit, grapes and oranges.[197]

The benefits of regularly consuming fruit are not limited to skin health. At the end of a meal, replacing the usual energy-dense sweet dessert or ice-cream with a fruit salad is one of the best strategies for keeping your body weight at bay. A half-cup scoop of chocolate ice-cream contains about 250 calories and one slice of sponge cake contains 240 calories, mostly made up of saturated fat and simple sugars with no fibre. In contrast, a whole cup of unsweetened raw strawberries and blueberries provides only 45 calories with 80 g (2.8 oz) of vitamin C (87 per cent RDA) and no fat. Or if you eat a large 200 g (7 oz) ripe mango, you will have consumed 130 calories, and 4 g of fibre loaded with 390 mcg of vitamin A (43 per cent RDA), 55 g of vitamin C (62 per cent RDA), and 2 mg vitamin E (15 per cent RDA).

Eating whole fruits as dessert also induces prolonged satiety because of the viscous gel-like gut environment produced by the fruit's dietary fibre, which delays gastric emptying and decreases the activity of enzymes digesting carbohydrates. Dietary fibre as I've said before may protect against weight gain also through modifications of the bacteria living in our gut.[198] One study reported that a group of bacteria, called Bacteriodates, that are typically abundant in lean people are also higher in people who consume fruits.[199]

BEST FOODS FOR A HEALTHY AND GLOWING SKIN

If you want supple skin that shines with health, then you should favour these foods and beverages.

Low-glycaemic fruits rich in vitamins and phytochemicals

Fruits loaded with vitamin C, quercetin, anthocyanins and proanthocyanidins promote radiant skin and help blemishes heal properly. The best sources are oranges, lemons, blueberries, blackcurrants, strawberries, kiwi fruits, papaya and apples. Vitamin C is needed to produce collagen, which strengthens the capillaries that supply the skin with oxygen and nutrients.

Vegetables rich in carotenoids

Carrots, sweet potatoes and pumpkin followed by broccoli, butter head lettuce, parsley, spinach, and watercress are rich in beta-carotene, while papaya, kale and spinach are loaded with lutein.[200] These compounds are powerful antioxidants that play a key role in protecting skin tone and health.

Cold-water oily fish, nuts, seeds and avocado rich in mono- and poly-unsaturated fats

Several human studies show that omega-3 fat intake makes our skin more resistant to sun damage by reducing skin inflammation and UV-induced gene mutation. As well, UV-induced redness is decreased.[201]

Green tea and other herbal teas

Data from animal studies suggest that certain phytochemicals of green tea may protect skin against UV damage, skin cancer and skin sensitivity.[202]

Regular consumption of fruit can also provide a wide range of essential vitamins that are required for the correct functioning of our cells. For examples, oranges and lemons are a very rich source of the antioxidant vitamin C.[203] Several bioactive molecules in fruits, such as carotenoids and fibre, may be implicated in the prevention of some cancers. In one epidemiological study, the consumption of yellow or orange fruits and vegetables rich in alpha-carotene during early adulthood has been associated with a reduced risk of breast cancer.[204]

Various other bioactive components, which are synthesised for protecting a plant against infectious diseases, pests and environmental stress, have been discovered in fruits. These phytochemicals seem to play a synergistic role in decreasing the risk of multiple human disorders, including cancers, cardiovascular diseases, hypertension and cognitive impairment.[205,206]

Fruit phytochemicals are primarily phenolic compounds. Each fruit contains some unique phenolic constituents in significant concentrations as well as in proportion to others.[207] For instance, wild blue- and blackberries contain the highest phenolic phytochemical content, followed by pomegranate, cranberry, blueberry, plum and apple, which might contribute to lowering inflammation.[208,209]

Pomegranate is very rich in polyphenols. The most abundant of these polyphenols is punicalagin, responsible for about 50 per cent of the juice's potent antioxidant activity.[210] Several studies have shown that pomegranate can potentially lower inflammation, blood pressure and artery plaque build-up.[211,212] Data from small clinical trials suggest consuming pomegranate juice may inhibit prostate tumour growth and lower blood prostate-specific antigen (PSA) levels,[213,214] but these results have not been confirmed in larger trials.[215]

FISH: SUBSTITUTE MEAT WITH FISH FOR THE GOOD OF YOUR HEART

Fish-eating Inuit and Japanese populations traditionally had lower rates of heart disease compared to meat-eaters living in the US and North Europe.[216] Other observational studies support these findings and suggest that regular fish consumption can protect the heart, especially in people at higher than average risk of coronary heart disease.[217]

Eating four or more servings per week of fish rich in long-chain omega-3 polyunsaturated fatty acids seems to lower the risk of having a heart attack by 22 per cent compared to people who consumed seafood less than once a month.[218] However, it is not necessary to eat four servings of fish every week. Several studies have shown that even consuming one to four servings of oily fish per month has a significant cardioprotective effect compared with no consumption.[219]

Fishes rich in long-chain omega-3 polyunsaturated fatty acids mainly inhabit colder water and include salmon, anchovies, herring, mackerel, tuna and sardines.

Not all fish products prevent heart disease, though. In the Cardiovascular Health Study, eating broiled and baked fish three or more time per week was associated with 49 per cent lower risk of dying for an heart attack and 58 per cent lower risk of sudden cardiac death.[220] However, eating fried fish or fish sandwiches was not associated with a lower risk of sudden cardiac death, and might even increase the risk of death; probably, because most commercially prepared deep-fried seafood is cooked in partially hydrogenated oils containing trans-fat.

Results from epidemiological studies also suggest that eating seafood is associated with a lower risk of ischaemic stroke when blood flow to the brain is blocked by a blood clot, but not of haemorrhagic stroke when a weak blood vessel bursts and there is bleeding in the brain itself.[221]

Common seafood varieties	EPA+DHA, mg per 115 g (4 oz)
Salmon: Atlantic, Chinook, caho	1200–2400
Anchovies, herring, shad	2300–2400
Mackerel: Atlantic and Pacific not King	1350–2100
Tuna: Bluefin, albacore	1700
Sardines: Atlantic and Pacific	1100–1600
Oysters, Pacific	1550
Trout: freshwater	1000–1100
Tuna: white (albacore) canned	1000
Mussels: blue	900
Salmon: pink, sockeye	700–900
Squid	750
Pollock: Atlantic, walleye	600
Crab: blue, king, snow, queen, Dungeness	200–550
Tuna: skipjack, yellowfin	150–350
Flounder, plaice, sole	350
Clams	200–300
Tuna: light canned	150–300
Catfish	100–250
Cod: Atlantic and Pacific	200
Scallops: bay and sea	200
Haddock, hake	200
Lobster	200
Crayfish	200
Tilopia	150
Shrimp	100
Shark	1250
Tilefish	1000
Swordfish	1000

Table 6: Seafood long-chain polyunsaturated fatty acid composition of different fish varieties. EPA indicates eicosapentaencic acid and DHA indicates docosahexaenoic acid.[222]

Multiple studies have shown that the fish fat omega-3 (eicosapentaenoic acid and docosahexaenoic acid) is responsible for many of these beneficial effects, because of its potent antiarrhythmic actions (i.e. they block the impulses that cause an irregular heart rhythm).[223] Results from large randomised clinical trials show that fish oil supplementation rapidly reduces fatal arrhythmias and sudden cardiac death.[224]

Several other mechanisms are responsible for the cardiovascular protective effects of fish oil. These include lowering blood triglycerides, decreasing blood pressure and inflammation, decreasing platelet aggregation (formation of clots in the arteries) and improving vascular function.[225] Fish is also one of the best sources of vitamin B12. It exceeds meat in its vitamin B12 bioavailability, and unlike red meat, its consumption is associated with a lower risk of colon cancer.[226]

EXTRA-VIRGIN OLIVE OIL: THE HEALTHIEST CONDIMENT

For centuries extra-virgin olive oil has been the main condiment and a source of fat and energy in the Mediterranean countries, home to some of the most long-lived people in the world. Olive oil is a nutritionally balanced and healthy condiment. Traditionally it is extracted from the ripe fruit of the olive tree without using chemical solvents or heat. Because of this the unrefined cold-pressed juice of these fruits is rich in unspoiled monounsaturated fats, vitamins and bioactive compounds that are so beneficial to our health. Of course, the better the quality of the olive fruit and the faster the juice is cold pressed, the higher the quality and taste of the oil produced.

I use only first cold-pressed extra-virgin olive oil to dress my salads, raw or roasted vegetables, legumes and pasta sauces. When I am in a hurry, one of my favourite, yet simple to prepare dishes, is garlic, olive oil and chilli pepper spaghetti. Because of its rich and unique flavour, extra-virgin olive oil is the best condiment; it makes any dish taste better, even a simple slice of bread. As a snack, my son loves to eat a couple of slices of whole-wheat bread sprinkled with extra virgin olive oil and a few drops of organic soy sauce.

The mixture of phenolic compounds contained in extra-virgin olive is responsible for its fruity, pungent and slightly bitter taste and for its aroma. More than 30 phytocompounds have been described, the most important being oleuropein, tyrosol, and hydroxytyrosol. The fresher the olive oil, the higher the concentrations of phytocompounds.

One hundred grams (3½ oz) of extra-virgin olive oil (about 7 tablespoons) contains up to 25 mg of alpha-tocopherol and 1–2 mg of carotenoids, which are both potent antioxidants, as well as 20–500 mg of oleuropein and 98–185 mg of phytosterols.[227] These compounds provide several beneficial effects, including: reduction of plasma triglyceride and markers of oxidative stress and increased levels of the good HDL-cholesterol.[228,229] Extra virgin olive oil phenolics modulate important enzymes that inhibit molecules that are contributors to inflammation and thrombosis.[230]

Newly pressed extra-virgin olive oil also contains a molecule called oleocanthal that prevents blood clots. We can immediately taste if olive oil contains oleocanthal by its pungency: the stinging, peppery sensation that we can detect in our throat. Once we begin to appreciate the health benefits of this spicy kick, it is difficult to imagine life without it. Oleocanthal has a structural profile strikingly similar to that of ibuprofen, the medicine used as an analgesic and to reduce inflammation and platelet aggregation.[231]

Consuming 50 g of extra-virgin olive oil every day (which contains approximately 9 mg of oleocanthal), is equivalent to taking a baby aspirin, which is important for the prevention of heart disease, and potentially of cancer and Alzheimer's disease.[232-235]

Nonetheless, we have to keep in mind that one tablespoon of olive oil also contains approximately 120 calories. If we over-consume olive oil, without balancing it out with the proper amount of physical activity, we will gain weight. The effects of overweight and of the excessive accumulation of abdominal fat on chronic inflammation, oxidative stress, insulin sensitivity and metabolic health in general will overcome the beneficial effects of the polyphenols contained in olive oil.

WHAT SHOULD WE DRINK?

Nothing can beat a fresh glass of spring water for quenching our thirst. It is the best beverage to hydrate our cells while providing a range of essential minerals and oligo-elements. But these qualities can be further improved by pouring hot or boiling water over tea leaves or other herbal plants. A range of powerful bioactive compounds can be released and absorbed when we consume herbal infusions.

Depending on the season, I like to make different types of tea and herbal infusions. During the hot summer months, I prefer to drink peppermint tea because of its refreshing properties; during the cold winter periods, I enjoy thyme with some ginger or cloves. Green tea, on the other hand, alternated with infusions of sage or rosemary, is a staple all year long.

Several studies suggest that coffee is also healthy if consumed within limits. Epidemiological studies suggest three to four cups a day achieves the largest risk reduction for cardiovascular and cancer outcomes.[236]

Green and black tea (*Camellia sinensis*)

Tea originates from the dark-green leaves of a type of camellia bush that grows mainly in tropical and subtropical climates. A good cup of tea is one of life's pleasures, but accumulating data suggest that this revitalising drink may have much greater healing properties. There is evidence that tea, especially green tea, can help guard against cancer and heart disease.[237,238]

Tea's health properties are predominantly linked to a family of phytochemicals known as catechins; the main one being epigallocatechin gallate (EGCG), which typically comprises 60 per cent of the catechin content in a cup of green tea.[239] Studies of EGCG, epicatechin and other flavonoids show they have powerful pharmacological effects (both on cultured cells and in animal models of disease) against the toxic effects of free radicals. They also possess potential anti-inflammatory and anticancer properties.[240,241]

Both green and black tea have been shown to prevent cancer in a variety of animal models, including cancer of the skin, lung, mouth, oesophagus, stomach, colon, pancreas, bladder and prostate.[242,243] A very small clinical trial suggests that green tea catechins might work also in humans by preventing precancerous prostate lesions from turning cancerous.[244] Catechin may work by promoting self-destruction of tumour cells while sparing nearby healthy cells.

Drinking black and green tea has also been shown to reverse the beginnings of plaque build-up in the arteries (endothelial dysfunction) of smokers and in patients with coronary artery disease through its antioxidant effects.[245,246]

Herbal teas

Herbal teas, also called tisanes, are made by infusing or boiling in hot water the leaves, fruits or other parts of plants, including chamomile, sage, rosemary and a host of others. Each one of these plants contains bioactive compounds with potential pharmacological effects.

Everybody knows chamomile tea for its relaxing and calming effects, and several randomised clinical trials have demonstrated its modest but significant effects on anxiety and sleep disorders.[247-249] One of my favourites is sage tea, with its delicate, tangy flavour with some bitter notes. However, sage tea should not be drunk during pregnancy.

Other herbs, plants and spices that I also enjoy making tea with are thyme, peppermint, hibiscus, echinacea, rooibos, passionflower, rose hip, anise, cinnamon, ginger and ginseng. Each one of these plants is loaded with a long list of different bioactive compounds. Some have other healthy goodies that have not been tested yet. The fact that they have not been studied does not mean that we should refrain from consuming these herbs. Indeed, I experiment and change the mix as much and as often as possible, because biodiversity (remember?) is the key to health.

HOW MUCH SHOULD WE DRINK?

One of the great urban myths is that we should drink at least 5 litres (1.3 gallons) of water a day if we want to stay healthy. There is no evidence to support this claim. In reality, unless we have a serious medical condition, for instance a high fever or a psychiatric disease, we should just drink when we are thirsty.

A study published in the prestigious journal *Proceedings of the National Academy of Sciences* has shown that our brain is pretty good at judging when we are dehydrated and how much we should drink. Indeed, the motivation to drink is closely regulated, as under-drinking or over-drinking can both cause negative health effects.

In healthy humans, certain brain areas (those controlling our emotions) are activated when we drink in response to feeling thirsty, but immediately after thirst has been quenched, other brain regions kick in to stop the drinking response.[250] Interestingly, the volume of fluid consumed approximates the fluid deficit, suggesting that these brain circuits are important to prevent people from drinking too much water, which could result in dangerously low blood sodium concentrations, possibly triggering the swelling of the brain. This study also reported that drinking to satisfy thirst was perceived as a pleasurable sensation; in contrast, drinking excess water was felt as an unpleasant emotion.

CHAPTER TEN

FOODS TO ELIMINATE OR DRASTICALLY REDUCE

At least 60 per cent of calories in the average Western-style modern diet come from 'ultra-processed' foods that have been designed to be highly palatable, convenient and affordable, and to have a long shelf-life.

Studies indicate that these industrially processed foods are major contributors in driving the pandemic of obesity, type 2 diabetes, cardiovascular disease and other diseases, including cancer, that are spreading at an alarming pace around the world.

These are not natural foods; they are 'industrial' foods often modified by chemical processes with many synthetic additives that are then assembled into ready-to-eat or ready-to-heat hyper-palatable food and drink products. Typically, they contain refined flours, hydrogenated oils, high-fructose corn syrup, sucrose or artificial sweeteners and salt, together with a range of preservatives, artificial flavours, colours, emulsifiers and other cosmetic additives.

If you want to stay healthy you should eliminate these foods from your diet. Data from two large independent epidemiological studies published in the *British Medical Journal* suggest that even a small consumption of ultra-processed food is associated with an increased risk of mortality, and a higher probability of developing heart disease, stroke and cancer, in particular breast cancer and colon cancer.[1-3]

Mortality increased by 18 per cent for each additional serving of industrially processed food consumed. In these studies, ultra-processed foods were classified as:

- mass produced packaged breads and buns

- sweet or savoury packaged snacks

- industrialised confectionery and desserts

- sodas and sweetened drinks

- meat balls, poultry and fish nuggets, and other reconstituted meat products transformed with the addition of preservatives other than salt (for example, nitrites)

- instant noodles and soups

- frozen or shelf-stable ready meals

- other food products made mostly or entirely from sugar, oils and fats, and other substances not commonly used in culinary preparations such as hydrogenated oils, modified starches and protein isolates.

WHY ARE ULTRA-PROCESSED FOODS BAD FOR YOU?

Multiple factors are responsible for the detrimental effects of ultra-processed foods. These include that they may:

- contain high concentrations of empty calories, in particular saturated and trans-fat, salt, added sugars or high fructose corn syrup

- be low in vegetable fibre, vitamins and phytochemicals

- contain high levels of potentially carcinogenic molecules, including acrylamide, heterocyclic amines and polycyclic aromatic hydrocarbons.[4] This applies to some products only

- contain food additives that are legally authorised, but controversial. Examples are sodium nitrite in processed meat, titanium dioxide as a whitening agent, talc and carbon black.[5] Some studies suggest they could have a potential detrimental or carcinogenic impact

- be packaged in material that releases carcinogenic and endocrine disruptors such as bisphenol A (BPA), into the food.[6]

Childhood, adolescence and early adulthood, are highly susceptible periods for the accrual of damage caused by these highly processed foods and for the development of obesity. For instance, in a randomised clinical trial at the National Institutes of Health in Bethesda, in the US, 20 weight-stable young non-obese individuals were chosen to consume either an ultra-processed or an unprocessed diet for two weeks, followed by the alternate diet for another two weeks. The two diets were designed to contain the same amount of calories, macronutrients, sugar, sodium and fibre, and the volunteers were instructed to consume as much or as little as desired.

The results of this study were shocking: the people who ate the ultra-processed diet consumed on average 510 kcal per day more and gained about 1 kg (2 lb) of body weight in only 14 days; while the people consuming the unprocessed food *lost* 1 kg (2 lb) of body weight.[7] One kilogram (2 lb) in two weeks may not seem much, but over a year it means a weight gain of 24 kg (53 lb). A 1.8 m (5 ft 9 in) tall, fit boy who weighs 75 kg (165 lb), could escalate from a BMI of 23 to one of 30.5 in less than a year. The dire consequences of this weight gain on the risk of developing some of the most common and debilitating chronic illnesses, have already been explained in Chapter 4.

SUGARS: NOT SO SWEET RESULTS

The added sugars found in highly processed foods and sweetened beverages increase the probability of developing obesity, diabetes, cardiovascular disease, some types of cancer and of course dental caries. When drinks and foods have these sugars added, it increases the calorie intake without contributing any of the essential nutrients. Eating these foods makes it almost impossible for people to meet their nutrient needs for vitamins and minerals while staying within calorie limits.

What are added sugars?

Examples of added sugars listed as ingredients in processed foods and drinks include corn syrup, high-fructose corn syrup, malt syrup, corn sweetener, white and brown sugar, glucose, fructose, dextrose, lactose, maltose, invert sugar, molasses, sucrose, trehalose and turbinado sugar.

How much sugar is too much sugar?

The American Heart Association recommends that children should not consume more than 25 g (about six teaspoons) of added sugar per day and that sugar should not be given to toddlers younger than 24 months.[8] My belief is that soft drinks, candies, and other sweets and sweetened foods rich in added sugars and HFCS have no place in our homes. When children are hungry and they open the pantry or the refrigerator, and they do not find these unhealthy products, they will not be able to eat them. Instead they will choose a healthy piece of fruit or a carrot.

SOFT DRINKS AND SODAS

Although people are gradually becoming aware of the detrimental health effects of consuming soft drinks or heavily sweetened sodas, this knowledge does not seem to block them from buying bottles of these unhealthy sugar-sweetened beverages and putting them in the fridge for their children to drink. So probably I need to explain a bit more about these drinks and how bad they are for your, and most importantly, for your kids' health.[9]

Most of these soft drinks are made with a processed, concentrated, high fructose corn syrup (HFCS) or a combination of artificial sweeteners and additives. HFCS has become popular as an ingredient in soft drinks and an additive to many industrial sweet and savoury foods, because it is cheaper, easier to use and sweeter than table sugar. HFCS, a concentrated form of sugar (a combination of one molecule of glucose and one of fructose), has been heavily implicated in the growing epidemic of obesity, metabolic syndrome and type 2 diabetes.[10,11,12]

Data from a large epidemiological study suggest that every can of soft drink consumed by children translates into a 60 per cent increase in their risk of becoming obese.[13] In contrast, other studies have shown that reducing their consumption is associated with a lower body weight.[14,15]

Fructose has been shown to be particularly harmful, because it causes insulin resistance and can lead to fatty liver.[16-18] In animal studies, fructose intake is associated with altered intestinal flora, increased gut permeability and liver inflammation.[19]

Long-term consumption of artificially sweetened beverages has also been associated with an increased risk of developing cardiovascular disease, stroke and cancer, especially pancreatic and colon cancer.[20-22] A new study published in *Science* shows that even moderate consumption of soft drinks containing HFCS contributes directly to the development of colon cancer.[23]

Is it okay to drink 'diet' soda?

Unfortunately, the answer seems to be no. 'Diet' soft drinks are essentially a mixture of carbonated water, artificial or natural sweeteners, colours, flavours and other food additives. High-intensity sweeteners commonly used are aspartame, saccharin, sucralose, acesulfame potassium (Ace-K) or Stevia. These chemical compounds are 200–13,000 times sweeter than regular sugar.

Even though these drinks contain no calories, sugar, fat or protein, a growing body of scientific evidence suggests that drinking 'diet' soft drinks may also be associated with an increased risk of obesity and metabolic syndrome. A study published in *Cell Metabolism* has demonstrated that sustained sucralose intake stimulated hunger, and as a consequence increased food consumption, leading to obesity.[24] It seems that certain areas of the brain detect a discrepancy between the dietary sweetness and energy intake, stimulating a fasting-like state and a sensory and behavioural response that forces people to increase calorie consumption.

SALT: SNEAKY SODIUM

Sodium is found in table salt and occurs naturally in very small concentrations in some foods as well. However, 70–80 per cent of the salt most people consume every day is hidden in processed and packaged foods. Industrial bread, cheese, processed meats, potato chips, sauces, spreads and even breakfast cereals are the main culprits. A small bag of chips contains 170–210 mg of sodium, two slices of a typical industrial bread can contain up to 270 mg of sodium, one serving of cottage cheese 450 mg and one can of vegetable soup can hide a whopping 640 mg of sodium.

How much salt should you consume?

According to the guidelines of the World Health Organization (WHO) and the Institute of Medicine (IOM), adults and children aged 14 years and older should consume no more than 6 g of salt or 2300 mg of sodium per day, which is about 1¼ teaspoons of ordinary table salt. That is a maximum. An 'adequate' intake set by WHO and the National Health and Medical Research Council of Australia is 2.3 g of salt or 920 mg of sodium per day, that is nearly a third of the maximum amount.[25]

But in Western countries, and even more so in China and Japan, many people consume at least 10 g of salt every day. Unless you stop eating industrial highly processed food products like potato crisps and other salt and sodium laden foods it will be almost impossible to cut out salt from your diet. Carefully read the labels of the products you buy. And better still learn to cook most of your meals at home by using a variety of fresh whole minimally processed foods.

You also need to avoid adding too much salt to your food when cooking or adding salt as a condiment to your food (a good pinch of salt contains approximately 400 mg of sodium). Instead, use spices and culinary herbs, and not salt, to maximise the taste of your dishes if you want to reduce the risk of developing salt-related, serious diseases.

> ## CALCULATING SALT CONTENT
> Many food labels only state the sodium content. To convert sodium to salt, we need to multiply the sodium figure in milligrams by 2.5 and then divide by 1,000.
>
> Example: how much salt is there in one can of vegetable soup containing 640 mg of sodium?
>
> 640 mg x 2.5 = 1600 mg of salt, then divided by 1,000 = 1.6 g salt

It is well accepted that consuming too much salt increases blood pressure in people with or without hypertension.[26] In the INTERSALT study, the risk for developing hypertension over three decades of adult life was tightly related to dietary sodium excretion.[27]

The DASH-Sodium (Dietary Approaches to Stop Hypertension) trial also found a significant direct relationship between salt intake and increased blood pressure.[28] Several other studies have demonstrated that a modest salt reduction can lower systolic and diastolic blood pressure levels by 5.4 and 2.8 mmHg, respectively, in hypertensive individuals, and by 2.4 and 1.0 mmHg in people with normal blood pressure.[29,30] A new human study suggests that high salt intake can even promote inflammation.[31]

Finally, two large randomised clinical trials have found a direct relationship between sodium intake and total mortality over a period of 23 to 26 years, even at the lowest levels of sodium intake.[32,33]

DIET, SALT AND BLOOD PRESSURE

For the great majority of individuals living in Western countries, blood pressure (especially systolic blood pressure) increases with age. However, this is not an inevitable pattern of 'normal' human physiology, because the blood pressure of people living in traditional rural areas and eating calorie- and salt-restricted, fibre-rich diets remains low and flat during the entire lifetime.[34]

In support of these observations, we found that calorie restriction with an adequate intake of all the essential nutrients lowers blood pressure to super-physiologic values (i.e. below 115/75 mm Hg) even in healthy non-obese young men and women.[35,36] The blood pressure among a group of people practising calorie restriction with optimal nutrition was in the 110/60 mmHg range even in those aged more than 70. There are multiple mechanisms behind this powerful effect, but having low abdominal fat is a major contributor.

However, this is not sufficient on its own. In my studies at Washington University, we observed that elite athletes who are very lean because of high levels of exercise still experience an age-related increase in blood pressure. The problem is that many of these athletes consumed a typical Western diet, rich in processed and salty foods with a very limited intake of fibre and potassium-rich vegetables.

Should you totally give up salt?

Absolutely not. Sodium has many important biological functions, such as maintaining blood and cellular volume and pressure, and transmission of nerve impulses.

Most importantly, a healthy diet that does not include the use of iodised salt cannot meet the daily requirement of iodine (150 mcg/day). Iodine is a mineral that is essential for the production of thyroid hormones, and for the prevention of thyroid diseases. It is a critical micronutrient in the human diet, something our bodies can't synthesise, so we must rely on food to obtain it. In Australia and in many developed countries, it's been added to salt (in the form of potassium iodide) for many years. It is also mandatory in many developed countries to fortify common commercially made foods such as bread.

But even in a highly developed country such as Australia, a national survey has found mild iodine deficiency in a subpopulation of individuals.[37] It has long been known that mild iodine deficiency during pregnancy and breastfeeding can affect the brain development of unborn children and infants, and potentially lead to a reduced intelligence quotient and attention deficit and hyperactivity.[38-40] Unfortunately, these commercial products are often baked with refined flours (and potentially with a large set of other unhealthy ingredients and chemicals).

My advice is to buy only iodised salt and use this at home to cook your food and dress your salads. On average 5 g of iodised salt (close to a teaspoon) meets the 150-mcg recommended daily intake of iodine, but if we want to reduce our salt intake close to the recommended 2.3 g per day, we should also consume foods that are naturally rich in iodine. Examples are dried seaweeds (range 65–680 mcg per 100 mg), marine seafood (range 50–100 mcg per 100 mg) and very small amounts of cheese and milk (range 80–170 mcg per 250 ml (8½ fl oz) depending on the amount of iodine in supplements given to dairy cows).

If you are pregnant, breastfeeding or considering pregnancy, talk with your doctor about an iodine supplement.

MEAT: IS IT GOOD OR BAD FOR YOUR HEALTH?

For many people, meat is considered a staple food, with some eating either beef, chicken, lamb, pork, ham, salami, bacon or sausages daily, often several times a day. A selection of fried bacon, sausages, scrambled eggs, ham and cheese is typically served as an English or full American breakfast in many hotels. It may be followed by a hamburger or meat sandwich (you can choose between ham, turkey, chicken or roast beef) for lunch and often roasted or sautéed meat (usually chicken, pork or beef, sometimes fish) for dinner.

Americans eat more meat than anyone else in the world. In 2016, the average American consumed around 97 kg (213 lb) of red meat, followed by 95 kg (209 lb) in Australia, 86 kg (189 lb) in Argentina and 69 kg (152 lb) in Europe.[41] Per capita meat consumption has also increased dramatically in many other countries as well. Since 1961, meat consumption in China has grown approximately 15-fold and in Brazil four-fold. This alarming trend has dire consequences not only for human health, but also for environmental health and animal welfare.

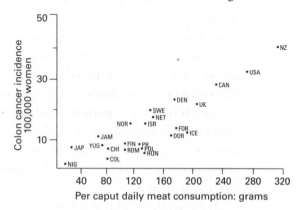

Figure 15: Correlation between meat intake (g per person per day) and incidence of colon cancer in women in 23 countries.[42]

How much meat should we consume?

A growing body of evidence suggests that we should limit red meat consumption to no more than 350–500 g (11–18 oz) a week; very little, if any of it should be processed meat.[42] How much is 350 g (12 oz) of red meat? Well, that is about how much one medium fillet steak and one lamb loin chop weigh.

WHAT IS RED MEAT?

Red meat is defined as beef, veal, pork, lamb, mutton, horse, goat meat and that from any other mammal.

WHAT IS PROCESSED MEAT?

Processed meat is defined as any meat preserved by smoking, curing, fermenting or salting, or with the addition of chemical preservatives. Examples include bacon, salami, sausages, hot dogs or processed deli or luncheon meats.

If you eat a Western-style diet you will most likely eat way more than that every week and it is time to cut down your consumption. Here is why.

According to the World Health Organization, processed meat is a Group 1 carcinogen, which means that the evidence for processed meats causing cancer (especially colon, rectum and gastric cancer) is very strong.[43] Red meat has been classified as a Group 2A carcinogen, a probable cause of cancer.

The estimated risk of developing colon cancer increases by 17 per cent with each 100 g (3½ oz) of red meat consumed each day.[44-46] The risk associated with eating processed meat is even higher: for every 50 g of processed meat eaten per day, the risk of colon cancer increases by 18 per cent.[47]

Accumulating data suggest that red meat consumption may also be associated with an increased risk of developing pancreatic and prostate cancer, while processed meat might increase the risk of stomach cancer.[48,49]

Excessive meat consumption is also implicated in cardiovascular disease, obesity and type 2 diabetes.[50-53] This may explain why data from a recent epidemiological study published in the prestigious *British Medical Journal* suggest that an increase in red meat consumption, especially processed meat, is associated with a 10 to 13 per cent higher risk of death.[54]

What about the quality of the meat we eat?

Around two-thirds of domestic animals are raised in factory farms and treated and traded as mere commodities. These industrial systems favour high production and low-cost above all else, and force billions of animals to live in unfair, smelly, dirty and precarious conditions.

These animals cannot freely walk in the sun, breath fresh air and eat naturally abundant food. They are brought up in confinement at high stocking densities. For example, millions of chickens are confined to battery wire cages, and calves and pigs in metal stalls or windowless sheds. These alienated, stressed and suffering creatures will never nurture and enjoy their offspring, build nests, dig around in the soil, or live a natural life. Moreover, these unnatural overcrowded living conditions, the poor quality of food they consume and the extensive use of antibiotics (as growth promoters and for the prevention of infections) have huge consequences on the quality of meat, milk and eggs produced and consumed by billions of unaware people.[55-59]

If consumers were shown how farmed animals were reared, they might never eat their meat, milk and eggs again. I suggest you watch two excellent documentaries on this topic: *Dominion* and *Slaughterhouse*. We urgently need a food and farming revolution – one that drastically reduces the overconsumption of cheap, mass-produced and unhealthy meat and animal products, and favours the production and consumption of small quantities of ethically sourced high-quality animal products, respectful of the welfare of animals and of the health of our planet.

What's so bad about red meat?

Meat and all the fat from animal products are very rich in saturated fatty acids. Lard, sausages, salami and fatty cuts of beef, pork and lamb contain very high concentrations of these fatty acids, but also dairy foods, including butter, cream, ghee, regular-fat milk and cheese and the skin on chicken provide a substantial load of saturated fat.

Heart disease is still the leading cause of mortality for both men and women. Having a high blood cholesterol level is one of the main risk factors in promoting atherosclerosis (fatty deposits in the arteries), which is the underlying cause of approximately 90 per cent of cases of heart attacks, 60 per cent of strokes, most cases of heart failure, peripheral arterial disease and vascular dementia.[60] As we have already discussed, both epidemiological and clinical trials have demonstrated that one of the most important determinants of blood cholesterol levels is our intake of saturated fatty acids.

Animal products, particularly red meat, are also a rich source of l-carnitine and choline, which get metabolised by the gut microbes to produce a metabolite called TMAO. Elevated levels of TMAO induce inflammation and increase platelet aggregation that can lead to heart attacks and strokes in humans, and might also be involved in the development of obesity and type 2 diabetes.[61] Processed meats are typically very high in salt, which as we have already discussed increases blood pressure and the risk of heart attacks and stroke too.

Several mechanisms are also responsible for the cancer-producing effects of red and processed meat:

- Red meat contains a high concentration of heme iron which, when broken down in the intestine, promotes the formation of highly carcinogenic molecules, called N-nitroso compounds; heme iron also increases oxidative stress that damages the DNA by increasing the rate of mutations.[62]

- Red meat is also very rich in a molecule (sialic acid) that when incorporated into human tissues, elicits a powerful immunological and inflammatory reaction, which promotes a five-fold increase in carcinoma incidence.[63]

- Over 95 per cent of human exposure to dioxins and dioxin-like compounds (pollutants and by-products of industrial processes) occurs via the ingestion of meat, eggs, dairy products and fatty fish.[64] Since dioxins are fat-soluble, they accumulate in fatty tissues of animals that eat contaminated feed or graze on polluted soils.[65] Data from epidemiological and experimental animal studies have demonstrated that dioxin-like compounds are carcinogenic.[66-68] These highly toxic chemical compounds also damage the immune system, interfere with our hormones and cause reproductive and developmental problems.[69]

- The way meat is cooked can increase the risk of developing certain cancers. When meat is cooked at high temperatures, and it is blackened or charred (for example on a barbeque), high concentrations of heterocyclic amines (HCAs) and polycyclic aromatic hydrocarbons (PAH) are formed that are potent and harmful mutagenic molecules.[70] They are rapidly absorbed and diffused in our body; they can even be found in hair strands.[71]

- Meat processing, including curing with sodium nitrates or smoking, induces the creation of carcinogenic molecules, called *nitrosamines*, that have been shown in animal experiments to be the most broadly acting and most potent group of carcinogens.[72,73]

Finally, another link between cancer and the consumption of meat and other animal products is their high load of protein and specific amino acids (i.e. sulphur and branched chain amino acids). These trigger cancer-producing pathways, and inhibit the ability of certain immune cells to recognise and destroy malignant cells before they develop into tumours.[74-76]

The total protein intake in the typical Western diet is on average at least 40 per cent higher than it needs to be. An average American man consumes no less than 90 g (3 oz) of protein per day, 60 per cent or more of which is animal proteins. This is important because we have shown that protein restriction or the substitution of plant protein for animal proteins markedly inhibits prostate and breast cancer growth.[77,78] More recently, it has been shown that moderate protein restriction enhances the capacity of the immune system to recognise and kill tumour cells and powerfully decreases tumour growth.[79-81]

SHOULD WE ALL BECOME VEGETARIANS?

No, it is not necessary to become a vegetarian. Consuming small portions of high-quality meat a few times a month is okay, unless someone has strong ethical reasons for not doing so. However, before we buy or consume meat the next time, we should ask ourselves two questions:

1. When was the last time I ate meat? Do I really need to eat meat today?
2. Where is this meat coming from? What has the animal been eating? How has it been raised?

EAT WHOLE FOODS, NOT SUPPLEMENTS

The human body is a sophisticated machine that needs the right amount of calories, protein, fibre, vitamins, minerals and trace elements; neither too much nor too little. Supplements cannot replicate all the complex but balanced array of vitamins, phytochemicals, minerals and oligo-elements contained in whole foods.

In the 1980s and 90s some studies on cells and experimental animals did show a protective effect of supplementation with vitamin C, vitamin E and beta-carotene against cardiovascular disease, dementia and cancer. In those years there was great enthusiasm among researchers around the world, who continued to publish batteries of scientific articles on the miraculous effects of antioxidant supplementation in non-human experimental models.

Then, the first large double-blinded randomised clinical trials with thousands of participants taking these vitamins were launched. In these trials neither the participant nor the researcher knew whether the pill contained vitamins or placebo. The results of this and many other very expensive studies were all negative.[82] No protection against a wide range of chronic diseases was established. Some clinical trials have even found that high doses of beta-carotene and vitamin E can cause detrimental effects, including increased mortality, cancer and haemorrhagic stroke.[83-84]

Does this mean that beta-carotene, vitamin E and selenium are bad for our health? Absolutely not! These vitamins, as well as many other phytocompounds, in the right concentrations (those found in natural foods), have a synergic action whose effect depends on the context, and most likely also on the composition of the gut microbiota.[85,86]

Vitamin and mineral supplements should never be used as a substitute for a healthy and well-balanced diet, unless prescribed by your doctor for a specific health condition.

PART IV

PHYSICAL EXERCISE AS A DAILY MEDICINE

SCIENCE-BASED SECRETS TO STAYING FIT AND HEALTHY WITH EXERCISE TRAINING

CHAPTER ELEVEN

MAXIMISING HEALTH THROUGH PHYSICAL EXERCISE

There are plenty of good reasons to be physically active, apart from being fitter and looking better. Much like the air we breathe and the food we eat, movement is essential for our health.

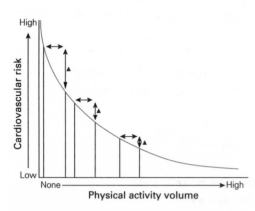

Figure 16: Relationship between physical activity and cardiovascular risk. A similar increase in physical activity yields different risk reductions across the activity spectrum. Physical inactivity is associated with the highest risk, whereas high aerobic exercise volumes are associated with the lowest risk.[1]

Over thousands of years, we evolved to engage in relentless physical activity. There were no cars, elevators, drinking water or gas heating at home, or a supermarket down the road. Food was scarce, and our great-grandparents or ancestors had to walk several hours a day to get from one settlement to another to find food, water and firewood to cook and to heat their homes. There were no tractors with powerful ploughs, trucks and mechanical shovels. Brute physical strength was necessary to hunt, till the land, lift and carry heavy objects without the aid of modern machines.

In other words, our bodies have developed, over thousands of years of evolution, to function optimally with daily physical exertion. We are metabolically and genetically programmed to operate at our best with constant and regular physical activity.

Not surprisingly, several epidemiological studies have shown that physically active individuals are healthier and live longer than sedentary ones.[2] Inactive people have a much higher risk of morbidity, disability and mortality.[3] As shown in figure 16, data from many epidemiological studies suggest that the steepest decrease in the risk of developing cardiovascular disease takes place at the lowest levels of physical activity.[4]

It is important to fix in our mind a key concept: even small amounts of physical activity are beneficial to our health, and a decline in the risk of developing multiple chronic illnesses and disability starts by simply getting moving.[5]

PHYSICAL INACTIVITY: THE BIGGEST PUBLIC HEALTH PROBLEM OF THE 21ST CENTURY

To exemplify the importance of maintaining an active lifestyle, new studies suggest that prolonged periods of inactivity – for instance, the number of hours per day spent in a sitting position to watch television or work at a computer – are associated with an increased risk of developing and dying from cardiovascular disease, cancer (breast, endometrium, ovary and colorectal) and diabetes mellitus regardless of the degree of obesity and the number of exercise sessions held during the week.[6,7]

It is of paramount importance, therefore, in order to improve our metabolic health and reduce the risk of dying prematurely, to move as often as possible, to take frequent breaks at work and limit the amount of time we spend in a seated position.[8-10]

Every week we should all try to incorporate as many structured exercise sessions as possible. Ideally, we should all be able to find at least 30 minutes a day to work out, but if this is not possible, even multiple small bouts of at least ten minutes of leisure-time physical activity, spread throughout the day, are sufficient to provide some metabolic and psychological health benefits.[11,12] Additional paybacks can come from engaging in more vigorous and prolonged aerobic exercise or short bouts of high-intensity interval training during the weekend.[13]

HOW MUCH EXERCISE DO WE NEED?
According to the 2018 Physical Activity Guidelines Advisory Committee Scientific Report[14] to achieve substantial health benefits, we should undertake:
1. at least 150–300 minutes a week of moderate-intensity, or 75–150 minutes a week of vigorous-intensity aerobic physical exercise, or an equivalent combination of moderate and vigorous-intensity aerobic training
2. muscle-strengthening activities of moderate or greater intensity that involve all major muscle groups on two or more days a week.

THE 2,500-YEAR HISTORY OF SPORTS MEDICINE

That regular physical exercise is key for promoting health has been known since ancient times, although our ancestors did not know the biological processes responsible for its beneficial effects.

Susruta, a famous Indian clinician, who lived around 600 years BCE, was the first to prescribe exercise for the treatment of chronic afflictions and the 'preservation' of better health. He wrote: 'Diseases fly from the presence of a person habituated to regular physical exercise', but he also stated that 'Exercise should be taken every day, but only to half the extent of the patient capacity as otherwise it may prove fatal'.[15] Before prescribing exercise, he added, doctors should consider the age, strength, physique and diet of their patients. Susruta believed that exercise training was important to keep the body strong, compact and light; to enhance the growth of muscles; to improve digestion and complexion; and to reduce senility.

In ancient China, during the era of the Yellow Emperor (1050–256 BCE), doctors prescribed moderate exercise for its strengthening and health effects.[16] Two important precepts of ancient Chinese medicine were 'Water which flows never becomes putrid' and 'A moving door hinge cannot be eaten by worms'. Lu Jiuzhi, a doctor of the Qing dynasty, in his book entitled *Treatise on Disease of Excessive Comfort* wrote:

> *Ordinary people are often reminded of the diseases induced by excessive effort, but not of those caused by laziness, which are much worse. Preventing excessive comfort of body and mind is essential to preserve health and live a long life.*

In the West, Pythagoras (570–490 BCE) was the first scientist from ancient Greece to advocate daily exercise for health promotion. He did not believe that maladies were the result of the gods' spells, but, rather, due to disharmony of body elements. To re-establish harmony and achieve a healthy state, he believed that a daily regimen of healthy diet, exercise (including long walks, running, wrestling and boxing), music and meditation was necessary.[17] Hippocrates, the famous Greek physician and father of Western medicine, who lived between 460 and 377 BCE, said:

> *If we would be able to provide everyone the right amount of exercise and nourishment, nor too little or too much, we would have found the road to health ... food and exercise, while possessing opposite qualities, yet work together to produce health.[18]*

Then during the Dark Ages of the Medieval period, this empirical knowledge faded away. It was erroneously thought that exercise was *bad* for health, because the heart had a finite number of beats over a lifespan. Increasing heart rate, therefore, was accelerating and exhausting the finite potential and length of life. Only at the beginning of the 20th century did modern science begin to rediscover and elucidate the importance of exercise in boosting health. However, the first studies on its preventive mechanisms only date back to the second half of the 20th century.

I was lucky to train and work with one of the world's pre-eminent exercise physiologists, Professor John Holloszy, who made important contributions to sports science and the effects of training on numerous metabolic and hormonal pathways, and heart health.[19]

John told me that when he started working in this field in 1960, many scientists, including his mentor, the 1947 Nobel Prize winner Carl Cori (1896–1984), believed he was wasting his time. Exercise was thought to have nothing to do with health. But John was persistent in his endeavours, and during the 1970s and 1980s designed and conducted a long series of experiments to elucidate how exercise brings specific health benefits.

In the following chapters, I will clarify how different types of physical activity improve health and reduce the risk of developing chronic diseases. An understanding of cause and effect between physical events and biological adaptions is extremely important to maximise health benefits and reduce the hazards of pseudoscientific beliefs that are still surprisingly widespread in our culture – even among public school teachers, journalists and some health professionals. For example, one of these scientifically unsupported beliefs, as I will discuss later, is that exercising hard can compensate for the unhealthy food people consume every day. This is wrong: exercise cannot, and must not, be a substitute for a healthy diet!

CHAPTER TWELVE

BENEFICIAL EFFECTS OF AEROBIC EXERCISE

One of the ways to improve both our physical and psychological health is to train the cardio-respiratory system, our heart and lungs, by using a range of aerobic exercises.

Examples of aerobic exercises, or 'cardio' as it is often called, are brisk walking, jogging, running, cycling, skiing, skating, dancing, aerobics and swimming, but also team games with a ball and circuit training. Basically, all those that get our heart and sweat glands pumping.

Examples of aerobic activities to achieve exercise guideline recommendations:
Moderate-intensity aerobic activities you can do to achieve more than 150 minutes a week include:

- brisk walking
- cycling (less than 16 km/h)
- water aerobics
- tennis (doubles)
- volleyball
- ballroom dancing
- raking the yard.

Vigorous-intensity aerobic activities you can do to achieve more than 75 minutes a week include:

- uphill walking or race walking

- running or jogging

- cycling (at more than 16 km/h)

- tennis (singles)

- strenuous fitness class

- aerobic dancing

- heavy gardening (digging/hoeing).

During these rhythmic and repetitive activities involving primarily the large muscle groups of the lower limbs, the heart rate and breathing rate are increased for extended periods. This supplies the muscles with nutrients and oxygen to produce energy, so that the movement may continue. It is an astonishing mechanism!

Similar to how a car engine is powered by its cylinders, the mitochondria in our muscle cells act like combustion chambers. The fuel (consisting of carbohydrates and fats that are stored as glycogen in our muscles and liver, and triglycerides in fat cells) and oxygen that is extracted from our lungs interact to produce energy, which contracts the muscles and keeps us moving.

The faster the rate at which we move, the more oxygen and energy substrates that are required for combustion within the mitochondria. Therefore, the heart and the lungs must work faster to bring oxygen and nutrients to the muscles.

BURNING CALORIES WITH ENDURANCE EXERCISE

Amazingly, if we keep training regularly, both the *number* and *activity* of mitochondria within our muscles rise. So, there is an increase in the number of cylinders and therefore in the power produced.

This was one of the most notable discoveries of John Holloszy back in 1967.[1] Of course, a car with more cylinders will consume even more gasoline. And it is precisely for this reason that undertaking aerobic exercise for at least 30 minutes, three to five times a week, or better still every day, will help to burn more fat stored in our body that will be transformed into energy by the growing number of mitochondria.

A trained master athlete with a VO_2 max (a measurement for the maximum amount of oxygen a person can utilise during intense exercise) of 5 litres per minute is estimated to burn nearly 1100 calories during an hour of a moderate to intense workout. A sedentary person with a VO_2 max of 1.6 litres per minute in the same time will burn only 360 calories, less than one third (see figure 17).

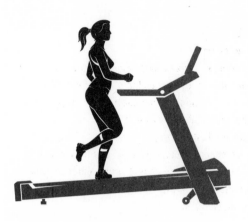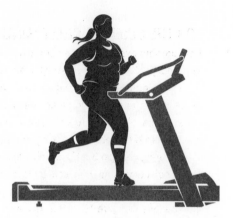

Athlete
VO$_2$max 5L/min
Can easily expend 18 kcal per minute
or 1080 kcal per hour

Sedentary
VO$_2$max 1.6L/min
Can *only* expend 6 kcal per minute
or 360 kcal per hour

Figure 17: Relationship between VO$_2$ max and energy consumption in elite athletes and sedentary individuals

However, for that same sedentary person, three months of regular moderate to intense aerobic exercise training typically increases VO$_2$ max by 15 to 25 per cent, and may improve by 50 per cent over a two-year period depending on one's initial fitness level. This indicates that the aerobic capacity of previously sedentary people improves rapidly and steadily. This improvement eventually levels off as we approach our 'genetically determined' maximum.

Even more extraordinary, after five to ten days of aerobic training there is a twofold rise in aerobic mitochondrial enzymes which coincides with increased mitochondrial capacity to generate energy, so that in just a few weeks the capacity of muscle mitochondria to *produce* the energy storage molecule adenosine triphosphate (ATP) can increase by 50 per cent.[2]

Even in elderly men and women, a program of moderate aerobic training induces a 20 per cent increase in the number and enzymatic activity of muscle mitochondria and therefore in the consumption of calories in just nine months.[3] This is awesome, because it means that aerobic exercise training makes us more efficient and our ability to burn calories greatly improves. If the VO$_2$ max increases from 1.6 to 2.6 litres per minutes, you burn 590 instead of 360 calories every hour of aerobic exercise training.

Simply put, you will be able to burn 1 kg (2 lb) of fat (which contains about 7,000 calories) in 12 days, instead of 20. Additionally, because of the increased enzymatic mitochondrial activity, you will withstand more aerobic exercise, with prolonged effort, without accumulating lactic acid. Lactic acidosis is responsible for the unpleasant sensation of muscle soreness and burning, rapid breathing, and eventually nausea and stomach pain, which is experienced with strenuous and prolonged exercise.

FOR THE SCIENTIFICALLY MINDED

How aerobic exercise lowers blood glucose levels

The biological mechanism through which aerobic exercise lowers blood glucose levels is twofold. First, the reduction of abdominal fat increases the circulating levels of the insulin sensitiser hormone adiponectin, and reduces inflammation and insulin resistance, which leads to an increase in the flow of glucose from the blood into cells, where it is used to produce energy or transformed into glycogen.[4-7]

Second, a single bout of aerobic exercise sharply increases a glucose transporter on the cell membrane of muscle cells (called GLUT4), which helps to pump glucose from the blood to the mitochondria for energy production, therefore reducing circulating glucose levels (Figure 18).[8,9] It is an amazing mechanism!

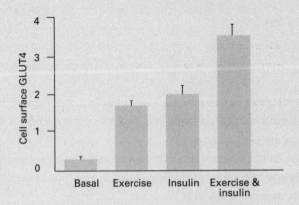

Figure 18: Increase in cell surface GLUT4 with exercise and insulin stimulation

Half an hour of moderate-intensity aerobic exercise is sufficient to increase the number of these transporters on muscle cells independent of the amount of exercise. It is as if more doors and windows were opened to get the supply of glucose into the cells. The good news is that moderate-intensity aerobic exercise increases insulin sensitivity more than vigorous-intensity aerobic exercise provided that total energy expenditure remains constant.

However, this effect is transient. After only 24 to 48 hours of inactivity, these doors and windows close (GLUT4 disappears within the cell) – even in highly trained athletes. This is why it is essential to exercise at least every other day, if we want to keep this valuable acute mechanism working at lowering blood glucose and insulin levels.[10]

Importantly, the lower blood insulin level also reduces the risk of cardiovascular disease and many common cancers.[11]

AEROBIC EXERCISE AND TYPE 2 DIABETES

The benefits of aerobic exercise training, however, are not restricted to burning calories and the control of body weight, but encompass the prevention of high blood glucose and type 2 diabetes as well.[12]

My group has repeatedly demonstrated that even in non-obese people aerobic exercise is the *most powerful* intervention to improve insulin sensitivity and glucose tolerance (the impairment of both are strong predictors of progression into type 2 diabetes). Aerobic exercise is even more potent than calorie restriction.[13,14]

Data from a large clinical trial show that walking for about 18 km (11 miles) per week, only 2.5 km (1.5 miles) each day, is very effective in improving oral glucose tolerance despite a relatively modest 2 kg (4.4 lb) reduction in body fat. The data suggest that walking 18 km (11 miles) per week may be virtually as effective as a more intensive multi-component intervention (diet- and exercise-induced weight loss) for preventing the progression to diabetes in individuals affected by prediabetes.[15]

Another clinical study published in the *New England Journal of Medicine* has shown that a combination of exercise training and diet can reduce the risk of developing type 2 diabetes by a whopping 58 per cent, compared with a 31 per cent decline in diabetic patients receiving the drug metformin.[16] Data from a randomised clinical trial indicate that diabetic patients exercising five to six times per week were able to eliminate glucose-lowering medications in 56.3 per cent of cases compared with just 14.7 per cent of the control sedentary group.[17]

ENDURANCE-EXERCISE TRAINING IMPROVES CARDIOVASCULAR HEALTH

Besides the positive effects of walking, running or swimming on blood glucose and insulin levels, these exercises also have beneficial effects on other cardiovascular risk factors.[18-19] For instance, endurance-exercise training, when combined with weight loss, increases plasma levels of the good cholesterol (HDL-cholesterol) and reduces triglyceride levels.[20,21]

Regular endurance training also decreases systolic and diastolic blood pressure, both during rest and submaximal physical activity.[22] The largest reduction occurs in systolic blood pressure, especially in patients with hypertension.[23]

Aerobic exercise also improves how we process glucose,[24] contributes to a reduction in body weight and inflammatory markers,[25] and has a beneficial effects on cardiovascular health, including improved arterial function and parasympathetic tone.[26-28] Not surprisingly, the odds of having a heart attack or a stroke are lower in people who do regular aerobic physical exercise.[29]

TIP: Accumulating data suggest that exercise intensity is more important than quantity in increasing the ability of HDL-cholesterol to move cholesterol from the artery to the blood. As I will explain later, an increased capacity of HDL particles to remove cholesterol from arteries (called reverse cholesterol transport) is associated with a much lower risk of heart disease, independent of the blood level of HDL-cholesterol.[30]

AEROBIC EXERCISE HELPS TO REDUCE CANCER RISK

Epidemiological studies suggest that aerobic exercise training is associated with a reduced risk of developing at least 13 different cancer types, but in particular breast, colon and endometrial.[31,32]

It can even help in improving the prognosis after being treated for breast, colon and prostate cancer.[33-35] People who had tumours of the colon or breast, and exercise regularly, die less of recurrences or metastasis.[36] Breast cancer studies suggest that 30–40 minutes per day of brisk walking can reduce mortality by 50 per cent.[37,38]

The mechanisms are complex and not yet entirely clear, but it seems that the reduction of abdominal fat and insulin levels play a key role. As previously discussed, an excessive accumulation of fat in the belly causes insulin resistance. Insulin inhibits the liver production of certain proteins, which normally bind to growth factors and hormones (e.g. IGF-1, testosterone, oestradiol), increasing their bioavailability and function.[39-41]

Obesity in women contributes to higher levels of oestrogens also because of the increased activity of an enzyme called aromatase that converts testosterone into oestradiol. This may explain why some women with premenopausal and postmenopausal breast cancer respond differently.[42]

As our knowledge of the mechanisms linking nutrition, exercise and cancer biology improves, we should be able to move from a one-size-fits-all approach to prescribing specific modes, amounts and intensity of exercise in combination with targeted nutritional manipulations. The individualised prescription will depend on the type of cancer and genetic and metabolic background of the individual.

CURIOSITY: BREATHING BEACH AIR MAY BENEFIT LUNG CANCER PATIENTS

Surprisingly where we exercise might have additional beneficial effects. Walking or running on a beach, for example, seems to be the best. It has been shown that sea spray air contains a range of microbiota and biogenic molecules that in human lung cancer cells inhibits some key gene pathways, potentially inducing the death of cancer cells.[43]

EXERCISE TRAINING PROTECTS MEMORY AND PREVENTS BRAIN FOG

Exercise training has profound effects on brain health, helping protect memory, enhance attention, thinking skills and the ability to process information both in young and older adults.[44]

The deterioration of brain structure is typical of ageing, but performing high levels of exercise seems to attenuate the age-dependent degeneration of grey and white matter in the prefrontal and temporal cortex, areas that regulate working memory and executive functions.[45] Data from a randomised controlled trial have shown that one year of aerobic exercise training can even *increase* the volume of the hippocampus (an area of the brain involved in memory consolidation), leading to improvements in spatial memory, a form of memory responsible for the recording of information about one's environment and spatial orientation.[46] In other words, exercise training powerfully *counteracts* the brain fog that comes with age and helps prevent cognitive decline.

Practising regular aerobic exercise has also been shown to reduce mental stress, anxiety and neuroticism, ameliorate symptoms of depression, and improve mood, self-esteem and self-concept. In particular, there is one factor called brain-derived neurotrophic factor (BDNF) that seems to be responsible for some of these beneficial effects. This exercised-induced hormone is as powerful as some antidepressant drugs in protecting against depression, but without side-effects.[47-49]

CHAPTER THIRTEEN

STARTING OR IMPROVING AEROBIC-EXERCISE TRAINING

Several factors affect our endurance-training response, including the initial level of aerobic fitness, the training intensity, its frequency and duration.

The good news for those who are sedentary is that the degree of improvement is much higher in someone who has a low VO_2 max prior to starting the exercise program than in individuals with high aerobic capacity.

For instance, it has been shown that sedentary people affected by heart disease can increase their VO_2 max up to 50 per cent, whereas training in normally active, healthy men improves VO_2 max only by 10–15 per cent.[1]

For people who have been inactive for a long time, I suggest a two-step approach. At the beginning, start by breaking up prolonged sitting with short sessions of light-intensity physical activity – for example, by doing some housework or by working at a standing workstation or walking around for a while. Climbing just 70 flights of stairs a week (ten per day) seems to lower average mortality risk by 16 per cent.[2] As a second step, as you get fitter, reallocate the time you employ in light-intensity physical activity to time spent in purposeful moderate- to vigorous-intensity exercise (e.g. sustained walking, jogging, biking, swimming).

TRAINING INTENSITY

A key factor that impacts our body's physiologic response to endurance exercise training is the *intensity of overload*, or in other words, how hard we work to perform the activity.

Percentage maximal heart rate	Percentage VO$_2$ max
50	28
60	40
70	58
80	70
90	83
100	100

Table 17: Relationship between percentage maximal heart rate and percentage VO$_2$ max

The VO$_2$ max test is the gold standard to establishing training intensity, but its use is impractical, time-consuming and expensive for everyday use. A useful substitute is monitoring our heart rate during exercise. In fact, maximal heart rate (max HR) and VO$_2$max are correlated in a predictable manner independent of age, sex, race, fitness level or training mode as shown in table 17.[3]

Note that there is roughly an 8 per cent error when we estimate the percentage of VO$_2$ max from the percentage of max HR. The relationship between the percentage of max HR and VO$_2$ max is about the same for arm or leg activities among healthy subjects of normal weight as well as obese people and patients affected by heart disease. However, exercises that use predominantly the arms result in lower max HR than exercises that use the legs.

How do you calculate your maximal heart rate?

To quickly calculate your maximal heart rate, subtract your age from 220. For example, if you are 50 years old, subtract 50 from 220 to get a maximal heart rate of 170.

A more accurate formula to estimate maximal heart rate is the following:[4]

$$\text{max HR} = 206.9 - (0.67 \times \text{age, years})$$

For example, for someone who is 50 years old: 206.9 – (0.67 x 50) = 173.4 max HR.

For obese men and women with body fat above 30 per cent, a modified formula applies:[5]

$$\text{max HR} = 200 - (0.5 \times \text{age, years})$$

In this example for an obese person who is 50 years old: 200 – (0.5 x 50) = 175 max HR.

As shown in figure 19, in general for most healthy men and women, it is sufficient to exercise at a heart rate of between 55–70 per cent of maximum (i.e. a 50-year-old man or woman should maintain a training heart rate of between 100–126 beats per minute), which allows them to talk while exercising. To achieve positive endurance-exercise training outcomes, it is not necessary to exercise so strenuously that it causes discomfort like abnormally rapid breathing and soreness (caused by lactic acid).

These easy and simple formulas, however, are not the ultimate test to figure out your heart-rate training zone, because they consider only your age. A more sophisticated fitness indicator is the Karvonen method, which was devised by a Scandinavian physiologist. This is a mathematical formula that helps you to better determine your target heart rate, because it takes into account not only your age but your resting heart rate as well. The formula suggests you should train at a heart rate equivalent to 60 per cent of the difference between resting and maximum heart rate.[6]

The Karvonen formula to calculate training heart rate is the following:[7,8]

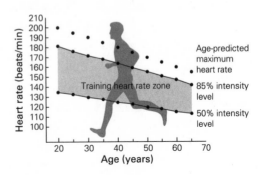

Figure 19: Heart rate zone training

$$HR_{threshold} = HR_{rest} + 0.60 \, (HR_{max} - HR_{rest})$$

For example, if you are 50 years old and your resting heart rate is 60, according to the Karvonen formula your ideal heart rate during exercise training should be 128 beats per minute: (60 + 0.60(173.4 − 60).

RESTING HEART RATE

You first need to measure your resting heart rate (just after you wake and are still in bed). The normal resting heart rate for adults ranges between 40 and 100 beats per minute. In healthy people, a lower heart rate at rest implies more efficient heart function and better fitness. For example, a well-trained athlete might have a resting heart rate close to 40 beats per minute.

How do you measure your actual heart rate?

Place your index and middle fingers together on your wrist, just inside the joint and in line with your index finger. Once you find your pulse, count the number of beats for a minute or over 15 seconds and multiply by four. A heart rate monitor can be used to get a more accurate measurement, and various apps can also measure heart rate.

As your aerobic fitness increases, though, your submaximal heart rate declines by approximately 10–20 beats per minute at any given level of oxygen consumption. Therefore, as you become fitter, it is necessary to periodically increase the intensity level to achieve the desired training heart rate.

For instance, if you are sedentary, you should start training gently just by simply walking. As your aerobic fitness improves, to maintain the same relative exercise intensity, you should start to walk briskly, and when this activity becomes comfortable, you should intermittently incorporate some jogging during your walking sessions.

As you get fitter, in order to achieve your targeted heart rate, it will be necessary to jog or run continuously. Once you have attained this level of fitness, 20 to 30 minutes of continuous activity at 70 per cent max HR should suffice to stimulate an adequate training effect in most healthy people.

> TIP: Not all types of exercise are the same: at maximum heart rate, for instance, running burns 21 per cent more fat than cycling.[9] But, if we maintain constant exercise intensity, duration, and frequency, the training response of different type of exercises that involves large muscle groups is more or less the same. Running, cycling, rowing, swimming, skating, rope skipping, bench-stepping and stair climbing all provide excellent 'overload' for the aerobic system.[10-12]

TRAINING DURATION AND VOLUME

In general, longer exercise duration can be exchanged for lower exercise intensity. For example, we can jog or run at 60 per cent max HR for 45 minutes, instead of exercising at 70 per cent max HR for 20–30 minutes. This has been shown to achieve similar aerobic improvements.

But a limit exists, beyond which increasing the duration and volume of exercise we perform does not translate into greater aerobic improvements and may even cause detrimental effects. For instance, in one test in young swimmers it was found that training for three hours instead of one and a half hours per day did not result in any significant improvement in swimming power, endurance or performance time.[13] Other studies have shown that both running long distances each week and training at high intensity are associated with an increased risk of injury to muscles, bones and knee cartilage.[14,15]

A study in Copenhagen that followed 1000 joggers aged 20 to 80 for 12 years, showed that less than 60 to 140 minutes per week of light jogging is necessary to reduce mortality. Increasing the workout to between two and a half to four hours per week did not cause a further decrease in mortality. Indeed, those who were performing high intensity jogging for prolonged periods were as likely to die prematurely as sedentary people.[16] Similarly, a study by the Cooper Institute showed that intense training for seven minutes a day is sufficient to decrease the risk of cardiovascular mortality, and that higher levels are not associated with additional benefits.[17]

TRAINING FREQUENCY

Data from multiple studies suggest that training frequency (how often we exercise) is not as important as training intensity or duration for improving aerobic capacity

(VO$_2$ max). Exercising two or four days a week, if the duration and the intensity remain constant for each training session, seems not to be associated with significant differences in VO$_2$ max.[18,19]

However, improving aerobic capacity may involve different training requirements than maintaining it. In one study of 12 young men, a ten-week exercise program consisting of running for 40 minutes, six days a week and interval training by cycling, increased VO$_2$ max by 25 per cent. However, during the 15-week maintenance program, those who were randomised to exercise two days per week maintained their gains in VO$_2$ max just as much as those who exercised four times a week, despite up to two-thirds reduction in training frequency.[20]

Similar results have been shown for training duration on maintenance of improved aerobic fitness.[21] Using the same protocol, reducing training duration from the original 40-minute sessions to either 26 or 13 minutes per day caused a similar maintenance of VO$_2$ max, despite a two-thirds reduction in training duration. Nevertheless, if the training intensity *decreased* at the same time, it significantly reduced aerobic capacity, indicating that intensity plays a key role in maintaining aerobic capacity.[22]

In terms of heart health, some studies suggest that training frequency has beneficial effects, while others suggest how many times we exercise per week contributes considerably less than either intensity or duration of effort.[23] However, if we decide to train at a lower intensity, then to retain the beneficial effects it is essential to increase the frequency that we train from: two days to five days a week. This is especially necessary for increasing energy expenditure and improving insulin sensitivity. Training only one or two days a week generally does not result in any significant change in energy balance and body weight or belly fat.[24]

HIGH-INTENSITY INTERVAL TRAINING: HOW AND WHEN?

To achieve significant weight loss and maintain good health through endurance exercise, we need to complete multiple sessions of aerobic exercise every week. For example, we should exercise three or four days a week with a single rest day separating workout days. Each session should last at least 60 minutes and the exercises should be performed at sufficient intensity to expend 300 calories or more.

If we need to train for no less than one hour (90 minutes if we walk slowly), three or

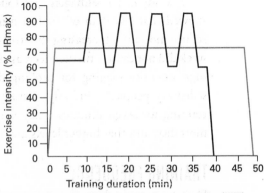

Figure 20: Example of high-intensity interval training (HIIT) versus moderate-intensity continuous training (MICT) protocol.[25]

four days a week, it can be challenging to make time for all this exercise. It's easier for retired people to find the time, but for those who work, it can be a real issue to find 45 to 90 minutes every day or even every other day.

A great way to get around this problem is to incorporate two sessions of high-intensity interval training (HIIT) into our weekly routine. With this method of training we alternate short periods (e.g. four minutes) of high intensity work at more than 80 per cent of maximum heart rate with recovery periods of three minutes at low intensity (see figure 20).

Another more intense version is sprint interval training. For instance, for 60 seconds, run, cycle or swim as fast as possible, then walk, cycle or swim very slowly for four minutes. At the beginning, repeat this four times, and then as fitness improves, increase to five or six repeats, which means a training session is only about 20 to 30 minutes.

The remarkable thing is that HIIT and sprint interval training seem to produce greater or comparable metabolic benefits as do long sessions (45 to 90 minutes) of low- to moderate-intensity continuous aerobic exercise. Performing HIIT only two days per week improves cardiorespiratory fitness (VO_2 max) to a similar extent to training five days a week.[26,27]

Some studies even suggest that HIIT is more powerful than moderate-intensity, continuous endurance exercise in improving cardiorespiratory fitness, especially in those people with 'low trainability' (i.e. people who see smaller improvements, or have these improvements take longer to occur).[28]

Performing 10–15 minutes of HIIT or sprint interval training two or three times per week can also help us to lose weight or maintain our ideal body weight, because we keep burning fat even after finishing training for at least 24 hours beyond the end of the exercise session.[29]

The potential beneficial effects of HIIT are not limited to cardiorespiratory fitness but are extended to heart health as well. HIIT programs seem to improve insulin sensitivity, blood pressure and heart function to a greater or comparable extent to moderate-intensity, continuous endurance exercise.[30-32]

In a clinical trial of diabetic patients, six sessions of high-intensity interval training for two weeks were sufficient to reduce blood glucose levels and blood pressure.[33] These beneficial effects seem to be linked to the increased number of mitochondria and glucose transporters GLUT4 (see page 153), which doubled in the muscle after a short session of high-intensity interval training.[34]

Depending on how well the program has been designed, HIIT has been reported to result in higher levels of enjoyment than long sessions of moderate-intensity training.[35]

TIP. A few minutes of intense bouts of stair climbing, at short intervals throughout the day, can enhance your cardio-respiratory fitness as much as sprint interval training by cycling. In one small clinical study, VO$_2$max increased by 12 per cent in sedentary volunteers who performed a 3 × 20-second stair climbing protocol (i.e. vigorously climbing stairs for only 20 seconds, three times per day) for three days a week for six weeks.[36] Therefore, in the morning, at lunch, and during your coffee or bathroom break, it is a good idea to climb as fast as possible a three-flight stairwell, knowing that this will deliver an effective workout. No need to find time to go to the gym, everybody can improve their fitness, wherever they are, and at any time.

USE IT, OR LOSE IT

Data from multiple studies have shown that when people stop exercising, they lose the positive benefits of metabolic, physiologic and performance capacity very quickly. This phenomenon is called *detraining*. Seven to 14 days of detraining is sufficient to significantly decrease both metabolic and fitness health benefits.

For instance, 20 consecutive days of bed rest results in a 25 per cent reduction in VO$_2$max and cardiac output. Maximum aerobic power declines on average 1 per cent every day. Within a few months, you fully lose several of the benefits of endurance training. For elderly people, for example, four months of detraining can completely abolish their exercise-induced cardiovascular improvements.

Even among highly trained professional athletes, the beneficial effects of training can be transitory and reversible. This is why athletes must undertake an exercise program several months prior to the beginning of the competitive season and keep exercising at a moderate level even during off-season. But what is most important is that just ten days of detraining in elite athletes causes a significant worsening of glucose tolerance and a major increase in insulin levels in response to a glucose load (see figure 21).[37] This is bad

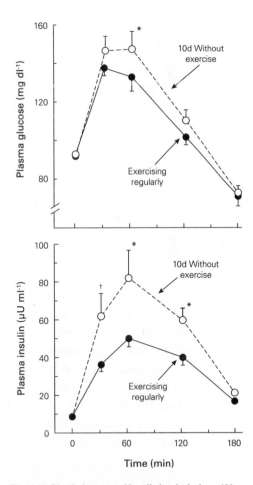

Figure 21: Blood glucose and insulin levels during a 100-g oral glucose tolerance test in 14 master athletes 16-18 hours after a usual training session when they were exercising regularly and after no exercise for ten days.[38]

because, as I have already explained, high blood insulin is a key factor implicated in pathogenesis of cancer and accelerated ageing.

HOW MUCH EXERCISE IS TOO MUCH?

Having a passion for something undeniably good sometimes defeats its own purpose when it is taken to extremes. It can lead to injury rather than good health. Some people overdo how much they exercise.

A recent meta-analysis of the results of six studies suggests that mortality risk declines progressively with increasing physical activity, up to a maximum of one to two hours per day of moderate exercise training, with no additional benefits for longer durations or higher intensity levels.[39] In contrast, multiple studies have shown potentially adverse health outcomes in people who are overtraining, especially marathon runners, triathletes, cross-country skiers and cyclists.[40,41]

Excessive exercise is associated with heart problems, including exercise-induced elevations in cardiac troponin levels;[42] post-exercise cardiac dysfunction;[43] accelerated coronary artery calcifications;[44] and evidence of cardiac fibrosis and patchy lesions of the heart.[45] It also increases the incidence of dangerous irregular heart rhythm problems (arrhythmias), including atrial fibrillation.[46-49] In particular, myocardial fibrosis, which may increase the risk of fatal arrhythmia, has been detected in 12 to 50 per cent of endurance athletes. The number of years of training, the number of hours performing high-intensity exercise and the number of completed marathons correlated with the degree of fibrosis of the heart.[50,51]

In the studies that we have conducted on master athletes in my laboratory at Washington University in collaboration with John Holloszy, we noted that during the VO_2 max test, many of the older master athletes, who have been running an average of 50 to 80 km a week for many years, experienced abnormally elevated blood pressure and dangerous arrhythmias. Moreover, many complained of joint pain and knee problems, and some of the older athletes had had their knee or hip replaced because of degeneration.

Most likely, a U-shaped relationship exists between physical activity and health, with sedentary lifestyle at one end of the U-curve and large volumes of high-intensity endurance exercise at the other, both of which increase cardiac damage.

Based on the available information, healthy people performing low- to moderate-intensity (heart rate between 55–70 per cent of the maximum) aerobic exercise experience the lowest risk and a higher metabolic benefit.

Simply put, we can walk, cycling at low speed or dance for as long as we want. However, most likely the health benefits are already maximised when we reach 100 minutes per day of leisure-time activity.

For daily strenuous activities (more than 80 per cent of the maximum heart rate), I believe that it is unsafe to perform large volumes of strenuous endurance-exercise training for longer periods of time on a regular basis.[52,53] Studies have shown that small doses of five to ten minutes a day of high-intensity exercise are generally sufficient, and further extending the high-intensity workout does not induce additional benefits, and in some people may cause irreversible health damage.

Preliminary data from my laboratory suggest that nutrition may influence the metabolic and cardiovascular response to vigorous exercise training. It would be important to conduct well-performed clinical studies to elucidate the role of calorie and protein intake, and diet quality, in modulating inflammatory and pro-ageing pathways during intense and prolonged exercise training.

It will also be key to establish the potential protective effects of nutrient-dense and balanced diets against the harmful acute and chronic effects of vigorous exercise training. Studies comparing athletes who are omnivores with vegetarian or vegan athletes found no difference in fitness, but we do not know if there are long-term health differences.[54,55]

CHAPTER FOURTEEN

FORTIFYING MUSCLES AND BONES: THE SCIENCE OF STRENGTH TRAINING

As we age it's normal to lose muscle mass, and consequently muscle strength.[1]

The problem is that muscle mass and strength are important for bone health and our ability to perform a range of daily activities, like climbing stairs, carrying shopping bags, lifting or pushing heavy objects. If over the years, we lose too much muscle mass, we are in danger of becoming frail and dependent on others to assist us, even with simple everyday activities like walking, dressing and bathing.

A sedentary lifestyle is a powerful risk factor for muscle and bone loss. Whenever we are forced to spend long periods in bed because of illness or when we break a bone and have to wear a cast for weeks, we lose a considerable amount of muscle and bone mass. Fortunately, it has been shown that physical activity in general, but most specifically muscle-strengthening exercises, can help us to counteract the loss of bone and muscle mass and strength.[2-4]

Moreover, in experimental models, both aerobic and resistance exercise training in old animals has been shown to be instrumental for muscle repair in response to trauma or muscle damage. Basically, exercise training powerfully activates stem cells within the wounded muscle, leading to regeneration of the damaged tissue.

Examples of muscle-strengthening activities are sprints, 100-metre (or 100-yard) running and jumping, all activities characterised by intense but brief efforts (a few seconds). However, among the best-known muscle-strengthening activities is weight-lifting, which in its extreme version is called bodybuilding. With resistance training the body's muscles are forced to work or hold against an applied force or weight (resistance exercise). You don't have to go to a gym or have a personal trainer to do resistance training. You can easily do this at home or in the office with some small weights, elastic bands or simply using your own body weight for resistance (for example, push-ups).

Weight-training improves strength and muscle power by both increasing muscle mass and training muscle fibres to contract simultaneously and in a coordinated way.[5]

The beneficial effects of weight-training can be instrumental in weight loss, because it increases resting metabolic rate,[6,7] which can enhance the fat-burning effects of aerobic exercise.[8] For instance, in a six-month randomised clinical trial of previously sedentary overweight and obese adolescents, a combination of endurance and resistance exercise training resulted in a significantly greater reduction in waist circumference than endurance exercise alone.[9] This successful exercise program consisted of four sessions per week; in each session, participants gradually increased from 20 to 45 minutes of aerobic exercise on treadmills, cross-training machines or exercise bikes with a progressive rise of intensity (from 65 to 85 per cent of maximum heart rate). Resistance-training consisted of seven exercises using weight machines or free weights, progressing from two sets of 15 repetitions at moderate intensity to three sets of eight repetitions at maximum resistance.

Resistance exercise is also very important for preventing osteoporosis (bone loss typical of ageing) and enhancing bone strength. The muscles are attached to bones by tendons. When we contract them, we create an immense force that concentrates on the bone's structure. For example, when we balance on one foot, the muscles contract and are estimated to generate a force equal to 2.75 times the weight of the person (see figure 22). For an individual weighing 70 kg (154 lb) that means 192 kg (423 lb) concentrated on the femur (thighbone). It has been calculated that standing on one foot for one minute generates the same amount of workload that we can get walking for about 53 minutes.[10] This translates into a powerful bone growth stimulation and applies to all the muscle groups.

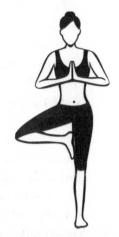

Muscle- and bone-strengthening exercises can be performed using weights or our own body weight in a range of movements and positions, including those practised during yoga or tai chi. Training with small weights is also indicated in elderly and frail individuals. These exercises, by strengthening the muscles of the legs as well as those of the shoulders, arms and back, can substantially decrease the likelihood of their falling and being hospitalised in nursing homes.[11]

Figure 22: Balancing on one foot for improving bone strength and balance.

INTENSITY, FREQUENCY REPETITIONS AND REST PERIODS

Usually, a well-designed weight-training workout program should allow you to gradually increase:

- intensity, i.e. how much weight or force you can lift or generate
- repetitions, i.e. how many times you lift a weight or do a push-up
- sets, i.e. the number of cycles of repetitions that you are able to complete.

Ideally, you should train two or three times per week, with a variety of exercises that stimulate all the major muscle groups (abdomen, chest, back, shoulders, arms, hips and legs). Because muscular strength and mitochondrial function (see page 151) peak in late afternoon,[12,13] when possible, it's a good idea to do these muscle-strengthening activities later during the day.

When starting out it's better to learn how to use your own body weight as a tool of resistance. Mastering key bodyweight exercises will improve strength, stability, mobility and motor control of all the major muscle groups. As you progress and gain strength, you can start using free weights, and if you want to go to a gym you can use other more sophisticated machines to continue challenging your muscles and increase your strength and resistance.

If the primary goal is to increase muscle mass, then it is better to use heavier weights, but with a lower number of repetitions. But if the goal is to tone up muscles and increase the control and coordination of muscles, then, use lighter weights, but with many repetitions. For instance, young and healthy people, who want to gain muscle mass, can repeat a single movement from six to eight times per muscle group, at 60 to 80 per cent of one-repetition maximum, for three or more sets. 'One-repetiton max' is the term for the most weight that an individual can possibly lift for one repetition. For those who are only interested in health and endurance, it is advisable to reduce the load at 40 to 60 per cent of one-repetition maximum, and perform one to three sets of 12 to 16 repetitions (this is appropriate for the elderly too). For burning fat, do one to three sets of 10 to 12 repetitions using enough weight so that you can just complete the repetitions. The ideal rest period between two sets is 45 seconds to two minutes.

While lifting weights (including using your body as a weight) it is essential to exhale as you lift to prevent an excessive and dangerous rise in blood pressure. It is also recommended that you do the exercises slowly and carefully, checking the movement both during concentric (weight-lifting), when you exhale, and eccentric (lowering of the weight), when you inhale. In particular, it is essential to check your posture. Poor posture may result in serious damage to your muscles, spine and joints. It is also important to rest for 48 hours between sessions to allow your muscles to recover, grow and strengthen.

MAKE A START WITH 15 MINUTES OF A BODY STRENGTH TRAINING PROGRAM AT HOME

No matter how old or fit you are, everybody should perform some strength-training exercises, ideally three to four times a week for maximum benefits. We don't need to spend hours at the gym to see results, it takes only 15 minutes to complete a full-body strength-building workout. It can be done at home, in the park or at an outdoor calisthenics gym, where there are pull-up bars, low bars, an abs bench or double parallel bars. Some of these exercises can be done even in an office, as a break from our screens. Here are some examples of exercises that I do regularly.

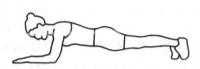

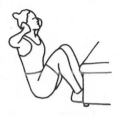

Plank
Support your body with your forearms and toes. Hold yourself flat, squeeze your gluts to stabilise your body. Hold for 20 seconds. Don't hold your breath. As you get better at this extend the time you hold the position.

Bent knee sit up
Lie on the floor with your knees bent and your feet tucked under a heavy piece of furniture. Clasp your hands behind your head and slowly exhale as you gently raise your body. Pause and while you inhale lower your body. Repeat.

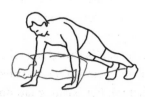

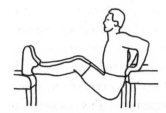

Push-up
Support your body with your arms stretched out straight, in line with your shoulders, and feet close together supported on your toes. As you inhale lower your body to nearly touch the floor. Exhale as you push up from the ground until your arms lock. Repeat.

Bench dip
Place the palms of your hands on a large chair, fingers forward and legs out straight on another chair. As you inhale slowly lower your body to give it a stretch, only until your forearms are level with the chair. Exhale as you push your body back to the starting position. Repeat.

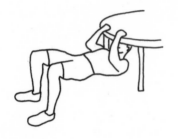
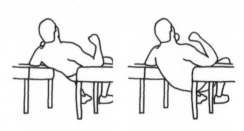

Pull-ups
Lie on your back under a coffee table. Place your feet flat on the floor, knees bent. Hold the table with an underhand grip. Exhale as you use your arms to pull yourself up off the floor. Inhale as you lower yourself to the starting position. Repeat.

Shrug
Position your body between two chairs with your feet on the floor and the back of your arms resting on the chairs. While exhaling squeeze your shoulder blades together raising your chest. As you inhale slowly lower yourself to the starting position. Repeat.

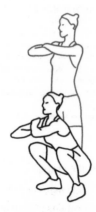
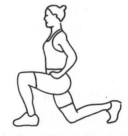

Squat
Place your feet shoulder width apart. Focus on keeping a straight back and not pitching forward during the squat. Bending at the hip and knees lower into a squat, keeping your weight on your heels. As you inhale go as low as possible, then rise to the starting position. Repeat.

Lunge
Stand with your feet in line with your hips. Take a step forward with your right leg. Lower your body until your right thigh is aligned with the floor. Press into your right heel to drive yourself back to the starting position. Repeat for left leg.

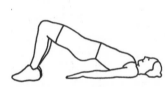

Bridge
Lie on your back with your palms facing down and knees bent at 90 degrees. Raise your hips while you slowly exhale. Hold the bridge for a moment than inhale as you lower to the starting position. Repeat.

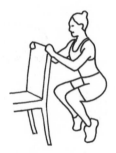

Calf squat
Holding the back of a chair, stand with your weight on your toes and inhale as you lower to a squat position with knees bent 90 degrees. Then lower your body at the ankle to feel a good stretch. Exhale as you raise your body onto your toes and hold for one second. Repeat.

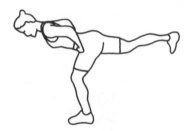

Leg lift
Stand with both feet shoulder width apart. While you are exhaling, lift your right leg up behind you. Making sure the rear leg stays in line with your torso, bend over at the waist while shifting your weight back and looking down. Keep your chest up. Keeping a strong low-back arch, descend until your hamstring range of motion runs out. As you inhale, reverse the motion back to the starting position. Repeat for left leg.

EXERCISE IS NOT A SUBSTITUTE FOR HEALTHY EATING

There is a gym culture that suggests physical exercise and muscle mass building are a panacea for all ailments. Food is just a source of energy and proteins to feed hungry muscles. The mantra is eat plenty of protein for strong muscles and carbohydrates for energy. There are all sorts of formulas: up to 2 g of protein (such as whey protein) for each kilogram (1 g per pound) of body weight, and 1 to 1.5 g of carbohydrates per kilogram (½ to ¾ g per pound) of body weight soon after exercising. Each personal trainer has their own recipe. This obsession with building big muscles is leading some fitness fanatics to consume massive amounts of proteins from eggs, meat and dairy products for breakfast, lunch and dinner in addition to all sorts of protein supplements.

According to this simplistic vision, all this food will ultimately be burned to produce energy or muscle growth. However, the ability to convert dietary protein into muscle during resistance exercise is limited. Well-conducted clinical studies have clearly shown that postprandial muscle protein synthesis is maximised when we consume approximately 30 g of dietary protein with every meal. Quantity depends on age and body weight: young people aged 18–37 years require 0.25 g for every kg of body weight (18 g per pound), while people older than 55 years need 0.40 g/kg (28 g per pound) with every meal.[14] Protein consumed in excess of this amount will not be incorporated in the muscle, but oxidised.[15] Preliminary data suggest that the protein excess stimulates the IGF/mTOR pathway, which in turn can promote cancer and ageing.[16]

Remember: our body is not a furnace. The quality of the food we eat provides the bricks that help to build and maintain all our cells, our organs, including our brain, heart and muscles. We cannot build a racing car with poor quality materials and hope that the car will withstand the stress of time.

In some yet to be published studies that I have conducted with John Holloszy at Washington University, indications show people who do vigorous exercise and eat a diet that resembles the modern healthy longevity diet (see Chapter 9) have a much better cardiometabolic profile than those who train but follow the usual Western diet.

A growing body of scientific studies also indicates that the quality and quantity of food we consume deeply influences the metabolic response to exercise. For example, data from a small but well-designed, randomised clinical trial indicate that a diet rich in high-glycaemic foods suppresses the beneficial effects of endurance exercise on glucose effectiveness through increased concentration of blood free fatty acids.[17] Glucose effectiveness is the ability of glucose per se to stimulate its own uptake into the skeletal muscle and to suppress its own liver production; this is a powerful marker of progression into type 2 diabetes. A high-glycaemic index diet also prevents the exercise-induced increase in fat oxidation and utilisation regardless of energy expenditure.[18]

In contrast, individuals eating a low-glycaemic index diet during exercise training experienced higher cardio-respiratory fitness (VO_2 max), lower blood pressure and lower insulin and improved fat utilisation during exercise. Some of these beneficial adaptations took place as early as seven days after the beginning of the exercise training.[19] These and other data indicate that dietary carbohydrate quality during exercise training must be carefully considered to improve metabolic outcomes.

A growing body of data even suggests that amino acid supplementation may cause adverse health effects. High doses of branched-chain and sulphur amino acids stimulate signalling pathways that are known to induce insulin resistance, accelerate the ageing process and promote cancer (see page 69 high protein diets promote disease and ageing).[20,21] Moreover, L-carnitine, a supplement taken by some athletes, increases the blood concentration of TMAO (see page 90) that might increase the risk of developing a heart attack or a stroke, independent of other classic cardiovascular risk factors.[22]

CHAPTER FIFTEEN

POSTURE, BALANCE AND FLEXIBILITY: THE ESSENTIAL EXERCISES

Posture, balance and joint flexibility are often overlooked when people talk about exercise programs, yet the health effects of poor posture, lack of balance, joint misalignment and stiffness affect many aspects of our daily life and contribute to a great deal of disease and disability.

PAIN AND JOINT DEGENERATION

One of the first complications of poor posture is neck pain, as well as shoulder and back pain. If we have poor posture, it will over time create stress and pressure on our muscles and joints, which eventually will trigger inflammation and chronic pain. Continuous stress of the joints will result in painful degradation of the tissues surrounding them, including degenerated cartilages, herniated discs and aggravated nerves.

For instance, if we have rounded shoulders (often caused by sitting at a desk all day), the curvature of our neck is affected. To be able to look straight ahead we are forced to hyperextend our neck and contract the muscles of the cervical spine (neck region) and shoulders. If this muscle contraction persists over time, chronic neck pain can result into muscle-tension headache, sometimes accompanied by nausea, dizziness and tingling in the hands. These are the same symptoms that we would experience after whiplash in a road accident.

Also a curvature of the spine (scoliosis), a flattening of the lower back (flat back syndrome) or an excessive curvature (hyperlordosis) from bad posture may cause a decrease in the movement of the diaphragm, lumbago (lower back pain), damage to the spine and intervertebral discs, and in extreme cases disk hernias with compression of the nerve roots and sciatica. Changes in the position of the hips and joint misalignment can also affect the knees and hamstrings. Over time, these abnormal postures cause structural damage, skeletal muscle strength deterioration and inflammation, which transform acute lumbago into chronic low back pain.

Chronic low back pain is a debilitating and serious medical condition. An estimated 12 to 15 per cent of all annual healthcare visits are due to low back pain.[1] The direct medical cost of low back pain in the US alone is estimated at around US$85 billion, which increases to between $100 and $200 billion if we take into consideration lost productivity.[2]

> NOTE: Being overweight and obese are major contributors to the development of chronic lower back pain and other mobility impairments, leading ultimately to physical disability.[3]

WHY GOOD POSTURE IS VITAL

When we sit in a fixed position for long periods of times, many bad things happen, including a flat back (reduced physiological lordosis), a hunchback (increased thoracic kyphosis) and a reduced spectrum of movements of the hips and knees.[4] What follows are some other problems you may experience.

Restricted breathing

A main complication of poor posture is restricted breathing. When the muscles of your back weaken and the shoulders bend forward, inevitably the movement of the ribcage and the ability to breathe is deeply compromised. Breathing becomes shallow and frequent and this has serious consequences for your metabolic, cardiovascular and psychological health.

These alterations increase the risk of developing abnormal respiratory function (bad ventilation and oxygenation of the lungs) and reduced thoracic pump efficiency, which cause problems of stagnation of the blood and lymph in the lower part of the body. Additionally people who for reasons of work or due to idleness, weakness or disease remain in static positions for long periods tend to have a higher risk of disk degeneration. This is because maintaining healthy discs in our backs depend on us changing our posture often. The nourishment of intervertebral discs relies on a sponge or pump mechanism (i.e. through pressure fluctuations with change of posture).

It's clear, therefore, why it is important for our health to maintain good posture and to change it as much as possible.

Increasing risk of bone fractures

Posture also affects your balance, and therefore the risk of falling and fracturing your bones. More than 90 per cent of hip fractures, which are associated with a 30 per cent increased mortality in one year, are the result of a fall due to a lack of balance.[5]

Poorer quality of life

Chronic and persistent neck, back, hip or knee pain can heavily influence your quality of life. Suffering pain limits your ability to move and has serious psychological consequences as well.

If we think about it, posture says a lot about a person's way of being in the world. Dr Daniel Raggi says:

> *Posture is the expression of our personal experience, of our education and cultural background, of the memory of our physical and emotional trauma, of our lifestyle and our stress level, of the nature of our work to which we are subjected over time. Posture is the way we breathe, how we stand, how we deal with ourselves and other people. Our posture is an expression of our history.*

Our poise, our physical bearing (that is the way we appear in time and space), and our dynamic presence (that is the way we carry our self and occupy the space) are important components of our personal power or charisma (the word derives from the Greek 'gift of grace'). It draws attention to us and influences those around us. A good bearing and posture echoes a good state of mind.

WHAT IS THE CORRECT POSTURE?

The ideal posture is achieved when the upper and lower body are perfectly aligned with the centre of gravity, the neck well centred on the shoulders, which should be relaxed and upright, the chest open, the abdomen flat and the pelvis, thighs and legs firmly on the ground below.[6] The weight of the entire body should not be on the heels or the balls of our feet, but should be distributed evenly on both feet.

Try to stay straight, with a unifying sense of expansive lift and lightness, even as you walk and sit down. There are immense benefits to learning the art of staying harmoniously upright or maintaining a balanced posture during movement.

How to diagnose a bad posture

First, check the soles of your shoes. If they are more worn at the front, back or on the sides there may be a postural problem. Then, stand with your back against the wall. Slightly open your legs (feet in line with your shoulders), rest your buttocks and shoulder (keeping them low) against the wall, in order to 'open up the chest'. Now check if your head touches the wall. If it does not touch, there is a cervical vertebrae misalignment. Now, try to correct your posture by touching the wall with your head, stretching your neck, bending your chin slightly forward, without forcing. It is useful to imagine a wire from the base of the neck lifting you up: while the back of the neck elongates and the chin drops forward. Now breathe using your diaphragm. This is the correct posture.

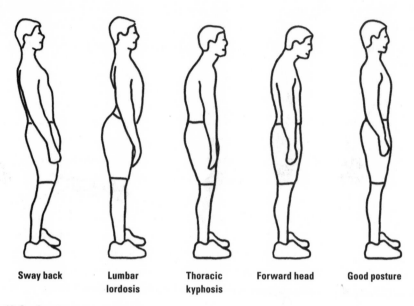

| Sway back | Lumbar lordosis | Thoracic kyphosis | Forward head | Good posture |

Figure 23: Good posture versus poor posture

What should you do to improve your posture?

There are many interventions such as exercise programs that will help to improve your posture. Later, when I discuss yoga, and describe some positions (asanas), we will come back to your posture. One of the many benefits of practising yoga is the strengthening, toning and harmonisation of all the different muscle groups, resulting in improved balance and posture.

But it is not necessary to learn and practise yoga to benefit from the positive effects of stretching and other flexibility exercises. It has been shown that stretching, before and after each session of aerobic or high intensity training, increases the oxygenation of the muscles, and the fluidity, sensitivity and ease with which we carry out movements.[7] The effects are very fast. It takes five weeks of a stretching program of 60 minutes per week, divided into multiple sessions, to improve posture, balance and flexibility. Muscle stretching is helpful even after long periods spent sitting, both for children and adults. Following are some examples of simple stretching exercises.

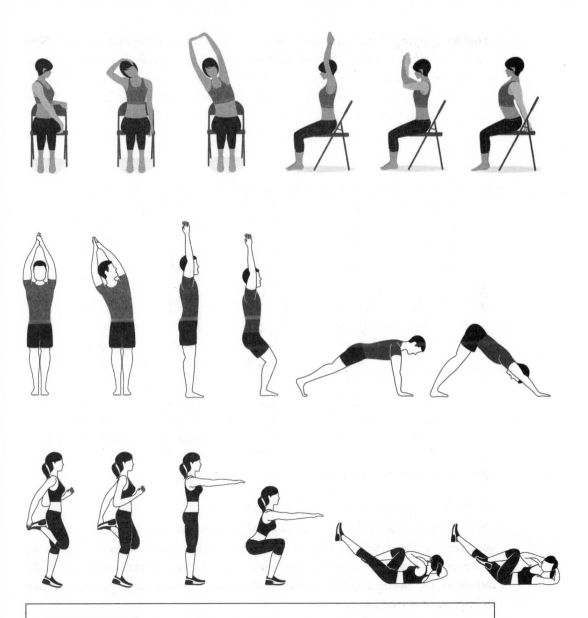

STRETCHING TIPS

- Always stretch within your comfortable limits – never to the point of pain.
- Take your time. Long sustained stretches reduce muscle tightness.
- Regularly stretch, you will feel better for it.
- Hold each stretch for at least 15 seconds.
- Breathe normally as you stretch, don't hold your breath.
- Stretching helps build back and neck muscle strength to support good posture.
- Stretching increases flexibility and movement of the joints.

CHAPTER SIXTEEN

HATHA YOGA, TAI CHI AND MARTIAL ARTS: EAST MEETS WEST

Hatha yoga, tai chi chuan (tai chi for short) and other martial arts such as taekwondo, aikido, judo and karate are ancient disciplines developed in the East with the aim of integrating and improving the physical and psychological health of practitioners.

In yoga as in martial arts, positions have been skilfully designed to exercise each muscle and tendon of the body, to improve coordination, balance and posture, and to increase agility and flexibility, while providing some muscle-strengthening and light-intensity aerobic activity in one package. These exercises do not need any equipment, because our body provides the weights and counterweights. Nevertheless, their primary benefit, as we will see later, is that they train and discipline both mind and spirit, especially when we combine them with certain meditative and breathing techniques.

TAI CHI

The ancient Chinese martial art of tai chi is based on the Taoist concept of yin and yang, the eternal union of the opposites. Over the centuries, it has evolved into a refined form of meditation and breathing exercises, combined with large, slow and circular exercise movements, similar to a silent dance. When engaging in this dance, it is important to free your mind from extraneous thoughts, focusing on performing gentle and harmonious movements, synchronised with a very deep breathing. Synchronising breath and movements enhances awareness of your internal state, which translates into an increased capacity to listen and respond to the signals that the body sends to the mind and the soul.

Careful and regular practice of these exercises makes the body more agile, balanced and harmonious, improves blood circulation and reduces psychological stress. The effects of tai chi have recently been tested in some scientific experiments and it has been shown that regular tai chi practice improves posture and balance,[1,2] and therefore is instrumental in reducing the risk of falls and bone fracture.[3,4] Another clinical study has shown that just three months of bi-weekly tai chi practice significantly improves symptoms of fibromyalgia, a condition that causes widespread pain and tenderness in the body.[5,6]

YOGA

The word 'yoga' means unite, tie together, subduing, channelling and focusing. It is an ancient Indian discipline, one of the six orthodox doctrines (darśana) of the Hindu religious philosophy. There are different forms of yoga, but let's concentrate on Hatha yoga or the 'yoga of strength'. The main purpose of Hatha yoga is to improve health, and fortify and discipline the body and mind in order to enhance our meditative abilities. Bellur K.S. Iyengar (1918–2014), who was one of the world-leading experts in this discipline, said:

> *Meditation must begin with the body. The practice of Hatha yoga*
> *helps the lazy body to become active and vibrant. Transforms the*
> *mind, making it harmonious, and helps to keep the body and mind in*
> *harmony with the soul, so that the three can be merged together. Our*
> *body is the vehicle of the self, which, if not checked in his desires, hinders*
> *the real meditation.*

According to Swami Vivékananda (1863–1902), Indian poet, philosopher and mystic:

> *Our body is like a boat that will help us to travel to the other side of*
> *the ocean of life. For this reason, it is essential to take care of both mind*
> *and body.*

From a purely physical point of view, the practice of Hatha yoga consists of a series of exercises (called asanas) designed to train every muscle of the body and to balance the agonist and antagonist muscles as they interact, so that the body as a whole becomes stronger, more resilient and balanced.

Controlled clinical trials have confirmed a set of specific asana exercises practised for six months can reduce chronic low back pain, and improve joint flexibility, balance and vitality.[7-10] Other clinical trials have shown that regular yoga practice reduces some biomarkers of inflammation[11] and improves arterial function, a well-known marker of cardiovascular health.[12]

When you practise yoga and have a good teacher, these asanas, which have been designed to strengthen and balance all muscles, should rapidly improve your posture, and increase flexibility, agility, coordination and body-mind balance. The movements should be purposely slow, supple and harmonic. It is helpful to envision a three-dimensional view of your body moving fluidly and well aligned in the surrounding space. The mind should remain alert, attentive, focused on the perfect execution of the synchronous movements and your breathing rhythm. In doing so there will be no need to banish extraneous thoughts, which disturb the mind, because you'll be perfectly focused in the present.

The implementation of these asanas, however, should not be conceived as a form of acrobatic gymnastics, but as an opportunity to listen to your body, to perceive points of tension, pain and also realise your limitations.

Yoga exercises also encompass relaxation poses. When you perform relaxation and meditative asanas (e.g. Padmasana, Savasana, Makarāsana, Vajrasana and Siddhasana), you focus on your breathing, trying to synchronise its pace with the movements of the abdomen, which must move smoothly like a bellows. Especially during relaxing yoga poses, train your mind to focus and control your breathing rate and form, which should be deep and rhythmic. When you inhale the air through the nose – very slowly – you should inflate the abdomen, while when you breathe out you should flatten it.

Regular yoga practice has been shown to have beneficial psychological effects by diminishing stress and anxiety, increasing sleep quality, and enhancing emotional and spiritual wellbeing.[13-16] Preliminary data from a small randomised clinical trial show that in healthy older adults, without any cognitive impairment, eight weeks of yoga practice results in a significant improvement in the ability to maintain focus and accurately retrieve information from working memory under stressful conditions that require more cognitive resources.[17] Following are examples of asanas that I practise regularly.

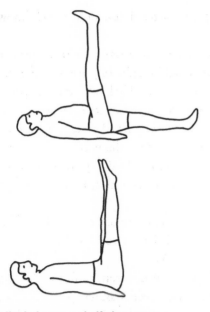

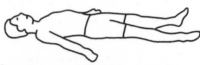

Savasana or corpse pose
Lie flat on your back while relaxing you
body and mind. Close your eyes and
focus on breathing naturally, and practise
eliminating tension from your body.

Ardha-halasana or half plow pose
Lie flat on the floor with arms at your sides.
Using your abdominal muscles, slowly lift
your right leg until it is perpendicular to the
floor. Hold for a moment then gently lower
your leg to the floor. Repeat with the left
leg. Then slowly lift both legs until they are
perpendicular. Gently lower them to the
floor.

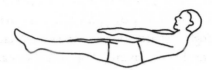

Naukasana or boat pose
Lie flat on the floor with feet together and
arms at your sides. Keeping your arms
straight and fingers outstretched towards
your toes. Inhale and as you exhale, lift your
chest and feet off the floor, stretching your
arms towards your feet. Hold and slowly
return to the starting position.

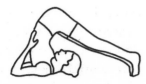

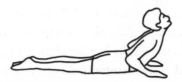

Halasana or plow pose
Lie on your back with your arms beside
you, palms down. As you inhale, lift
your feet off the floor, raising both legs
vertically. Continue to breathe normally, and
supporting your hips and back with your
hands lift them off the ground. Allow your
legs to sweep over your head until your toes
touch the floor. Hold the pose and let your
body relax. After a few seconds gently bring
your legs down while exhaling.

Bhujangasana or cobra pose
Lie on your stomach and place your
forehead on the floor. Keep your feet hip-
width apart and tops of your toes pressing
the floor. Place your hands under your
shoulders, keeping your elbows close to
your body. Exhale as you lift your upper
body, hold, then inhale as you lower your
upper body to the floor.

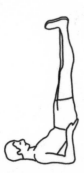

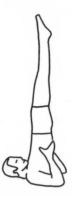

Viparitakarani or leg up the wall pose
Lie supine, feet together and hands beside the body. Exhaling, slowly raise your legs perpendicular to the ground. Raise the lower portion of the trunk by pressing your hands under your hips and using your elbows as a fulcrum. Keep the trunk in a slanting position, the legs upright and the back and the neck well-rested on the floor.

Savangasana or supported shoulderstand
In this pose follow the same steps for Viparitakarani but straighten your back. Your back is supported by your hands. Lift your trunk higher while your hands reach lower down your trunk towards your head. Your legs should be vertical. Hold for 5 minutes. Gently lower yourself by reversing the steps.

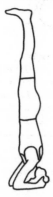

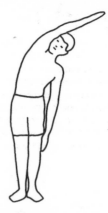

Sirsasana or supported headstand
Use a folded blanket to form a pad. Kneel on the floor, clasp your fingers together and set your forearms on the floor, elbows at shoulder width. Set the crown of your head on the floor. Snuggle the back of your head against your clasped hands. Inhale and lift your knees off the floor. Walk your feet closer to your elbows. Exhale and lift your feet away from the floor taking your feet up. As your legs rise to perpendicular hold for 10 seconds to start with. Graduallly build towards 3 minutes then 5 minutes.

Ardha kati chakrasana or standing side bend pose
Stand straight with feet together arms beside you. Lift your right hand up straight above your head. Breathe in and imagine being pulled up by your hand. Bend leftwards from your waist, sliding your right hand down against your body. Hold for a few breaths and then release. Repeat with your right hand.

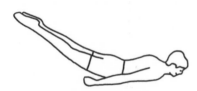

Shalabhasana or locust pose
Lie on your stomach with your arms at your
sides. Inhale and raise your legs. Hold
and relax.

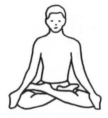

Lotus pose
Sit on the floor with your legs straight out
in front of you. Bend the left knee and hug
it to your chest. Lean back slightly and bend
the right leg and lift the left leg in front of
the right.

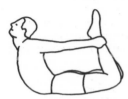

Dhanurasana or bow pose
Lie on your stomach with your arms at your
sides. Exhale as you bend your knees, reach
back with your hands and hold your outer
ankles. As you inhale lift your thighs, head
and chest up drawing your hips off the floor.
Hold and then relax back to a prone position.

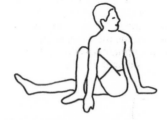

Vakrasana or half spinal twist
In a sitting position, bend your left leg and
place the left heel near your buttock. Place
your left hand and right hand on the floor
near your right thigh. Inhale and while
exhaling twist your trunk and neck to the
right, keeping the spine straight and looking
back over your shoulder. Hold and breathe
normally. Return to sitting by reversing the
steps. Repeat from the opposite side.

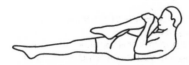

Pavana-muktasana or wind relieving pose
Lie on your back stretching your legs out
straight. Bend your right knee and hold it
with your hands, pressing it towards your
abdomen. Breathing out, lift your head and
touch your knee with your chin. Breathing in,
then stretch your legs straight again. Repeat
with your left leg. Then with both legs.

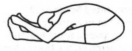

Paschimothanasana or seated forward bend
Lie flat on your back with legs close
together. Slowly raise your head, chest
and trunk until you are sitting up. Exhaling
slowly bend forward until you grip your
toes. Hold this position for 10 seconds then
slowly return to the upright position. Inhale.
Lie back and relax.

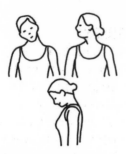

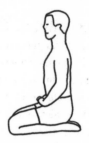

Brahma mudra
Sit comfortably with good posture. Face forward, inhale slowly as you turn your head to the right. Exhale slowly and turn your head slowly to the left. Return to facing forward. As you slowly exhale tip your head down, bringing your chin towards your chest. Return to facing forward. Slowly tilt your head back, then bring your head back to facing forward. Repeat all the four steps.

Vajrasana or thunderbolt pose
Kneel down and stretch the lower legs backwards while keeping them together. Gently lower your body so your thighs rest on the calf muscles. Place your hands on your knees and look straight ahead. Concentrate on your breathing. Hold for up to 5 minutes.

SLOW, DEEP BREATHING: A POWERFUL TOOL TO FIGHT STRESS AND ANXIETY

Acute stress is a key survival mechanism. If we encounter a barking angry dog on our path, without even thinking, our brain unconsciously detects it and the involuntary fight-or-flight stress response kicks in. Basically, our sympathetic nervous system is called into action, and energy is immediately converted to speed up heart rate and increase blood pressure, in order to deliver more blood and oxygen to the muscles, so that we can fight or flee as fast as possible. During a fight-or-flight response, the immune system is activated to ensure better protection against infections in case we are injured.

If occasional and short-term stress is good and potentially life saving, persistent stress and anxiety are very bad for us. Anxiety is a sensation of uneasiness and fear about the future (in the absence of a danger or hazard), complemented by a state of high arousal and augmented alertness.[18] A protracted state of heightened vigilance due to a high-pressure job, financial difficulties, challenging relationships and other day-to-day nerve-wracking situations can induce a chronic activation of the sympathetic nervous and cortisol systems leading to high blood pressure, inflammation, immune suppression and cardiovascular disease.[19,20] Preclinical studies indicate that chronic activation of the sympathetic nervous system can also accelerate ageing.[21]

HOW YOUR NERVOUS SYSTEM REACTS TO STRESS

The sympathetic and parasympathetic nervous systems are formed by a set of neurons and fibres that supply nerves to all our organs and glands, controlling the so-called vegetative functions, namely those that usually are beyond voluntary control. For example, stimulation of the sympathetic system in response to an imminent danger causes an abnormally fast heartbeat; constriction of blood vessels and a rise in blood pressure; increased air flow to the lungs (bronchodilation); constriction of the sphincters; and dilated pupils.[22] The body, in practice, is getting ready to fight or flee.

Conversely, when we are calm and peaceful the parasympathetic system prevails, which through the vagus nerve induces a reduction in heart rate; lowers blood pressure; increases salivary and gastric juices and bile secretion; increases intestinal motility; and dilates the blood vessels of the genitals and digestive glands.

In general, healthy people can handle repeated acute stress as long as there are sufficiently long stress-free periods, such as when the person is at rest. During these peaceful times, our parasympathetic nervous system is at work to dampen the fight-or-flight stress response and save energy. The activation of this component of the autonomous nervous system slows our pulse rate, lowers our blood pressure and promotes our digestive functions. This is called the 'rest and digest' response.

Breathing techniques, which are typically performed during yoga or deep meditation, can help increase the activity of the parasympathetic nervous system.[23] A series of studies have shown that slowing the respiratory rate from the typical 12 to 18 breaths per minute to five to six breaths per minute significantly reduces blood pressure in healthy individuals as well as in patients with hypertension and chronic heart failure. Stimulation of the parasympathetic system by slow breathing helps prevent short-term wide fluctuations of blood pressure.[24,25]

Data from experimental studies and clinical trials have also shown that this type of stimulation inhibits the production of TNF-alpha, a powerful pro-inflammatory cytokine,[26] and improves disease severity in patients with inflammatory disorders, such as rheumatoid arthritis and Crohn's disease.[27-30]

For many of us, deep (or diaphragmatic) breathing seems unnatural. However, it is an important skill we can all use: to learn to breathe slowly and deeply. To make a start, practise slow and deep breathing for five to ten minutes and then progressively increase to 15 minutes. It is important to find time to practise every day so that it becomes a regular part of your day.

Deep breathing exercise

The following steps will help you to practise slow diaphragmatic breathing:

1. Lie down on the floor, on your back, with the chest wide open and your arms and legs slightly apart. By making small adjustments, find the most balanced position. At least at the beginning, place your left hand on your abdomen: this allows you to feel your diaphragm's movements as you breathe.

2. Begin by observing your breath. Pay attention to the quality, symmetry and length of the inhalation and expiration movements, and to the intensity of the sounds produced by the air coming in and out of your nostrils. After a couple of minutes your breath should become slower and slightly deeper.

3. At this point, you should begin to take voluntary control of the velocity of the air coming in. Let the air slowly but effusively fill the lowest part of your lungs, while the abdomen moves out against your left hand.

4. Now, after a long slow smooth inhalation, when your abdomen is fully dilated, expire by engaging your abdominal muscles. Let them fall inward as you exhale slowly through your nose. At the end of the expiration, you should gently spread your ribs to allow for the next full soft inhalation.

5. Keep taking deep breaths in and out, feeling your stomach rise in and out, smoothly without interruptions. Your abdominal organs will be gently massaged by the contraction of the diaphragm and abdominal muscles. The movement of the abdomen and breath should be calm and natural, to draw a perfect circle. If you feel tension in your throat or temples, it means you are working too aggressively and should return to normal breathing until the tension subsides.

6. When you conclude your controlled-breathing session, you should return slowly and gently to a seated position, keeping your eyes closed and the mind calm. In this way you should retain the benefits of this peaceful and powerful practice.

It is an eastern tradition, during the last exhalations of a slow breathing session, to pronounce the mantra 'Aum' or 'Om'. You can try this too. With your eyes half closed, after having breathed all the air out, intone a few times the word 'aum' for the entire duration of the exhalation. If done correctly the sound creates a sweet but intense vibration that spreads to the brain from the larynx. When you reopen your eyes, it should feel like you have awakened from a deep sleep, with your mind clear and relaxed. Recent, but very preliminary research, using functional magnetic resonance imaging, suggests that the vibrations emitted with the pronunciation of the word 'aum' induce an inhibition of the activity of the limbic system, which is important for controlling our emotions.[31]

Once you have mastered this relatively easy deep-breathing exercise, and enjoyed its full benefits, you might consider learning the more sophisticated yogic art of controlled breathing or 'pranayama'. Pranayama consists of exercises that control the three stages of breath: a conscious, rhythmic and intense prolongation of inhalation, retention and exhalation. According to Patañjali, an Indian philosopher of the 2nd century BCE to whom we owe the codification and systematisation of the art of yoga, the practice of Pranayama is essential to achieve the control of the emotions, which brings mental stability and equanimity. In the Hatha Yoga Pradipika, one of the classical texts of yoga, it is written:

> *Breath is the key to self-realisation. When used correctly, the yogi can*
> *cross from the realm of purely physical development to that of the spirit*
> *and achieve the merging of the individual self with the universal soul.*

A regular practice of pranayama results in the acquisition of a tremendous willpower, which is essential to become a master of oneself. However, before we attempt it, Patañjali, the father of modern-day yoga, advises to strengthen our body and mind through an assiduous practice of the key physical asanas.[32] He also recommends that when we feel tension around our temples while practising pranayama, we should immediately revert to normal breathing.

FINAL RECOMMENDATIONS: EXERCISE PRECAUTIONS

Sedentary people should begin doing physical activity gradually. Then, they can slowly increase the length and frequency of the workout sessions as they become more able. It is not wise or advisable to start a program of exercise that involves long running sessions. Start with frequent short walks at a fast pace, and gradually increase the distance and speed.

The same principle needs to be applied to resistance exercise, yoga and tai chi, which as for all the other martial arts initially should be practised carefully and under the guidance of qualified instructors. Some asanas, such as the headstand and lotus positions, if performed incorrectly can cause damage to the joints, especially to the neck, back, knees and ankles. People affected by glaucoma should avoid inverted positions and those with osteoporosis should avoid forceful yoga practices.

If you are an adult who has never played sports, has begun to exercise again after years of inactivity or who has existing illnesses, it is recommended you consult a doctor first. Your doctor can rule out the presence of potential life-threatening illnesses (e.g. cardiac arrhythmias or hemodynamically significant atherosclerotic plaques that limit the flow of oxygen-rich blood to your heart and other parts of your body) or functional alterations (dissymmetry of the limbs or flat feet) that could make it dangerous or difficult. Your safety comes first!

PART V

PREVENTION

CHAPTER SEVENTEEN

TAKE PREVENTATIVE ACTION TO STAY HEALTHY

Smoking, alcohol, sun and even gum disease can affect your chance of living a long, healthy life. Limiting exposure to harmful substances like cigarettes may be obvious, but with other factors like the sun and alcohol it is a matter of striking the right balance.

SMOKING KILLS YOU AND HARMS YOUR LOVED ONES

It seems outdated to speak of the damage caused by cigarette smoke, but unfortunately too many people still smoke, damaging themselves and the loved ones living with them, because it has been clearly demonstrated that passive smoking is as detrimental as active smoking.[1] Children are particularly damaged by passive smoking. The functioning of the lungs of infants who have been exposed to tobacco smoke and nicotine, both during prenatal life and after birth, is compromised forever.[2] As they grow older, they will develop more respiratory infections during the winter, will lose valuable days of school, and take many antibiotics, which will alter the health of their gut flora. They will also have a higher risk of becoming ill with asthma.[3]

The scientific data are incontrovertible. Mortality among smokers is three times higher than in people who have never smoked, and smokers live on average 11 to 12 years less as shown in figure 24.[4] An enormous difference.

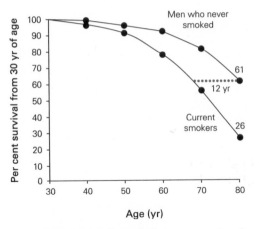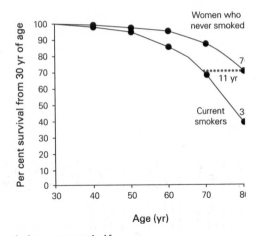

Figure 24: Comparison of mortality between current smokers and those who have never smoked.[5]

Not only will smokers live for a shorter time, but they will almost certainly suffer one of the many maladies that are caused by cigarette smoking. It is a lottery, no one knows which will appear first: lung cancer (the risk of developing lung cancer is about 25 times higher in smokers than in non-smokers); a heart attack; a stroke; or chronic obstructive respiratory disease.[6]

The carcinogenic substances that enter their circulation also increase the risk of developing many cancers of the oral cavity, pharynx, larynx, oesophagus, stomach, colon, pancreas, bladder, kidney, endometrium and breast.[7] However, the list of smoke-related disease doesn't end here, it continues to grow. A recent study on a population of about a million people followed for 11 years showed that smokers have a two-fold increased risk of dying from kidney failure, hypertensive heart disease, infections, and various other respiratory diseases. Even mortality from intestinal ischaemia (where blood does not reach the gut so it slowly dies) is six times higher.[8]

Many 'social' smokers believe that smoking one or two cigarettes every day is relatively safe, but a recent study published in the *British Medical Journal* suggests that smoking just one cigarette per day carries a risk of developing coronary heart disease and stroke around half of that for people who smoke 20 per day.[9] No safe level of smoking exists for heart disease and stroke.

Smokers need to abandon this unhealthy habit altogether, instead of cutting down.

The mechanisms through which cigarette smoking promotes illness and death are many and complex. I do not believe it is appropriate in this book to explain in detail what happens when people inhale cigarette smoke, but some notions are probably useful to understand the type of damage smokers are inflicting on themselves.

1. Smoke activates the immune cells that produce inflammatory molecules, called cytokines,[10] which increase the risk of forming atherosclerotic plaques, cancer cells and dementia. Chronic inflammation also accelerates the ageing process and causes fibrosis of virtually all tissues.

2. Cigarette smoking increases oxidative stress, which in concert with inflammation, alters the function of the arteries and the heart, and makes the platelets more likely to aggregate to form blood clots.[11] If a blood clot blocks an artery supplying blood to the heart or the brain, the downstream tissue dies.[12]

3. Smoking drastically increases the risk of cancer. Cigarette smoke contains a mixture of at least 250 chemicals known to be toxic or carcinogenic, which not only act locally, but because they are absorbed into the bloodstream, spread everywhere in the body. Sadly, an increased concentration of these smoke-related mutagenic substances can be found in the urine of those passively exposed to tobacco smoke as well.[13]

But if smoking is so bad – in many countries, 'smoking kills you' is written in large capital letters on each pack of cigarettes – why do people continue to smoke? There are social and imitation factors, especially among teenagers, but also biological reasons. Nicotine is a drug, which causes addiction and inhibits appetite. It has been clearly demonstrated that nicotine binds to specific receptors on some hypothalamic neurons, called POMC, whose activation induces a reduction of hunger.[14]

Smart and aware people, however, should not bargain the loss of 2 or 3 kilos of body weight against the risk, or rather the certainty, of developing one of the above-mentioned devastating diseases. As we have widely discussed, there are other healthier ways to lose weight!

Finally, remember that it is never too late to stop poisoning yourself with smoking. It has been shown that even people who have quit smoking at 50 years of age, live six years longer than those who continued smoking.[15] Nonetheless, it takes approximately 20 years to reduce the smoke-associated risk back to close to the normal risk of non-smokers.[16]

SUN EXPOSURE AND VITAMIN D: HOW, WHEN, WHERE AND WHY?

The advice from the American Cancer Society and other medical organisations is to avoid sun exposure from 10 am to 4 pm, or to cover yourself with clothes and sunscreen if you go to the beach or walk in the park on a beautiful sunny day.[17] The main reason for such drastic recommendations is to reduce exposure to the sun's ultraviolet (UV) rays, which increase the risk of skin cancer.

Exposure to the sun for decades, typically among sailors and outdoor workers, is the usual cause of the most common skin cancer. Occasional exposure with severe sunburn, typically among people with fair skin and especially children, is associated with the rarer, but more malignant, melanoma.

However these strict recommendations do not take into account that skin exposure to sunlight stimulates the production of a very important vitamin, vitamin D. UV (B) radiation penetrates the skin and converts cholesterol into vitamin D3. The liver and kidneys transform this biologically inert form of vitamin D into an active molecule, called 1,25-dihydroxyvitamin D, that the body can use to promote calcium absorption, bone health and many other vital health functions.[18]

If we avoid the sun as the guidelines insist, then, the only alternative is to take vitamin D supplements daily or to consume foods naturally rich in vitamin D like cod liver oil. Not my favourite!

Yet accumulating data suggest that there are many other positive effects of sun exposure, not just the synthesis of vitamin D. A growing body of evidence indicates that sunlight may play a key role in improving immune function and in reducing the risk of developing a series of inflammatory and autoimmune diseases, such as psoriasis, multiple sclerosis and asthma.[19,20] Sun exposure also has positive effects on psychological wellbeing by increasing the production of endorphins.[21] Endorphins are molecules structurally similar to the drug morphine that boost pleasure and feelings of euphoria.

A recent provocative study conducted in Sweden even suggests that the mortality of people who avoid sun exposure is almost twice as high of those who get regular sun.[22,23]

Skin colour, melanin, vitamin D and sun exposure

For centuries, people from all over the world have lived outdoors and worked several hours a day in the hot sun without sunscreens. People lived most of their lives in the same latitude that they and their forefathers were born in. Skin colour is the result of that evolution. People whose ancestors lived in tropical or subtropical regions have darker complexions than those who live above the 35° parallel.

Skin colour depends on the levels of a pigment called melanin, a natural sunscreen that protects cells from the damage of overexposure to UV rays. The dark skin, rich in melanin, of Africans is so efficient at absorbing UVB rays that it reduces the production of vitamin D3 by 93 to 97 per cent, the same effect we can get with a SPF-15 or 30 sunscreen.[24]

The benefit of a pale skin for individuals who live in areas with little sun, however, is precisely to allow more UV rays to penetrate, resulting in more production of vitamin D3, which is necessary for calcium absorption and bone health, among other things. In fact, several studies have demonstrated that vitamin D plays a key role in the prevention of osteoporosis.[25] Vitamin D deficiency is also implicated in chronic pain.[26] Pain patients with vitamin D deficiency require twice the dosage of pain medication as those who are not deficient.[27]

Accumulating data suggest that vitamin D may also play a role in the prevention of cancer, multiple sclerosis, type 1 diabetes, rheumatoid arthritis and Crohn's disease.[28] A low concentration of vitamin D in the blood, for example, is associated with a greater risk of colon cancer, especially when combined with a low intake of calcium,[29] although trials have not made clear why that is.[30] Vitamin D deficiency also has important effects on brain development and mental health. One study found that mice with low levels of vitamin D have a significantly less developed cerebral cortex.[31]

Professor Michael Holick, one of the world's leading experts on vitamin D, believes that inadequate sun exposure has become a major public health problem, and there needs to be an immediate change to the current sun-avoidance, public health guidelines.[32] He thinks, and I agree with him, that we should get enough sun exposure (or vitamin D supplementation when the sun isn't available) to maintain a serum 25-hydroxyvitamin D level of at least 30 ng/ml. To achieve this level we should expose our arms and legs, and if possible also the abdomen and back, two or three times a week to direct sunlight, until the skin gets a little red. This mild redness should be enough to increase our blood concentrations of vitamin D to a level similar to consuming 15,000 to 20,000 units of vitamin D.[33] How many minutes we expose ourselves to sunlight to produce enough vitamin D clearly varies depending on the time of day, season, latitude, cloud cover and type of skin complexion.

In early summer a person with a fair skin who lives in New York should expose their arms and legs (face and hands are not enough) to the midday sun for approximately five to 15 minutes, two or three times a week, to meet the weekly requirement of vitamin D. After 15 minutes, if we want to continue staying in the sun, we should cover our exposed skin with a sunscreen (at least SPF 15), in order to prevent premature ageing of the skin and reduce the risk of skin cancer. Sunburn is to be avoided at all costs!

During the winter, and also in the summer in the early morning and in the late afternoon the UVB rays are almost completely absorbed by the ozone layer of the atmosphere. Unless we live nearer the equator, we need to take a vitamin D supplement to avoid a deficiency during the long winter months. To attain a serum level of at least 30 ng/ml would require taking 2000 IUs of vitamin D daily, which would be equivalent to 25 per cent of the body surface exposed to a mild reddening dose of sun, two or three times a week. Just to be safe it is a good idea to ask your doctor to measure serum 25(OH) vitamin D levels once a year, for instance, at the end of the summer when the blood levels should peak.

It is not true that we can easily meet the needs of vitamin D with food. Fatty fish, like salmon, and sun-dried mushrooms contain small amounts of vitamin D. But even if we consume foods enriched with vitamin D (for example fortified milk or juices) we still will not be able to cover more than 10 to 40 per cent of our daily requirement.

NUTRITION AND SKIN CANCER

What we eat could be very important for the prevention of skin cancer. A recent study published in the *New England Journal of Medicine* has shown that daily supplementation with nicotinamide (vitamin B3) can reduce by 23 per cent the risk of a recurrence of skin cancer in high-risk patients who have had two skin squamous cell carcinomas in the previous five years.[34] Vitamin B3 is found at high concentrations in fish, brown rice, peas and avocados.

Numerous studies suggest that the risk of melanoma is also influenced by dietary habits: it is lower in those who eat lots of vegetables, fruit, fish and foods rich in vitamin A, C, D and E.[35] Therefore, it seems that what we eat plays a fundamental role, independent of sun exposure, to protect or increase the risk of neoplastic transformation of certain cells of the skin. Further research is needed.

ALCOHOL: THE GOOD, THE BAD, AND THE UGLY

That heavy alcohol consumption is linked to poor health is an undisputed fact.[36] It is also a major cause of fatal traffic accidents, violent crimes, injuries, depression and suicide. Heavy alcohol users (who drink five or more drinks on the same occasion on five or more days in one month) have an increased risk of liver cirrhosis, pancreatitis, heart disease, stroke, dementia and cancer of the oral cavity, larynx, oesophagus and liver. They also have fertility issues including reduced sperm count,[37] and chronic sleep disorders.[38]

Moderate intake of alcohol is defined as the daily consumption of one drink for healthy women or one to two drinks for healthy men (reduced to no more than a single drink per day in men older than 65 years).

One drink is:

- 120 ml/4 fl oz wine
- 360 ml/12 fl oz beer
- 45 ml/1½ fl oz of 80 proof (40 per cent alcohol)
- 30 ml/1 fl oz 100 proof alcohol (50 per cent alcohol).

Some epidemiological data, however, suggest that moderate alcohol consumption may reduce mortality from heart attacks. A study, published in *The Lancet,* analysed data from 83 studies of almost 600,000 current drinkers without previous cardiovascular disease from 19 high-income countries. The results suggest that the lowest mortality risk for heart attack (myocardial infarction) was in those drinking around or below 100 g (3½ oz) of alcohol per week (equivalent to five to six glasses of wine or pints of beer). However, with other cardiovascular illnesses, including stroke, heart failure, fatal hypertensive disease, and fatal aortic aneurysm there was no safe level for alcohol consumption.[39]

The reality is that the scientific evidence linking daily light to moderate intake of red wine with a reduced incidence of heart disease is based mainly on epidemiological data.[40] Some randomised clinical trials have shown that moderate consumption of red wine or alcohol has a small, but significant effect in increasing HDL-cholesterol, in reducing fasting insulin, triglycerides, LDL-cholesterol and total cholesterol-HDL-cholesterol ratio.[41-43] However, well-conducted studies indicate that even moderate alcohol intake (8–21 drinks per week) is an independent predictor of enlargement and dysfunction of the heart's left atrium, which can lead to atrial fibrillation, a major risk factor for stroke.[44,45]

A direct relationship exists between elevated blood pressure and alcohol consumption, with no lower threshold: even light drinking seems to increase blood pressure. Data from randomised trials show that reducing alcohol intake can lower blood pressure by 3.3 and 2 mm Hg; the reductions seem to be similar in both people with normal blood pressure and people with high blood pressure.[46] In other randomised trials, drinking 200 to 300 ml (10 fl oz) of red wine per day resulted in a significant elevation in blood pressure in both men and women.[47]

The harmful effects of regular alcohol consumption, even in moderate quantities, aren't limited to the heart. The International Agency for Research on Cancer (AIRC) has classified alcoholic beverages as human carcinogens (group I). New studies suggest that drinking on a regular basis as little as one or two drinks per day increases the risk of cancer, in particular breast cancer[48] and colorectal cancer.[49] A study published in *Nature* demonstrates that acetaldehyde, a key metabolite of alcohol, damages chromosomes and mutates stem cells.[50] Alcohol also elevates blood testosterone and oestrogen concentration, which may further increase the risk of prostate, breast and endometrial cancer.[51-53]

To summarise, alcohol can act as a poison or a medicine, depending on the dose and frequency of its consumption. My advice is to not consume alcoholic beverages on a regular basis, but enjoy them intermittently in small doses, which may have a favourable effect. I love drinking one glass of excellent red wine – a full-bodied, velvety and round Shiraz with lovely tannin and dark fruits is my favourite – or a cold Hefeweizen beer with meals, two to three times per week, especially in the company of friends.

BRUSH YOUR TEETH REGULARLY: GUM DISEASE CAUSES SYSTEMIC INFLAMMATION

Poor dental hygiene causes aesthetic problems and is also associated with chronic inflammation and heart disease. It's not just a matter of preventing dental cavities, but most importantly inflammation of the gums.

Periodontal, or gum, disease is responsible for persistent bad breath, and for at least one-third of adult tooth loss. If you don't brush your teeth regularly, at least every 24 hours, dental plaque accumulates. The accumulation of this film of saliva and bacteria along the gum line causes irritation and inflammation, because of the damaging toxins produced by the bacteria. If your gums bleed when you brush your teeth, it means that you have ongoing gingivitis, which will only get worse unless the dentist manually removes the hardened plaque (tartar) from your teeth.

Initially, you will notice only some parts of the gums swelling, but with time the situation can degenerate, and the reversible gingivitis will become periodontitis, with potential loss of teeth. Clinical signs of periodontitis are:

- Gum margins recede and detach from the teeth with formation of gum pockets where bacteria can accumulate and destroy your teeth and the underlying bone.

- Gingival retraction (the tooth looks longer).

- Teeth become loose, begin to move in the most extreme cases, and may fall out.

The real problem is that the chronic gingivitis is caused by activated immune cells that produce inflammatory substances.[54] These molecules can penetrate into the blood vessels and cause systemic inflammation,[55] which is a powerful risk factor for the development of atherosclerotic plaque, which hardens and narrows your arteries.[56,57] A recent study showed that periodontitis consistently increases the risk of heart attack by 50 per cent, independent of other risk factors such as smoking and diabetes.[58] Mechanical removal of tartar significantly reduces blood C-reactive protein levels, a marker of inflammation,[59] demonstrating a cause-effect relationship.

Although gingivitis and periodontitis are more common in adults, they can also affect children, so it is essential for kids to be taught to brush and floss their teeth every day.

How you brush your teeth is also important. Many people just give their teeth a quick scrub before leaving home in the morning, or a hurried brushing before collapsing into bed at night. However, this is not enough to decrease your risk of developing cavities or getting gingivitis. In order to really see substantial results, you should brush your teeth for two minutes in the morning and again at night before going to bed. Brush from the front to the back, moving from the right side of your mouth to the left, or vice versa. Make sure to clean not only the outer, but also the inner surface, and finally the chewing surface.

Using an electric toothbrush provides better oral health results than regular manual toothbrushes. My son Lorenzo loves using his electric toothbrush with technology that allows him to see where he is brushing and adjust his technique to never miss a zone. The built-in two-minute timer also helps him to brush just the right amount, with a timer for each zone of his mouth.

Flossing your teeth once a day to remove the food trapped between them is equally important. Despite all this, we all still need to go to the dentist twice a year to remove any tartar that is difficult to reach or that we have missed.

CHAPTER EIGHTEEN

THE IMPORTANCE OF HEALTH SCREENING

Undergoing periodic check-ups and screening is important, even for people who are apparently in good health, and do not have any signs or symptoms of disease.

Regular health checks and blood tests can identify metabolic alterations early on, which if left untreated can lead to potentially deadly chronic illnesses. Tests can identify early signs of disease (for instance a precancerous cervical lesion, a colon polyp, a small breast cancer mass), that can be addressed with an early and much less invasive treatment. This, in most cases, drastically reduces the risk of serious complications and death.

Independent of our lifestyle (such as what we eat, how active we are, if we smoke cigarettes), having regular physical examinations, blood tests and prevention screening is important to maximise our chance to live a long and healthy life. Table 8 shows how frequently and at what age different tests are recommended.

As we will see, though, our age, lifestyle, underlying health, family history of illness and other important factors need to be taken into consideration. These might considerably impact the check-ups and screening procedures we undertake and how often.

It is essential to periodically ask your doctor to measure a number of cardiometabolic markers, which have been shown to predict the risk of developing heart disease and stroke, such as your BMI, blood pressure, cholesterol, glucose, white cell counts and C-reactive protein, and triglycerides (see appendix).

WHAT TESTS DO WE NEED AND WHEN?

	19-26 years	27-45 years	45-59 years	60-64 years	65+ years
BMI & waist circumference	Regular screening for all adults				
Blood pressure	Once every 2 years for blood pressure (BP) <120/80 mmHg, or every year for systolic BP of 120–139 mmHg or diastolic BP of 80–89 mmHg				
Cholesterol	Regular screening for men over 35 and women over 45 For high risk men and women screening starts at age 20				
Fasting glucose	Regular screening for adults, especially if BP higher than 135/80 mmHg				
White blood cell count & C-reactive protein	Regular screening for adults				
Carotid IMT	For high-risk people screening starts at age 35*				
Aortic aneurysm				Once in men aged 65–75, especially if smokers	
Eye exam	Depending on symptoms and risk*			Every 1-2 years	
Colorectal cancer	Not routine except for people at high risk*		Colonoscopy at age 45 and then every 10 years; or annual faecal occult blood tests; or CT colonography every 5 years		
Breast cancer (women)	Mammography & MRI in high-risk women only, starting at age 30*		Mammography every year age 45–55; every 2-year from 55+;		
Prostate cancer			PSA screening starts at 45–50 years depending on risk*		
Testicular cancer	Clinical testicular exam at each health maintenance visit				
Lung cancer	Low-dose helical CT scan in current or former smokers aged 55–74 years in good health, with at least a 30-pack a year history of smoking				
Cervical cancer	Women aged 21–29: pap smear every 3 years Women aged 30–65: pap smear with HPV testing every 5 years				
Skin cancer & melanoma	Every 3 years total skin exam*		Annual total skin exam*		
Bone mineral density (BMD) test (women)	Bone mineral density (BMD) testing for women younger than 65 years, but at high risk of bone fractures*		Provide BMD testing		
HIV infection	One time screening age 16–65; every 3–5 years if at high risk; annually if at very high risk; screen all pregnant women				

BP=blood pressure; IMT=intima-media thickness; MRI=magnetic resonance imaging; CT=computed tomography.
*discuss with your doctor risks, benefits, limitations and potential harm

Table 8. Suggested prevention screening exams for healthy adults

Other simple and inexpensive laboratory tests that should be ordered are: haemoglobin to exclude anaemia, transaminases to exclude liver disease, and blood urea nitrogen (BUN) and creatinine to dismiss the presence of renal disease.

Having a carotid intima-media thickness and echo cardio test from time to time is also a good idea, especially if your cardiometabolic risk factors are abnormal. Carotid intima-media thickness (IMT) is a non-invasive ultrasound parameter of early atherosclerosis. A positive association exists between IMT thickness and the risk of subsequent cardiovascular events in the general population, independent of all major cardiometabolic risk factors. An echocardiogram can detect early signs of a stiffening of the heart walls (diastolic dysfunction) and cardiac valve problems.

SCREENING FOR CANCER

Cancer is the second leading cause of death in many industrialised countries, but among women aged 40 to 79 and men aged 60 to 79 years it is the number one killer. An estimated 38 per cent of American women and 46 per cent of American men will develop a malignant cancer during their lifetime, and about 60 per cent of those diagnosed will die because of it.[1] As you can see in table 9, the earlier we diagnose the cancer, the higher the chance of surviving. Primary prevention with a healthy diet and regular exercise is crucial, but screening is extremely important as well.

	All stages	Local	Regional	Distant		All stages	Local	Regional	Distant
Breast (female)	90	99	85	27	Oral cavity & pharynx	65	84	65	39
Colon & rectum	65	90	71	14	Ovary	47	92	75	29
Colon	64	90	71	14	Pancreas	9	34	12	3
Rectum	67	89	70	15	Prostate	98	>99	>99	30
Lsophagus	19	45	24	5	Stomach	31	68	31	5
Kidney	75	93	68	12	Testis	95	99	96	74
Larynx	61	78	46	34	Thyroid	98	>99	98	56
Liver	18	31	11	2	Urinary bladder	77	69	35	5
Lung & bronchus	19	56	30	5	Uterine cervix	66	92	56	17
Melanoma of the skin	92	98	64	23	Uterine corpus	81	95	69	16

Table 9: Probability of survival at five years from time of diagnosis.[2]

Cervical cancer screening

A good example of the importance of screening in preventing death is cervical cancer. In the 1850s, cervical cancer was the most frequently observed malignant tumour in Western Europe, but organised screening with the Papanicolaou (Pap) smear test has resulted in a drastic decline in cervical cancer incidence and mortality over the past 50 years.

Cervical cancer is caused by a sexually transmitted infection with certain types of human papillomavirus (HPV) that can cause changes to cells in the cervix, and eventually develop into a malignant cervical tumour. This is why it is so important for sexually active women to start screening for cervical cancer beginning at age 21 in order to detect potential early precancerous cervical lesions. The US Preventive Services Task Force recommends that women aged 21 to 29 should undergo screening with cytology alone every three years; HPV testing should not be used in this age group.[3] In women who are 30 to 65 years old, instead, it is better to co-test with both an HPV and cytology test every five years. Woman who underwent HPV vaccination should continue the screening program regardless.

After age 65 women should stop screening if their cytology tests were negative for three times in a row or they had two consecutive negative co-test results within the ten-year period before ceasing screening. Once screening is discontinued, it should not resume for any reason, including having a new sexual partner. Other countries, for example Australia, have adopted slightly different screening protocols: the two-yearly Pap test for people aged 18 to 69 has been replaced by a five-yearly HPV test for people aged 25 to 74.

Cervical cancer, however, is not the leading type of cancer, at least in Western countries. The five most frequent type of male tumours are prostate, lung, colorectal, urinary bladder and skin melanoma, while in women the most common are breast, lung, colorectal, uterine corpus and thyroid.[4]

Colorectal cancer screening

Colorectal cancer, for instance, in both men and women is the second leading tumour and almost always develops from one precancerous polyp in the rectum or colon. With colonoscopy we can discover these precancerous polyps, which the gastroenterologist can remove before they transform into invasive and deadly cancers.

Faecal occult blood tests and colonoscopy can also help find a colorectal cancer at an early stage, before it starts to invade other tissue or, even worse, to metastasise to local and distant organs. As illustrated in table 9, the probability of survival at five-years free of disease is 90 per cent when the tumour is still localised, but only 14 per cent if at the time of diagnosis the tumour has already metastasised to other organs. Screening for colorectal cancer prevents 20–25 deaths per 1000 people screened.[5]

Breast cancer screening

Worldwide, breast cancer is now the most common cancer diagnosed in females and the leading cause of death from cancer among women. Regular screening means more women are diagnosed earlier and this has led to higher survival rates than women diagnosed later with more advanced breast cancer. The survival at five-years free of disease is 99 per cent for localised breast tumours, but only 27 per cent if metastases are already present at diagnosis. This is why it is essential for average-risk women to undergo regular screening mammography starting at age 45 years in order to detect as early as possible a potential malignant lesion. Women aged 45 to 54 years should be screened annually, while those aged more than 55 can transition to biennial screening, because breast cancer tends to grow more slowly after menopause. Indeed, the holiday time (i.e. the estimated period of time that a clinically asymptomatic breast tumour is detectable by mammography) is shorter among women in their 40s (approximately 1.7 years) than in those aged 50 to 59 years (3.3 years) or 60 to 69 years (3.8 years).

Women with a known BRCA mutation (or with a first-degree relative with a BRCA mutation) and other rarer, high-risk genetic syndromes or who had been treated with radiation to the chest for Hodgkin's lymphoma should undergo annual screening mammography and magnetic resonance imaging starting at age 30. In women aged 50 to 75, screening for breast cancer every two years is estimated to prevent about seven deaths per 1000 women screened. If screening starts at age 40, it could prevent one extra death per 1000 women screened.[6] This is why women aged 40 to 44 years should have an opportunity to begin screening before age 45 years, if they wish. It is also recommended that women should continue screening mammography as long as their overall health is good and they have at least ten years of projected longevity.

Prostate cancer and PSA screening tests

For men, one of the main health concerns is the development of prostate cancer. Prostate cancer is the most common cancer type in men in the United States and in many other industrialised countries, accounting for 20 per cent of new cancer cases and 10 per cent of cancer deaths.[7] While there is some debate about PSA screening – a test that measures the level of prostate-specific antigen (PSA) in your blood – these statistics show screening is valuable. In men aged more than 70 years it is estimated there is no benefit in screening for PSA. And in those aged 55 to 69 years, PSA screening prevents about 1.3 deaths from prostate cancer over 13 years per 1000 men screened and three cases of metastatic cancer per 1000 men screened, with no decrease in total mortality.

Let's make it simpler: of 1000 men aged 55 to 69 offered PSA screening, only about 240 got a positive result, which might indicate a potential diagnosis of prostate cancer; of these 240, approximately 100 got a positive biopsy with a diagnosis of malignant cancer. For men with low-grade prostrate cancer some countries, like Sweden and Australia, then advise an active surveillance approach to see if the cancer is slow growing and they therefore may avoid intervention. On average, 80 out of those 100 men decide to undergo surgery or radiation therapy (50 of whom will develop erectile dysfunction and 15 urinary incontinence). Of these men, only three will avoid cancer from spreading to other organs, while five will die from prostate cancer despite surgery or radiation treatment. In summary, out of 1,000 men offered PSA-based testing, only 1.3 men avoid death from prostate cancer.

Potential harms of PSA testing are:

- false-positive results with consequent psychological effects

- damage induced by trans rectal core needle prostate biopsy, including bleeding and infections

- over-diagnosis and over-treatment with surgery or radiation resulting in major side effects, including erectile dysfunction, urinary and faecal incontinence, and potentially death

- secondary cancers from radiation and chemotherapy.

Data from several clinical trials show that between 20 and 50 per cent of prostate cancer cases diagnosed through screening may be over-diagnosed.[8]

The problem is that it is still not possible to predict which men (who have been diagnosed with prostate cancer through screening) will benefit from cancer treatment, because we cannot differentiate tumours that are not growing or slowly growing from those that are aggressive and deadly. Indeed, a certain number of treated men may avoid death and disability from prostate cancer, but others would have died of unrelated causes before their cancer became serious enough to disrupt their health or reduce their lifespan.

Because of these results, the US Preventive Services Task Force has determined that the choice for men aged 50 to 69 years to have PSA-based screening should be an individual one and should include a discussion of the potential benefits and harms of screening. Those men who choose to be screened (after discussing with their doctor) should receive a PSA test with or without a digital rectal examination between age 45 and 50 (depending on the family history of prostate cancer). Men with PSA <2.5 ng/ml should repeat the test every two years, while those with PSA ≥2.5 ng/ml every year. For men with a PSA level ≥4.0 ng/ml a biopsy is recommended.

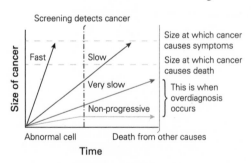

Figure 25: Overdiagnosis of cancer

BEYOND ACTIVE SURVEILLANCE AND WATCHFUL WAITING

Suppose you have decided to screen, and your PSA scores 2.5–4 ng/ml, or even worse, because of a high PSA the results of the bioptic material is a localised small (low volume) and slow-growing (low grade, e.g. Gleason score <6 and PSA <20) tumour. What should you do?

Active surveillance might be an option and indeed has become the dominant management for low-grade or well-differentiated prostate cancer in many countries. For example, 74 per cent and 50 per cent of men with low-grade prostate cancer in Sweden and Australia, respectively, have opted for active surveillance.[9] With active surveillance, the patient is followed closely (i.e. PSA tests every three to six months, digital rectal examination every six months, MRI scans, and biopsies at one and three years), and only if the cancer shows signs of faster or more aggressive growth, the patient will undergo surgical and or radiotherapy treatment.

Can we do anything more to lower the risk of being diagnosed with cancer or to slow the progression from a low-grade to a more aggressive tumour that will force us to undergo surgical or radiation treatment?

The answer is a definite 'yes'. As I have illustrated in the previous chapters of this book, changing your diet and exercise patterns can impact cancer progression and prognosis by controlling a cascade of metabolic, hormonal and immune modifications that reduce cell proliferation and mutations, and enhance the ability of certain specialised immune cells to recognise and kill cancer cells.

PART VI

OUR MINDS

SCIENCE-BACKED SECRETS TO PROMOTE EMOTIONAL, INTUITIVE AND CREATIVE INTELLIGENCE

CHAPTER NINETEEN

NOURISH YOUR MIND AND TRAIN YOUR BRAIN

The central pillar for the promotion of health in ancient medicine systems has always been the 'nourishment of the mind'.

One of the oldest and most important texts of traditional Chinese medicine, the *Yellow Emperor's Classic of Internal Medicine*, says, 'First of all it is critical to feed our mind', which requires that 'man challenges his intellect while remaining calm, optimistic and spiritually happy'. Only when 'a state of peace and tranquillity without avarice and wild passions' is achieved will 'the functions of the Qi (the vital life force) be harmonious, the inner vitality maintained and diseases prevented'. Similarly, a health cornerstone of the most famous medieval school of medicine in Europe, the Schola Medica Salernitana, was: 'Dispel the serious concerns, not to succumb to anger, and to maintain a happy and serene mind'.

Modern science has discovered that our brain is a wonderful organ, both dynamic and plastic, which has the ability to constantly learn new skills, integrate new experiences, and form and store long-term memories. Stimulating the mind with new tasks has been shown to improve brain function and help protect us from cognitive decline, just as physical exercise prevents the loss of bone and muscle mass. More recently, growing evidence indicates that our thoughts and emotions can also shape our brain function and structure. Negative emotions and persistent psychological stress also negatively impact metabolism and the function of all our organs, including the immune system. In experimental studies, mice that lived in environments enriched with cognitive stimuli were not only protected from brain atrophy and cognitive impairment,[1-3] but strikingly, lived longer.[4,5]

We also know that social relationships, emotional connections with family and friends, and feeling part of a community that shares its values, whether spiritual or philosophical, play a vital role in maintaining health and in promoting longevity. It is known that loneliness, solitude, depression and anger can induce a series of metabolic and inflammatory alterations that promote illness and accelerate the ageing process.

There is, nevertheless, a higher level of mental and consciousness development, which for now cannot be explored with the reductionist scientific analysis. It is not just a matter of intellectual stimulation, such as learning a foreign language, mastering a new musical instrument or solving a complex mathematical problem. There is something deeper. The ancient Hindu, Buddhist and Taoist philosophical doctrines teach us that, with our mind, we can explore ourselves and navigate within the depths of our conscious and unconscious world. Rabindranath Tagore, the famous Indian poet, philosopher and 1913 Nobel Prize for literature winner, wrote:

> *Most men are busy exploring the outside world, not knowing that the most beautiful trip we can take is the one inside ourselves.*

Along this line, more than 2000 years ago, Socrates, the most prominent exponent of the Western philosophical tradition, warned:

> *Can we possibly know what the art is that enhances man himself, if we don't know who we are? If we will know ourselves, we will perhaps understand how we should take care of ourselves, otherwise we will never know. [...] Knowing ourselves makes us free, while the opposite condition is that of slaves.*

Although there is still no scientific evidence to support my thesis (and perhaps there never will be), I believe that the root of all things that happen to us lies in one's own inner being. They are just the reflection of something that stems from our own soul. In the *Upanishads*, the mystical and philosophical culmination of the Vedas,* it is written:

> *Examine your thoughts, because they will become your words;*
> *scrutinise your words, because they will become your actions;*
> *check your actions, because they will become your habits;*
> *fix your habits, because they will form your character;*
> *control your character, for it becomes your destiny.*[6]

As I will explain, it is essential to control what we eat and do, because these things will form our thoughts and emotions. It is also important to cultivate the 'whole person' if we want to shape our destiny. We should learn to develop not only our brainpower,

---

* The Vedas are ancient Sanskrit texts containing some of the key philosophical concepts of Hinduism.

but also our emotional, intuitive and creative intelligence; our empathy and the interpersonal and social relations; and our body, psychic and spiritual awareness.

IMPROVING OUR BRAIN FUNCTION: COGNITIVE TRAINING

Cao Tingdong, the famous physician of the Qing dynasty, in his treatise entitled *Maxims of Gerontology* wrote:

> *The mind should not be idle, otherwise it will become like a dead tree and cold ash.*

He recommended 'use the brain regularly' and feed the mind with thoughts 'so that a sufficient amount of information and blood will reach the cortex and cognitive (thinking) abilities will not decline with age'. He believed that elderly people should never stop learning new things by convincing themselves that 'they are no longer capable of doing anything and they are of no use'. Old people, instead, should continue studying new things like learning to compose poems, drawing and painting or playing a new musical instrument.

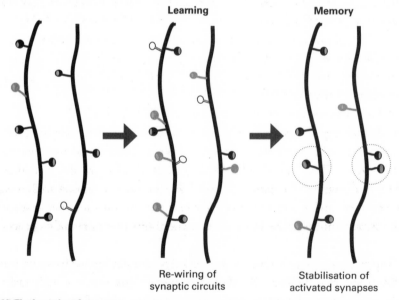

Figure 26: The formation of synapses

We now know that new cognitive stimuli and experiences (like learning to play a musical instrument) cause a rearrangement of the connections between nerve cells and the architecture of our cerebral cortex.[7] In simple terms, this means each experience, if repeated over time, induces the growth of new nerve protrusions (dendritic spines) and new neuronal connections called synapses (see figure 26). These form a network that connects more neurons, forming memory traces.[8] Several experiments have shown that even small modifications of these dendritic spines are associated with an improved ability to learn and store complex motor and sensory tasks.[9-11]

The formation and disappearance of these new synapses, however, is constantly evolving.[12,13] It is a very plastic phenomenon meaning that the brain has the ability to change throughout life. In laboratory experiments, mice exposed to rich environments were shown to undergo a rapid increase of the turnover of these synaptic protrusions. In contrast, exposure to monotonous and stimuli-poor environments inhibits the turnover and formation of new synapses.[14]

BRAIN PLASTICITY CAN IMPROVE INTO OLD AGE

This brain 'plasticity' – which is huge in children – fades with each passing year.[15] This is especially so when the intellect is not being stimulated with new ideas, concepts and experiences.[16] It is for this very reason that it becomes extremely important, as suggested by Cao Tingdong, many years ago, 'that the mind should not be idle'.

It has been scientifically proven, for example, that some training programs like doing sudoku, puzzles or computer games (cognitive training programs) are effective in improving cognitive function and memory, even in older people, probably through a strengthening of pre-existing synaptic circuits.[17] Sophisticated experiments with electroencephalogram (EEG) and functional magnetic resonance imaging (fMRI) have shown that undertaking new tasks and fresh cognitive stresses changes the electrical activity and metabolism of our neurons, and that these changes are held for long periods of time, even after the end of the cognitive training.[18-20]

What has emerged from recent clinical trials, is that these cognitive training exercises improve brain plasticity even in older people already suffering from the early stages of dementia. This suggests that healthy cerebral areas are able to compensate for the lack of activity of the damaged ones.[21] For instance, a clinical study involving 2832 elderly men and women showed that just ten training sessions resulted in a significant increase in cognitive skills, such as the ability to reason and to process data faster.[22]

The important message is that we should keep stimulating our brain by learning new tasks, skills and abilities. We should challenge our intellect with tasks that require the involvement of multiple brain areas. Learning a new language or a musical instrument could be a good start.[23]

You don't need to become a Mozart or Beethoven, but simply engaging different brain areas simultaneously will increase your global brain plasticity. When, for instance, you play the piano, this stimulates areas of the cerebral cortex that control auditory, visual, fine movements of the hands and feet, and reasoning functions, among others.[24,25] Other activities that stimulate your brain functions are dance, yoga, tai chi or playing chess.[26] Even learning to paint or sculpt promotes the formation of new neural circuits in many brain areas, and helps develop agility and hand-brain coordination, but especially creativity.[27]

FASTING AND ENDURANCE EXERCISE BOOST EFFECTS OF COGNITIVE TRAINING

Our neurons, like the rest of our body, suffer when we are overfed; they suffer uncontrolled excitation, which is known to damage multiple brain functions.[28] Experimental data show that reducing calorie intake, especially through fasting, and performing bouts of vigorous aerobic exercise, improves stress resistance and cognitive function, and lessens brain inflammation.[29]

Both fasting and exercise challenge our brain, which reacts by adapting stress response pathways that increase the production of certain brain proteins (i.e. neurotrophic factors), which in turn stimulates the growth of new nerve cells from stem cells in the hippocampus, and the formation and strengthening of synapses.[30] It is believed that fasting helps kick-start defensive mechanisms, which help offset the overexcited signals that epileptic brains often exhibit.[31]

Fasting can also promote DNA repair mechanisms and fuel the production of ketones, a major energy source for neurons. Ketones have been shown to reduce inflammation, oxidative stress and increase the efficiency of mitochondria in nerve cells.[32] Mitochondria (ATP-forming organelles) within our cells are essential for developing and maintaining the connections between neurons, thereby improving learning and memory ability.

PREVENTING COGNITIVE DECLINE

Nothing could be worse than losing our memory, slowly forgetting everything, including the names of our children and finally our own identity, as happens with dementia. The exact mechanisms leading to progressive memory loss and cognitive impairment are not known yet. Most importantly, we do not have medication or a cure for dementia, which starts with some memory lapses of recent events, personality changes (withdrawal), problems with organising or expressing thoughts, and progresses to increased confusion or poor judgment, and greater memory loss. In the most advanced stages, people lose their ability to communicate and need full-time daily assistance for eating, dressing and bathing.

The *Lancet Commission on Dementia Prevention, Intervention and Care* concluded that more than one-third of cases of dementia are potentially preventable by a suite of lifestyle interventions, of which nutrition, exercise and the prevention of obesity are key players.[33] Some prospective trials have shown promising cognitive outcomes from interventions that include various healthier diets and physical activity programs.[34] I personally believe that the percentage is greater than one-third, because at least 30 per cent of dementia cases are due to vascular dementia (blocked arteries leading to impaired blood flow to the brain) and the rest to Alzheimer's disease.

Let's keep in mind that whatever is bad for our heart is bad for our brain, because some of the same factors that promote heart disease (e.g. elevated blood pressure and arterial stiffness, high cholesterol, insulin resistance, type 2 diabetes, inflammation, oxidative stress and smoking) also increase the risk of developing Alzheimer's disease.

Also something that can be prevented is suffering one or more concussions which increases our risk of developing memory loss and dementia.[35] It is of paramount importance to protect our head from injuries by wearing a helmet whenever there is any risk (e.g. cycling, horseriding, skateboarding, skiing and many other sports).

A HEALTHY DIET HELPS TO PREVENT COGNITIVE DECLINE

Accumulating data suggest that healthy lifestyle modifications might have a positive effect on cognition even in older individuals who are genetically susceptible to dementia.[36]

For instance eating a healthy Mediterranean diet has been shown to reduce the risk of developing dementia, especially when associated with a reduction in calorie intake.

Obesity, type 2 diabetes and insulin resistance at midlife are powerful risk factors for subsequent insulin resistance, corresponding to a 40 per cent greater risk of Alzheimer's disease among people *without* type 2 diabetes, and doubling of the risk in patients with type 2 diabetes.[37] Insulin resistance inhibits cerebral blood flow, impairs glucose uptake in neurons, and increases the accumulation of toxic material in the brain. Obesity-associated inflammation augments the deleterious effects of insulin resistance.[38]

In humans, calorie restriction induces major improvements in factors strongly implicated in the development and progression of Alzheimer's disease, including insulin sensitivity, inflammation and oxidative stress, LDL-cholesterol, blood pressure and arterial stiffness.[39] An easier form of practising calorie restriction is intermittent fasting, which has also been shown to be successful in preventing cognitive deficits in mice and rats with a form of Alzheimer's disease.[40] A moderate reduction in protein intake has additionally been shown to improve age-related brain and cognitive changes.[41]

Further studies have examined the association between cognition and foods consumed, of which the most widely studied is the effect of the Mediterranean diet. There have been numerous observational studies and at least five randomised clinical trials examining the association between the Mediterranean diet and age-related cognition and Alzheimer's disease.[42,43] Overall, these trials showed improvements in some measures of cognition, and the Mediterranean diet reduced the risk of insulin resistance and type 2 diabetes in subjects with a higher adherence to a Mediterranean diet.[44]

PHYSICAL EXERCISE CAN HELP PREVENT DEMENTIA

Exercise has multiple benefits for the brain, including reducing stress, increasing neurotrophins, targeting inflammatory changes and improving vascularisation.[45] Data from two randomised clinical trials showed that six months of physical activity resulted in a modest but significant improvement in cognition in older people at risk of dementia, especially when combined with a healthier diet.[46,47] More recently, resistance training was found to improve cognitive function in older people with mild cognitive impairment.[48]

The good news is that the beneficial effects of regular physical activity on brain health can begin to accumulate in a short amount of time (as short as six months) even if started late in life, and these effects can be achieved with moderate levels of exercise. For example, the results of a six-month randomised clinical trial involving 60- to 79-year-old men and women demonstrated that aerobic-exercise training significantly increased grey and white matter volume in the prefrontal cortex.[49] This and other human studies show that aerobic exercise training can improve the function of the executive control network, so that our brain becomes more efficient, plastic and adaptive, which translates into better learning and performance.[50]

Another randomised clinical trial published in the prestigious journal *PNAS* shows that a seven-year aerobic exercise program increased hippocampal volume by 2 per cent, successfully reversing age-related loss in volume by one to two years.[51] The hippocampus is a key brain region involved in verbal memory and learning, and this explains why in this study spatial memory was significantly improved. This is consistent with observational data showing that older adults who are fit have larger hippocampal volumes.[52]

The mechanisms through which physical activity protect the brain and reduce the risk for cognitive impairment are not well known, but exercise training is known to augment the amount of blood flowing to the brain, in particular into the hippocampus.[53,54] For instance, it has been shown that walking at a fast pace for 50 minutes, three times a week for six months, can improve the neuronal plasticity and cognitive function even in patients with mild cognitive dysfunction.[55] We have discovered that when we exercise, the contracting muscle produces a hormone called cathepsin B that through the bloodstream reaches the brain. There, it stimulates the production of BDNF, a powerful neurotrophic hormone that promotes the growth of dendritic spines and new nerve cells from stem cells in some brain regions.[56] The result is an improvement of cognitive function and in the ability to memorise things.

QUALITY SLEEP LOWERS THE RISK FOR DEMENTIA

A growing body of evidence shows that adequate and uninterrupted sleep helps the brain repair itself. A good nights rest reduces cerebral inflammation and improves the function of brain cells (see page 218). Sleep plays a central role in many behavioural and physiological functions, including development, energy conservation, brain waste clearance, modulation of immune responses, cognition, performance and vigilance.

It is well established that disturbed sleep is highly prevalent in patients with Alzheimer's disease and plays a role in cognitive impairment.[57]

It is not surprising that sleep disturbance is also associated with diabetes, heart disease and stroke as well as cognitive dysfunction. 'Sleep disturbance' includes a range of issues, including abnormal sleep duration, fragmented sleep, poor sleep quality, insomnia and obstructive sleep apnoea. Importantly, increasing evidence suggests that sleep disturbance affects blood glucose.[58] A plethora of studies demonstrates that shorter sleep durations are associated with impaired glucose tolerance, as well as decreased insulin secretion and sensitivity.[59] Even in healthy people, resting only five hours per night for one week resulted in significantly reduced insulin sensitivity.[60]

Of concern is the fact that sleep disorders markedly increase in prevalence with ageing.[61] Up to 75 per cent of people over 65 years have obstructive sleep apnoea and 30 per cent report insomnia.[62] Hence, the importance of quality sleep in the prevention of dementia development. But more on that later.

THE IMPORTANCE OF STRONG SOCIAL RELATIONSHIPS

Active learning and strong social relationships are key weapons to fight cognitive decline. As we have already discussed, studies suggest that people who stay involved, keep their brain engaged and are willing to learn new tasks are better at processing information and have better memories. People who are curious and interested in many things tend to age much more slowly than people who become disengaged, isolated and refuse to try new things.

New data also suggest that participating in social activities, including cultural, artistic and sport activities, has a positive effect on brain function and lowers your risk of dementia.[63]

CHAPTER TWENTY

REST AND SLEEP QUALITY

While keeping our mind active and engaged is important for brain health, nonetheless we have to be careful to avoid overstimulation.

Excessive and prolonged mental work, similar to extreme physical exercise, is harmful. One of the tenets of traditional Chinese medicine is to balance 'activity with rest'. In the treatise *Medical Notes of the One Hundred Classical Schools* it is said that to preserve health, prevent sicknesses and promote longevity:

> *It is imperative to use both the mind and the body, alternate work with rest, and exercise with inertia. None of these activities must be neglected.*[1]

If we begin to perceive signs of mental fatigue (e.g. struggling to maintain concentration, experiencing drowsiness or blurred vision), we need to stop and rest, perhaps by taking a nap followed by a short walk. It is important to alternate mental with physical work.

That resting is vital to our health is further confirmed by the fact that we spend about a third of our life sleeping.

Li Yu, a doctor of the Qing dynasty, wrote: 'To stay fit we must give priority to sleep, which helps us regain the energy surplus'. He added: 'Sleep is the panacea that cures all diseases and saves thousands of lives'.[2]

We now know that just a few months of sleep deprivation can kill a human being. Patients suffering from a rare medical condition called 'fatal familial insomnia', develop a progressive inability to sleep that results in death in about nine months.[3]

Sleeping well every night is critical to health and survival, as much as the food and the water we ingest.

WHAT SCIENCE TELLS US HAPPENS WHEN WE FALL ASLEEP

With an electroencephalogram (EEG), we can measure the electrical activity in our brains.[4] When we are awake, for instance, and perform intellectual activities, low-voltage unsynchronised electric beta waves (8–30 microvolts) that occur with high frequency (13.5–30 hertzcycles per second) are typically detected. As soon as we fall asleep, the electrical brain activity progressively slows down.

Stage 1

During the first phase of sleep (stage 1 or NREM1), which normally lasts only a few minutes (typically less than ten minutes), the relatively unsynchronised beta brain waves are replaced by more synchronised and slower alpha waves with a frequency of 8–13 Hz, and then by theta waves with a frequency of 4–7 cycles per second. In this stage of very superficial, easily disrupted sleep, occasionally referred to as somnolence, the muscles are still quite active, our eyes roll around slowly and may open and close from time to time; breathing and heart rate start to slow down.

Stage 2

Then, we move swiftly into stage 2 (NREM2), during which muscles relax even further and our conscious awareness of the external world totally disappears. Neuronal background electrical activity in NREM2 is relatively low voltage with variable frequency, but close to theta waves (3–7 Hz), interspersed with short electrical spikes lasting 0.5–1 seconds (sigma waves) and K-complexes.

Stage 3

Finally, we move into stage 3 (NREM3), also known as delta or deep slow-wave sleep. During NREM3, we are even less responsive to the outside world: basically we are unaware of any sounds or other stimuli around us. In this stage, delta brain waves are synchronised and reach their maximum amplitude with a very slow speed (0.5–4 Hz). At this stage the metabolic activity and temperature of the brain, breathing and heart rate and blood pressure are drastically reduced. If we are abruptly awakened, we can remain in a dazed state for a few minutes, and may take up to 30 minutes before we can reach normal mental performance.

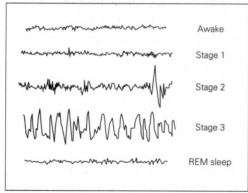

Figure 27: Stages of sleep

REM sleep

After NREM3, roughly between 70–90 minutes after falling asleep, we enter REM sleep, and we start dreaming. In fact, electrical waves at this stage are mixed but mostly alpha and beta types, typical of the awake state. During a night of 7–10 hours of sleep, we are typically going through four or six cycles of REM sleep, 80–100 minutes apart. As the night goes by, the length of the period in which we are in REM sleep increases and slow-wave sleep decreases. Normally, most of the deep sleep in stage 3 takes place in the early hours of the night, while REM sleep predominates in the last part, before awakening. This has implications for the timing of certain sleep disorders. For example, sleep walking (somnambulism) occurs during slow-wave sleep and therefore usually manifests in the first half of the sleep period.

BENEFITS OF SLEEP

Modern science has confirmed the importance of sleep in regenerating the brain and has started to explain the mechanisms. For instance, during deep slow-wave sleep there is an activation of functions that help the neurons to remove toxic metabolites, which have been accumulated during the day.[5] In addition, it seems that sleeping exerts an anti-inflammatory effect[6-8] and improves the efficiency of the immune system, reducing the risk of infections.[9-11]

Information processing and memory consolidation (particularly of things like facts and events) also takes place during this deep slow-wave sleeping period. Sleeping deeply helps us to consolidate in our memory all the key information that we have learned during the day.[12,13] If something important occurs during the day, our brain strengthens the experience (and related emotions) about this event overnight while we are resting.

During the first few hours of rest there is an activation of mechanisms that increase brain plasticity and the formation of new synaptic protrusions.[14] A new study suggests that delta slow-wave sleep improves the consolidation of long-term memory by inhibiting the dopaminergic activity of neurons. In contrast, an excessive excitement of neurons during wakefulness (beta waves) accelerates the oblivion of newly acquired information through an activation of dopaminergic activity.[15]

Sleep deprivation, and particularly disruption of slow-wave deep sleep, can disrupt the ability to encode and consolidate new memories[16-19] and impairs the strength and quality of learning.[20] In one study, research volunteers were asked to solve some mathematical problems, but concealed deep within the formula was a hidden rule.

Approximately 23 per cent of the volunteers discovered it. However, the number of subjects who were able to successfully solve the problem soared to 59 per cent in those who were allowed to sleep on it for eight hours,[21] suggesting that sleep sets the stage for the emergence of insight.

Simply put, if we do not sleep soundly, we fail to fix in our minds some of the knowledge we have acquired during the day. The sensory perceptions and notions that have been saved into the transitory memory (similar to the RAM memory of our computers) of an area of the brain called the hippocampus will be deleted, rather than being saved onto the hard disk of the brain.[22]

During sleep, and probably also during deep meditation, our brain behaves more similarly to our computer, that is, it is able to run multiple programs at once. Typically, our conscious awareness can concentrate on only one entity at a time. The magic moment that all of us experience when we have been trying hard to recall the name of a person and 50 minutes later it hits our mind is not fortuitous. Only during deep sleeping or meditation can we overcome this limitation, and the brake that limits our imagination comes off. Only then, the prefrontal cortex, which normally performs as a traffic controller, and consciously decides which thoughts or concepts are appropriate or forbidden, literally goes to sleep.

Howard Nusbaum, a neuroscientist at the University of Chicago, explains this concept better: 'if during the day we are looking for a new idea to solve a complicated problem or task, typically we keep ruminating, until most likely we end up using the most familiar one; but if we sleep, a better solution can materialize in our mind'.

In terms of stimulating creativity, the sensory experiences that stimulate our neurons every day – colours, smells, sounds, tastes and perceptions – if consolidated in our long-term memory (thanks to the slow-wave sleep), can suddenly emerge when needed in the form of flashes of intuition and creativity. Intuition, as we will see later, is that kind of instant knowledge that does not make use of reasoning or sensible information, and it is typical of artists and people of genius.

> TIP: Some new data suggest that, as with sleep, even short periods of wakeful rest can help consolidate our memories. When you are having a busy day at work, schedule 10–15 minute periods of rest during the day – to sit quietly and relax. This will certainly boost your mental performance and enhance your ability to master new information.[23]

SLOW-WAVE SLEEP DISRUPTION PROMOTES DEMENTIA

It is said that 'a good night's sleep refreshes the mind and strengthen the body, and a poor night's sleep can do just the opposite'. As already noted accumulating preclinical studies have started to support this old saying, and have shown that sleep deprivation and fragmentation not only harms the process of memory consolidation, but also increases the risk of developing Alzheimer's disease.[24]

In experimental mice, sleep deprivation acutely increases circulating amyloid beta and if the deprivation becomes chronic amyloid plaques and tau tangles accumulate.[25,26] Scientists have long associated accumulations of amyloid plaques and tau tangles with the development of Alzheimer's and other dementias.

In humans, it has been shown that one night of total sleep deprivation elevates soluble amyloid beta,[27] and a more recent clinical study on 17 middle-aged healthy adults without sleep disorders has shown that the disruption of slow-wave sleep induced an acute rise of amyloid beta in the brain.[28] In this study the disruption of slow-wave activity was achieved by delivering progressively increasing tones through earphones to the participants, so that they were forced out of slow-wave delta sleep. In the same experiment, it was shown that a more prolonged disruption of sleep quality, but not sleep quantity, correlated with a surge in another deleterious brain protein, called tau, which has been linked to brain damage.[29,30]

A GROWING NUMBER OF PEOPLE ARE NOT SLEEPING ENOUGH
- Approximately 35 per cent of adults sleep less than seven hours.
- About 48 per cent have trouble falling or staying asleep, one or more nights a week.
- Around 38 per cent unintentionally fall asleep during the day at least once a month.

Sleeping less than the recommended amount is linked to an increased risk of developing several chronic clinical conditions. For instance, sleep deprivation is associated with a higher risk of obesity, diabetes mellitus, hypertension and cardiovascular disease.[31-33] A lack of sleep has also severe consequences on mental health, because it is a major risk factor for stress, depression, burnout and anxiety disorders.[34,35] Finally, chronic sleep loss dramatically increases the risk of work-related injuries and accidents; it negatively impacts decision-making, productivity and creativity.[36,37]

HOW MANY HOURS SHOULD WE SLEEP?

There is no magic number of hours that works for everyone. Recent findings indicate that sleep need is under genetic control. The most important thing is that sleep should be deep and restful. We should be getting up in the morning regenerated, with a recharged and invigorated mind.

We know that babies sleep a lot: typically 16 to 17 hours a day, with a high proportion of REM sleep, which is thought to aid brain development. By age four, sleep duration has reduced to 12 hours, and then to 8 to 10 hours from ten years up.[38] A young adult sleeps on average 7 to 8 hours per day: 20–28 per cent in REM sleep, 4–5 per cent in NREM1, 46–50 per cent in NREM2, and 16–24 per cent in NREM3.

The duration of both REM and NREM3 sleep decline with the passing years. For instance, a three-year-old child spends about 17 per cent of the night in stage 3, which drops to a only 4.5 per cent in 70-year-old adults. Some studies even suggest that in some elderly people sleep in phase 3 and the corresponding delta activity are completely absent,[39] and it is becoming appreciated that this premature reduction in slow-wave sleep may be a 'biomarker' of premature brain ageing.

Interestingly, young people who sleep little (six hours a day or less) spend the same time in stage 3 sleep as those who sleep a lot (nine hours or more). They compensate by reducing the time sleeping in NREM1-2, while long sleepers spend more time in stage 2 and REM.[40] Studies conducted in those aged in their 70s suggest that individuals who sleep fewer hours tend to be more efficient and hard-working, while long sleepers are more anxious, depressed and isolated.[41]

HOW TO IMPROVE YOUR SLEEP QUALITY

As mentioned earlier, the number of hours we spend in NREM3 is a predictor of memory consolidation, brain health and regeneration.

Here are some tips to improve sleep quality:

Avoid using devices emitting blue light at night

Accumulating evidence suggest that *blue* light emitted from LED screens and other electronic devices contributes to the epidemic of sleep disorders and insomnia, because it disrupts the circadian rhythm of your brain. Data from a randomised clinical trial show that the use of blue light smartphones at night (from 7.30 to 10 pm) negatively influences sleep quality. The users of LED screen devices in this study had higher body temperatures and cortisol levels, and took a longer time to reach dim light melatonin onset.[42] A study published in *The Lancet Psychiatry* shows that people with disruption of circadian rhythmicity experienced an increased risk of lifetime major depressive and bipolar disorders, greater mood instability, higher neuroticism and unhappiness.[43] I recommend you switch off all electronic devices at least an hour before bedtime, and if possible to go to bed at more or less the same time every day.

Exercise training

Several studies have shown that exercise training increases the time we spend in deep sleep and the ability to memorise things.[44] In a clinical study of 12-year-old boys, two sessions of intense exercise (85–90 per cent of maximum heart rate) were sufficient to increase the time spent in NREM3, reducing NREM2 and the time required to fall asleep.[45] In another study, three weeks of daily 30-minute exercise training in the morning significantly increased the duration of sleep in stage 3 in a group of 18-year-old boys.[46] A similar beneficial effect of exercise on deep sleep was also noticed in another study conducted on elderly people living in a nursing home.[47]

Timing of exercise training seems to be important as well. Training hard in the evening has been reported to impair sleep quality.[48] Exercising during the morning enhances the following night's sleep.

Meditation and yoga

A growing body of evidence indicate that Hatha yoga with meditation can significantly improve sleep quality. In a large randomised clinical trial of 410 cancer survivors suffering from sleep disruption, a four-week yoga program consisting of two 75-minute sessions per week of Hatha yoga, breathing exercises (pranayama) and meditation resulted in improvements in sleep quality, and a 21 per cent reduction in the use of sleep medications.[49] The mechanism through which yoga improves sleep quality is not clear, but preliminary scientific studies suggest that 30-minute cycles of Hatha yoga practised twice a day (e.g. a series of yoga poses interspersed with relaxation asana) induce a significant increase in delta slow-wave sleep and a reduction of REM sleep.[50-52]

Learning

The intriguing thing that we recently discovered is that the duration and intensity of delta waves during NREM3 are an excellent marker of the daily amount of brain stimulation. It has been shown that learning a new visual-motor task causes a compensatory increase of delta waves in the cerebral area that had been previously stimulated by learning. This increase, in turn, causes a rise in the ability to remember the task.[53-55] In other words, a way to improve the quality of sleep is to keep the brain alert and active during the day by mastering new skills and concepts that stimulate the growth of new synaptic protrusions.

Listening to pink noise

Acoustic stimulation with pulses of pink noise, which closely mimic sounds found in nature, can increase slow-wave deep sleep activity and improve word-pair recall in young and older adults.[56] The frequency profile of pink noise (i.e. each octave carries an equal amount of noise energy) has the same fluctuations found in all sorts of natural phenomena, including waterfalls, heart beats, the firing of neurons, and even quasars. In a clinical study of 40 participants the exposure to pink noise significantly reduced brain wave complexity, while inducing more stable sleep time and improvement of sleep quality.[57]

CHAPTER TWENTY-ONE

MINDFULNESS MEDITATION: LEARNING TO LIVE IN THE PRESENT

We live in a world where many things are constantly competing for our attention and it's easy to be distracted and unfocused. We think that to be successful, we have to be busy all the time with as many tasks and projects as possible, rather than find time to rest and be absorbed by the beauty of simple things in life.

The word 'mindfulness', which has become extremely popular nowadays, is nothing but the translation of an ancient concept, rooted in the philosophy of Zen Buddhism. It means being conscious, focused and aware. Nyanaponika Thera (1901–94), a famous Buddhist monk, defines mindfulness as 'a condition of clear and unflinching awareness of what actually happens around and within us in the aftermath of the perception'.

According to Thich Nhat Hanh, poet, pacifist and one of the most important living Zen masters:

> *Mindfulness is the awakening of our consciousness in the reality of the present moment. The miracle by which we instantly recall our dispersed mind and we restore it in its entirety, so that we can live every single moment of our life.*[1]

In his book *Meditations*, the powerful Roman Emperor Marcus Aurelius, who was also a Stoic philosopher, recommended:

Manage any single action, word and thought as if at any moment life can end.[2]

Even the ancient Chinese doctors knew about the importance of awareness and attention. Cao Tingdong, in his book *Aphorisms on Gerontology*, wrote:

When we use our mind, let us not engage it simultaneously on multiple tasks; otherwise, the attention will be diverted, causing damage from overexertion. Let's focus only on a single goal at a time, so that we can avoid mental stress, because our attention is focalised and our mental activities concentrated.[3]

The first to use some of these philosophical concepts in Western medical practice was Jon Kabat-Zinn, a professor of the Massachusetts School of Medicine. In 1979 he founded a clinic for psychological stress management, and developed a program called *Mindfulness-based stress reduction*, readapting some Zen principles which highlight the importance of carefully observing all events, moment by moment, as they are, without filtering them through our mind, without labelling them as 'positive' or 'negative'. Meditation is a key part of mindfulness.

MINDFULNESS EXERCISES: THE ART OF NOW

Mindfulness exercises are based on two components:

1. focusing attention on the present moment (moment-to-moment awareness)

2. facing all new experiences with curiosity and open-mindedness, without judgment, without trying to change their meaning, even if they are perceived as unpleasant.

The purpose of the exercises is to get used to carefully observing, without filtering our feelings and thoughts, or judging or categorising them as good or bad. With practice we learn how to perform every action by focusing on the present moment, without lingering in the past or worrying about the future. Any time we feel distracted by the arrival of new images or thoughts, we refocus our attention on breathing, and go back to the observation of our breath, so we can be fully in the moment.

MINDFULNESS COMBATS 'CONSTANTLY THINKING DISORDER'

Too many people are unaware of how stress or anxiety works in their brain. They are constantly thinking even when trying to relax in bed. Their mind keeps 'going' and sometimes this obsessive thinking can drive them into a negative spiral, a dark hole. They fear every possible negative affect and that anything and everything could lead to failure or loss. They live their days not paying attention to what is happening within and around them.

Mindfulness can be instrumental in overcoming these harmful psychological processes. Experiments suggest that learning to observe our thoughts, instead of being carried away by them, improves awareness and subjective wellbeing. Negative emotions, moodiness, worrying and stress are reduced, while the level of self-esteem and life satisfaction are increased.[4]

The practice of mindfulness also has beneficial effects in preventing or addressing some more serious psychiatric conditions. The scientific studies conducted by Kabat-Zinn and other experimental psychologists have confirmed that the practice of mindfulness has positive results in the treatment of chronic stress, panic attacks, agoraphobia and depression.[5-9] These meditative exercises could also have a potential effect in treating insomnia,[10] bulimia[11] and fibromyalgia nervosa.[12]

INNER SERENITY TIME: HOW TO BEGIN

Starting to practise mindfulness on a regular basis is essential if we want to develop a state of inner calm and peace of mind. Learning to be aware enhances our self-care and self-respect, teaches us to treat ourselves with kindness, and is essential if we are to recognise that we are not our thoughts. We need to be able to observe whatever happens in our life from a wider perspective. This will change the way we live our life. People who develop such a state, when faced with stressful, sad or depressing experiences tend to be more resilient and not to be so easily discouraged.

Cultivating our emotional and psychological wellbeing is as important as promoting our metabolic and physical health. It reduces the risk of engaging in unhealthy behaviours, like getting drunk and over-eating. If we are metabolically healthy, we can better resist infections and other diseases. Likewise, if our mind is balanced and resilient, we won't be pulled down by adversities and negative experiences.

Meditation may cross-fertilise with diet or exercise training in promoting emotional stability and mood resilience via multiple metabolic pathways, including neurotrophic factors such as BDNF.[13-15] Body and mind influence each other.

Mindfulness can be taught and practised by anyone, even children. A pilot study in kindergarten children has shown that mindfulness caused a significant improvement in sociability, reduced aggression and selfishness, and an increased expression of gratitude, kindness to themselves and others, and a natural flair for goodness.[16] Students who have benefited from these programs seemed to also achieve at higher levels academically and experience less emotional distress. It is essential that our children learn to read and do maths, but also how to deal with their emotions, as do we all.

The mechanism through which these mindfulness exercises act is unclear, but it is not *only* due to relaxation, as some critics claim. In a study of 40 students practising a series of mindfulness exercises (20 minutes a day for an entire week), unlike simple relaxation, significantly increased the attention span and reduced conflict, anxiety, and symptoms of depression and fatigue.[17] Some preliminary data suggest that these exercises might also change the plasticity of certain areas of the brain,[18] enhancing the ability to process and store data.[19-21] Much more research is needed, but for now, we think that these exercises can modify the organisation of our mental processes by increasing introspection, self-control, self-understanding and self-acceptance.[22]

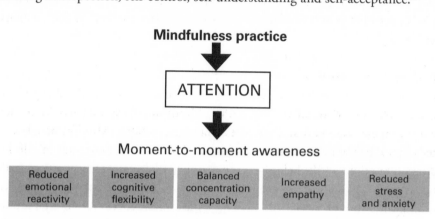

Figure 28: Mindfulness outcomes

TEN BENEFITS OF MINDFULNESS MEDITATION

Here are ten scientifically proven benefits of mindfulness meditation:

1. Enhanced concentration capacity. Most people lack the ability to focus on what's important and to let go of all of the internal and external distractions that are unrelated to the task at hand. Practising mindfulness can help you to improve this ability. One study showed that experienced meditators perform better on all measures of attention and have increased information-processing speed.[23] In another study, three months of intensive meditation training enhanced attentional stability.[24]

2. Decreased stress and anxiety. Stress is the physiologic reaction to a threat, while anxiety is a reaction to stress itself. Chronic stress and anxiety result in irritability, muscle tension, headaches, poor concentration and sleepless nights, and can also affect health by increasing blood pressure, heart rate and the risk of developing a heart attack. Performing regular aerobic exercise is very effective in reducing stress and anxiety, but mindful meditation has also been shown to decrease overall levels of tension and anxiety, elevate and stabilise mood, and improve sleep quality.[25,26]

3. Reduced negative thoughts. Cognitive rumination consists of repetitively thinking about the causes, consequences and symptoms of one's negative emotions without finding a solution.[27] When someone is depressed, the ruminative thoughts are usually about being inadequate or useless. The repetition and the sensation of inadequacy increase anxiety, which interferes with solving the problem. A study published in the prestigious journal *Science* has shown that people who spend their time ruminating over past or future events are much more unhappy than those living in the present and able to focus their attention primarily on the things they are doing.[28] Other studies have demonstrated that people who do mindfulness meditation ruminate less, an effect that is maintained even one month after the end of the meditation intervention.[29]

4. Reduced emotional reactivity. Fast recovery from emotional challenges and better tolerance to negative emotions, such as sadness, anger, disgust, guilt and fear, are emblems of sound mental health. Mindfulness training has been shown to improve these outcomes and increases emotional stability. Mindful people are in better control of their emotions. In one study, for instance, practising mindfulness meditation for eight weeks helped people to gain insight into their emotions and to reduce physical distress, anxiety and depression induced by watching sad movies.[30] Practising mindfulness teaches us to observe, face and govern our emotions and to become more capable at handling anxiety, fear, anger and other emotions that poison our wellbeing.

5. Increased flexible thinking. Cognitive flexibility is the capacity of our mind to adapt quickly and successfully to new and unanticipated environmental conditions. We can think of cognitive flexibility as being akin to changing gears in our car, but think of the gears as 'streams-of-thought' and the car as your 'brain'. If you are stuck in one gear and can't change it – your thinking is inflexible; your stream-of-thought cannot be upgraded or altered. However, if you can rapidly change the gear as needed, you possess greater cognitive flexibility. Practising mindfulness meditation reduces our emotional reactivity (our overreaction to events), but also increases our flexibility about the situation by disengaging the automatic previous learning and enabling new thinking in fresh ways.[31]

6. Enhancement of working memory. Working memory is similar to a computer's RAM memory and allows the brain to temporarily store and manage new information, while carrying out complex thinking tasks, such as learning, reasoning and comprehension. Improvements to working memory appear to be another benefit of mindfulness meditation. The improvement is pretty rapid, as only four days of meditation training have been shown to be sufficient to improve visual and spatial processing, working memory and executive functioning.[32]

7. Improved relationship satisfaction. Relationship satisfaction is the capacity to adapt well to relationship stress and the ability to share our thoughts and communicate our emotions with our partner, close relatives or friends. Mindfulness meditation can improve our capacity to express our emotions freely and in a more authentic manner. Practising it on a regular basis seems to enhance a couples' level of relationship satisfaction, closeness, acceptance of one another, and autonomy, while reducing relationship distress and conflict. People who practise mindfulness on a given day experience several consecutive days of improved levels of relationship happiness and less stress.[33] This leads to deeper and more meaningful relationships with our family members and friends.

8. Increased empathy. Empathy can be defined as the 'selfless' ability to understand another person's thoughts and feelings and behave in a more compassionate manner. Several scientific studies suggest that mindfulness meditation promotes our capacity for empathic understanding by enhancing unconditional, positive emotional states of warm-heartedness and compassion.[34] Neuroimaging studies suggest that meditation can increase activation of certain brain areas that control emotional processing and empathy.

9. Enhanced self-compassion. Mindfulness training also boosts self-compassion or self-love. By regularly practising mindfulness we can learn to act more kindly towards ourselves when encountering suffering and personal limitations, rather than disregarding them or damaging ourselves with excessive self-criticism. Individuals with self-compassion experience greater health, social connectedness, emotional intelligence and happiness, and less anxiety, shame and fear of failure.[35]

10. Improved quality of life. Mindful people tend to have greater intuition and self-insight, functions that improve wellbeing and quality of life. In a clinical study of primary care physicians, an abbreviated mindfulness-training course improved job satisfaction, quality of life and wellbeing, while reducing stress, attrition and the risk of job burnout.[36]

HOW NEGATIVE EMOTIONS AFFECT OUR WELLBEING

The detrimental effects of sustained negative emotions have been known since antiquity. Sun Simiao, a famous Chinese physician of the Sui and Tang dynasties, wrote in his book *Qian Jin Yi Fang* (*Supplement to the Formulas of a Thousand Gold Worth*) that:

A wise man should avoid surrendering to anxiety, anger, suffering and
unnecessary words. He should also try not to be impatient in satisfying
his own desires and avoid feeding feelings of hostility for prolonged
periods of time.[37]

Modern science has confirmed that persistent negative emotions and psychological stress, such as work and marital stress or caring for a sick relative, have harmful consequences on cardiovascular health.[38]

Anger and hostility also have negative influences on blood pressure, and on the function of the arteries and the heart. In experimental animals, chronic stress induces fibrosis of the heart and increased plaque formation in the coronary arteries.[39] Data from the prospective Atherosclerosis Risk in Communities Study (ARIC) show that people who get angry easily have a greater risk of dying from cardiovascular disease, independent of other classic cardiovascular risk factors.[40] And in the INTERHEART study, another large observational study, psychosocial factors (e.g. perceived stress, depression) were the third most important risk factors for heart attacks, after smoking and elevated cholesterol.[41]

Our 'negative emotions', like anger, grief and sadness, however, should not be ignored or bottled up. Emotional suppression results in amplification and the negative emotions get stronger. It is important, instead, that we learn to control our negative emotions with a mindful approach. When something makes us angry or anxious, we should take a pause and meditate. We should observe our emotions, delineate their contours, and then ask ourselves what is more important: the thing that makes us angry and nervous or our health? In an instant, if we are wise, these feelings should wear off.

Liu Yan Shi, a doctor in the Song dynasty, in his book *Speeches of Sun* tells the story of an officer called Lin Ying, who although he was 70 years old, looked like a man in his forties. When asked what his secret was, he replied:

The main thing is that I never get nervous about anything. Even if
I were running out of food tomorrow, I wouldn't worry about it.
Whatever happens to me, I gently cast it away from my thoughts and I
don't let it penetrate my heart, therefore feeling always quiet.[42]

In this respect, the Stoic philosopher and Emperor Marcus Aurelius, who was the most powerful man on earth during the 2nd century AD and controlled the life of millions of people, wrote:

When you find yourself forced, as it were into some confusion or
disturbance, by surrounding facts or objects, return into yourself as

speedily as you can; and depart no more from the true harmony of the soul, than what is absolutely unavoidable. You shall acquire greater power of retaining this harmony, by having frequent recourse to it.[43]

Persistent negative emotions and psychological stress also have a huge influence on metabolic and immune health. Acute mental stress causes an increased production of the stress hormone cortisol and a powerful activation of the sympathetic nervous system accompanied by a two- to six-fold increase in blood chatecholamines.[44] High cortisol and chatecholamines elevate blood pressure, increase inflammation and oxidative stress, and impair the function of the immune system.[45,46] Several studies have also shown that stress and negative emotions can have profound effects on several metabolic pathways that control glucose and energy levels as well as longevity.[47] For instance, mice with a deletion of the AC5 gene, in which the stress effect of chatecholamines is blunted, not only are protected against cardiac ageing and cancer, but live 30 per cent longer.[48,49]

Cultivating optimism

Of course, everyone experiences negativity, anger, jealousy, hate or frustration. Even 'negative emotions' have a role in our life. In *Tao Te Ching (The Book of the Way and Virtue)*,* the Bible of Taoism, Lao Tzu wrote:

Under heaven, all can see beauty as beauty, only because there is ugliness. All can know good as good, only because there is evil. Therefore, having and not having rise together, difficult and easy complement each other. High and low rest upon each other. Front and back follow one another.

However, negative emotions should not be allowed to dominate our life. We should try to balance them with 'positive emotions', such as positivity, enthusiasm, kindness and compassion. Maintaining a good mood and having an optimistic view of life is crucial for preventing disease and promoting health and longevity.

A study published in the journal *Circulation* demonstrates that optimism is associated with a reduced risk of developing cardiovascular disease and tumours, and of dying prematurely. In contrast, cynical and hostile people showed a higher risk of mortality, especially for cancer.[50]

But be careful of 'artificial optimism' promoted by a positivity culture that encourages limitless positive thought as the key to a happy life, and suggests we put

---

*   Stan Rosenthal's lucid and beautiful translation of the *Tao Te Ching* (1984) is my favourite. It can be found free online: http://enlight.lib.ntu.edu.tw/FULLTEXT/JR-AN/an142304.pdf

aside our feelings and emotions. This is not healthy either. Optimism should be based on the ability to deal with the world as it is, not as we *wish* it to be in an unrealistic way. We cannot disregard what happens in our life with its accompanying emotions by embracing false or fake positivity.

WHAT IS YOUR LEVEL OF MINDFULNESS?

Are you mindful? Do you live in the present? You can evaluate your state of mindfulness by using the questions of the MAAS (Mindful, Attention and Awareness Scale) designed in 2003 by Professors Kirk W. Brown of the Virginia Commonwealth University and Richard M. Ryan of the University of Rochester.[51]

Mindful, Attention and Awareness Scale questions						
How aware are you? Rate statements on a scale from 1 – almost always – to 6 – almost never						
1. I could be experiencing some emotion and not be conscious of it until sometime later	1	2	3	4	5	6
2. I break or spill things because of carelessness, not paying attention, or thinking of something else	1	2	3	4	5	6
3. I find it difficult to stay focused on what's happening in the present	1	2	3	4	5	6
4. I tend to walk quickly to get where I'm going without paying attention to what I experience along the way	1	2	3	4	5	6
5. I tend not to notice feelings of physical tension or discomfort until they really grab my attention	1	2	3	4	5	6
6. I forget a person's name almost as soon as I've been told it for the first time	1	2	3	4	5	6
7. It seems if I am 'running on automatic' without much awareness of what I'm doing	1	2	3	4	5	6
8. I rush through activities without being really attentive to them	1	2	3	4	5	6
9. I get so focused on the goal I want to achieve that I lose touch with what I am doing right now to get there	1	2	3	4	5	6
10. I do jobs or tasks automatically, without being aware of what I'm doing	1	2	3	4	5	6
11. I find myself listening to someone with one ear, doing something else at the same time	1	2	3	4	5	6
12. I drive places on 'automatic pilot' and then wonder why I went there	1	2	3	4	5	6
13. I find myself preoccupied with the future or the past	1	2	3	4	5	6
14. I find myself doing things without paying attention	1	2	3	4	5	6
15. I snack without being aware that I'm eating	1	2	3	4	5	6

The accompanying 6-point scale is 1 = almost always, 2 = very frequently, 3 = somewhat frequently, 4 = somewhat infrequently, 5 = very infrequently, and 6 = almost never.[52]

Table 9: Mindful attention and awareness scale questions

In the questionnaire above are 15 statements concerning everyday experiences. Using a scale of 1 – almost always – to 6 – almost never – score how frequently or infrequently you have each experience. Try to respond according to what really reflects your experience, rather than thinking about giving the 'best' answer. At the end of the test, calculate the average of the 15 score.

A high score indicates receptive attentiveness and more present awareness of experiences as they happen. A low score indicates an absence of attention and awareness of what is occurring in the present.

Everyone can benefit from mindfulness exercises to improve their level of attention and awareness and reduce their tendency to experience life on automatic.

MINDFULNESS EXERCISES

Setting up a life-altering meditation practice is easier than you might think. First of all, we can practise mindfulness at any time. For instance, I try to practice mindfulness as I walk to work or cycle in the park, while I am doing housework or mowing the lawn, so that attention and awareness increasingly become inherent modes of living my life, 'a mode of being'.

At the beginning, however, it may be a good idea to do these simple exercises in a silent place, seated on a chair or lying in bed. If possible, schedule a set time to practise each day; for instance, first thing in the morning, before starting your day.

You should begin by observing your breathing. For three minutes, focus your full attention on the air entering through your nose, your ribcage expanding and contracting, and the air flowing in and out your body. Observe without judging, be merely a spectator of your breathing. You do not have to change the rhythm. Remember that the goal is only to observe, without intervening.

If during this exercise, you realise that your mind is wandering, just be aware of this, and try to bring your thoughts back gently to paying attention to your breathing. The realisation that your mind was wandering is a good example of meta-awareness, a clear awareness of the moment-to-moment content of your consciousness.

Another mindfulness exercise that I love to practise is to observe nature. If you are in a garden or park, choose something around you to focus on, for example a bird, some leaves fluttering in the wind or a cloud moving across the sky. Look carefully for two or three minutes, without doing anything. Then relax and try to bring your mind into harmony with the object that you are focused on. It is like shining a lamp into a dark chamber. Your attention can be moved from one object to another and can be focused within as well as outside.

A third exercise is to pay attention to the sensations you experience when you drink or eat something like a piece of fruit. For instance, carefully observe a strawberry, how it has grown, its colour and shape. Appreciate its texture with your fingers, and bring it to your nose and notice its aroma. Take note of the thoughts that are evoked by touching or smelling the fruit. Then, put it to your lips and think about the feelings that come with it. Let it slip into your mouth and start to eat it gently and slowly, tasting and experiencing all the flavours that are released from the fruit. The same exercise can be done while sipping a cup of green tea, mint tea or a rosemary infusion. Try to analyse the different sensations, the varied aromas contained in these varieties of herbal teas arouse in you.

These incredibly easy exercises should make you more aware of just how often simple acts such as breathing, walking, eating or drinking are lived in automatic, without any awareness or connection to the experience.

Learning to 'live every moment of our life consciously' or 'mindfully' is an amazing way to rediscover the world, to experience everything in a revitalised way, as if it is the first time, with a childlike curiosity, taking nothing for granted.

Lastly, at the end of a mindfulness session, I always perform three to five minutes of deep diaphragmatic breathing (see page 186). Experimental data have shown that taking deep slow breaths has a pervasive calming effect.

Our grandmothers were correct when they told us to take a deep breath when we were upset. For the scientifically minded, deep breaths inhibit a tiny group of breathing-related neurons that communicate with the brain's arousal centre.[48] The inhibition of the arousal area results in the suppression of signals to numerous other portions of our brain that are responsible for vigilance and anxiety.

MINDFULNESS IS A PRECIOUS INSTRUMENT TO BOOST CREATIVITY

By learning to observe and perceive with attention all the things that happen around us – such as the shape, texture, smell and colour of a rose, or the feel of the air as it caresses our skin – we stimulate new synaptic connections that integrate and store new multi-sensory experiences and strengthen our brain plasticity.

As we travel through the world, observing with attention and curiosity all that we encounter on our journey, we accumulate in our brain an ocean of experiences, concepts, colours, sounds, scents and flavours. All of this information that is deposited deep in our minds forms the basis of our creative intelligence, and at the right time can be recalled, allowing us to create something unique and rare.

Steve Jobs, the founder of Apple, said:

> *Creativity is simply linking things. When you ask creative people how they have created something, usually they feel a little guilty because they do not know how to explain it. They simply 'saw' something. It becomes normal for them after a while, because they are able to connect the dots of all the experiences they have had and with those to synthesise new*

*things. People who have had few experiences, however, do not have
enough dots to be connected, and therefore end up with very flat and
banal solutions, because they lack a broad perspective. The greater our
awareness and understanding of human experience, the better the result.*

People who are distracted and unaware, miss the opportunity to connect with our
wondrous world, and therefore suffer the choices imposed by others, whether they are
vested interests and corporations that control information, or just those who prey on
our desires and fears.

Through the exercise of attention, awareness and consciousness, we become wiser
in choosing the lifestyle we need to keep us healthy and happy, in selecting the friends
with whom we can build a community and share positive values, and in connecting
with our precious environment and splendid planet.

CHAPTER TWENTY-TWO

FAMILY, HAPPINESS AND A FUTURE WITHOUT FEAR

Humans are social animals and congregate together in communities.

In the *I Ching* it is written:

> *Water flows to unite with water, because all parts of it are subject to the same laws. So too should human society hold together through a community of interests that allows each individual to feel himself a member of a whole. The central power of a social organisation must see to it that every member finds that his true interest lies in holding together with it.*[1]

The Indian sage Patañjali thought that the wise man, the one who is in search of insight and enlightenment, must learn to live in society as a happy, functional and useful individual in order to purify and to control his own mind.

THE IMPORTANCE OF FAMILY, FRIENDS AND COMMUNITY

Positive social relationships and friendship have been shown to play a key role in promoting metabolic, emotional and mental health.[2] The sense of belonging to a group is a fundamental psychological need for most.[3] In contrast, social isolation and lack of ties with other individuals are perceived as painful sensations.[4] Generally speaking, people connected into a rich social network of friends and relatives have lower levels of anxiety and depression, are healthier and have a lower mortality than those who are socially isolated. Other studies suggest that socially connected people have greater empathy for others and are more trusting and supportive.

One of the features of centenarians living in Okinawa and Sardinia is the strong sense of belonging to the family and to a broader social group of friends that supports and endorses uplifting thoughts and goals (see page 11). Not surprisingly, the premature mortality in happily married people is less than in unmarried ones.[5]

The mechanisms through which social relations seem to boost metabolic health are many. It turns out, for example, that the psychological wellbeing that we experience when we feel loved, inhibits inflammation and positively influences our immune response against infections.[6,7]

Multiple studies have shown that social isolation and loneliness are associated with an increased risk of mortality from heart attack. In an analysis conducted on 1290 patients who had undergone coronary bypass surgery, postoperative survival at 30 days and five years was much lower in those who had responded positively to the question, 'Are you lonely?', regardless of other cardiometabolic risk factors.[8] Part of the adverse effects associated with social isolation would seem to be linked to psychological stress and depression, which are potent risk factors for heart attack and stroke. These two conditions, increase inflammation and cause an increase in blood pressure and heart rate.[9,10]

Having many friends, and being a part of a community then, is important. Yet the *quality* of our friendships is also important. In the *I Ching* it is written:

> *In friendships and close relationships an individual must make a careful*
> *choice. He surrounds himself either with good or with bad company;*
> *he cannot have both at once. If he throws himself away on unworthy*
> *friends, he loses connection with people of intellectual power who could*
> *further him in the good.*

As social animals, we find positive friendships are a key to our wellbeing.

KNOWING OURSELVES: THE WAY TO DO IS BEING

Living longer by itself is of no importance to me. I have met many people obsessed with their body image and physical immortality. Some have even purchased an expensive life insurance policy to cover the cryopreservation costs of their whole body or 'neuro' (head only), hoping that, in the future, science will be able to revive them, so that they will live again.

But to what end?

What is the meaning of life?

Who are we? Why are we here and where are we going?

Where do we come from? What comes after death?

Do heaven and hell really exist?

Are we simply more evolved animals, who are born only to pass on our genes to future generations, but at the total and complete mercy of events, emotions, passions and instinctual impulses?

I personally believe that some people have completely misunderstood the real meaning of human existence, and do not comprehend the eternal laws that regulate all life in the Universe. This life, if properly lived, can be the gateway to self-realisation, freedom and enlightenment.

THE STREAM OF LIFE

Each one of us is born in a precise place and historical time, bound to an intricate net of biological, cultural, social and religious worldviews. As soon as we are born, the journey in our unique little world unfolds.

'Know thyself' was written in large letters on the portal of the Temple of Apollo built in the 7th century BCE at Delphi, one of the most important religious centres of ancient Greece. In this way, the pilgrims who entered the temple to interrogate Apollo's oracle were invited to reflect upon the importance of their 'inner search' for the ultimate discovery of truth and freedom.

To know ourselves, we need to understand who we really are, what our limitations, strengths, innate skills, and motivations and potentials are. A more in-depth understanding of our 'true self' can lead to greater self-awareness, self-esteem, self-acceptance and freedom. In contrast, a distorted vision of reality and of ourselves is one of the major causes of suffering, anxiety and discomfort that seriously affects people's daily lives and wellbeing.

MAXIMISING OUR POTENTIAL: LIVING ACCORDING TO OUR OWN NATURE

Knowing ourselves, our talents and natural affinities, concentrating on who we are and making the most of it is already a good start. According to the great Taoist philosopher Chuang Tzu, every living being is truly happy only when it manages to live in accord with its own nature. If we follow our nature, all is easy and unbarred; but if we fight against it, our life becomes painful and exhausting, similar to that of a man who rows against the current. In Chuang Tzu's book, Chapter VIII,* it is written:

---

* The *Chuang Tzu* has been translated into English numerous times, but there are two translations that I love and highly recommend: (1) the Burton Watson translation. Tzu, C. *The Complete Works of Chuang Tzu- Records of Civilization, Sources and Studies*, (Columbia University Press, 1968).; and (2) the selected translation of Fung Yu-Lan with the exposition of the philosophy of Kuo Hsiang. Chuang-tzu. *Chuang-tzu* (Chinese-English Bilingual Edition), Foreign Language Teaching and Research Press, (2012).

The duck has short legs, but if we try to stretch them, it will suffer. Flamingo legs are long, but if we try to shorten them by cutting off a piece, the animal will feel pain. We don't have to amputate what for natural order is long, nor stretch what is short.[11]

To live in accordance with our own nature, we need to accept our limitations and remove conflict within ourselves. Albert Einstein commented, 'Everyone is a genius, but if we judge a fish by its ability to climb trees, he will spend his whole life believing he is stupid'. If someone tries to be something they are not or struggles to achieve something entirely beyond their abilities or outside their control, they will end up miserable.

The problem is that most of our beliefs 'on what is good or bad' are not chosen, we are born into them. As soon as we enter this world, and probably even before for epigenetic reasons, our life starts to be shaped and influenced by a complex network of biological and cultural beliefs. We are children of particular people with distinct stories and behaviours, language, social class, education, profession, skills, religious and political attitudes. All these factors profoundly contribute to the development of our convictions and values, they create artificial layers of beliefs that deeply affect our identity and behaviours.

Influenced by American consumerism, for instance, more and more people nowadays embrace values such as individualism, competitiveness, materialism and self-gratification. This self-centred view of life increases people's vulnerability and instability, because when excessive importance is attached to material things, frustration and disappointment become more likely.

BEYOND THE SENSORY: FREEDOM FROM CULTURAL ILLUSIONS

Understanding who we are and what our intrinsic characteristics and qualities are is not easy. Our brains are powerful instruments that interpret the world around us. However, the perception of the world through the senses is often misleading. A stick dipped in water appears broken and partially bent, due to the different detour that light rays undergo passing from air to water. It is just an optical illusion. The moon appears larger when it is near the horizon, and smaller when it is above our head. This is not an optical, but a cognitive illusion. If we cross our index and middle fingers of one hand, eyes closed and rub with the fingertips the tip of our nose, after a few seconds we will perceive two nose tips. These and a thousand other illusory phenomena emphasise how the human perception of reality is interpretive in nature, and therefore subject to error. What we see, touch, smell, feel and taste is not reality, but an interpretation by our mind of the data supplied by the senses.

Many illusions are often produced by emotional, social and cultural factors. A dish that is not extremely spicy would be tasteless for an Indian or a Pakistani, but inedible for many American or north European men and women. Drinking an excessive quantity of alcohol is considered 'normal' in some societies, but a sin in others.

The fear or hatred for people with different skin colour or foreigners is formed by prejudice. Humans, in general, tend to overlook some aspects if in their culture they are considered taboo, or simply if they are not part of their culture; and they tend to magnify the role of facets that are considered as positive values by members of their community. Fashion and celebrity-media marketing communication are great examples of this phenomenon.

INTUITION: THE HIGHEST FORM OF INTELLIGENCE

But if our mind cannot, through the senses, perceive reality as it really is, how can we ever find our path in this world and understand what role we should play?

The word 'intuition', in fact, derives from the Latin *intueor* (composed of *in* 'inside' and *tueor* 'watch') and means 'observe deep within you', or also to 'immediately understand things without the need to make use of reasoning'. To know something intuitively does not mean to observe rapidly or carelessly. All the most beautiful works of art, the most elegant symphonies and revolutionary scientific discoveries arise from intuition.

Einstein, the physicist who theorised the principle of relativity with complicated mathematical formulas, was convinced of the importance of intuition, and said:

> *All the great scientific achievements resulted from intuitive knowledge, namely by axioms from which we make deductions ... Intuition is an indispensable condition for the discovery of these axioms.*

Developing our intuitive intelligence, to make our mind its own master, follows the same rules of exercise training. The more we exercise our abilities, the stronger they become. The only difference is that when it comes to training the mind, there is no limit to how far we can go and achieve. With this training comes a deep self-esteem and inner confidence. It's not the sort of confidence linked with career achievements, accumulation of wealth and power or finding a new partner. It's the fortitude that unlocks our inner strength, our intuitive mind.

Some scientific studies have shown that children who regularly practise martial arts or yoga are more alert, aware and disciplined, less aggressive, and have more self-esteem than those who participate only in conventional sports.[12] It has also been observed that the practice of yoga and martial arts, but not the standard physical training (e.g. running, biking), strengthens our executive functions.

The development of executive functions leads to improvements in our ability to:

- design and plan our actions into sequences of objectives to be achieved

- voluntarily inhibit impulses and irrelevant information and rapidly move our attention to other important information

- fluidly retain focus on a task or event for an extended period of time, without allowing other internal or external stimuli to interrupt the task

- change our behaviour as the conditions or tasks required of us change.[13]

The use of executive functions is also essential in all problem-solving activities, from the most difficult and theoretical (mathematical analysis or understanding of a philosophical text) to the social ones (relationships). Those who master these skills are more successful in defining their goals in life and in achieving them with more energy and a sharper focus.

What is important is to develop a deep understanding of how our body and mind work, to develop alertness, mental energy, sensitivity and the power of concentration, which can guide us towards the observation of our inner self. These qualities will help us to remove toxic influences from our lives, freeing up space for positive thoughts and actions. By practising these disciplines, we can also learn grace and self-control, flexibility and rhythmic endurance, promptness and patience, persistence and influence.

When I was a medical student, and I was practising Hatha yoga and Aikido for several hours every week, I gained a superior control of my emotions, and an undivided attention to details with a unique capacity to focus on the essential. These qualities were not only extremely helpful to pass my exams, but they also became instrumental for developing my career as a physician and a scientist. It is as if I have acquired a precious 'inner compass' that gives me internal guidance and confidence on how to live my life.

Aligning with the natural flow of life: The art of effortless action

Wu Wei is a key concept of Taoism that literally means 'non-doing'. In reality, I think that the true significance is 'aligning our thoughts and actions with the flow of life'. I personally believe that whatever we do in our life, it is of vital importance that we acquire that mysterious ability that some people call 'wisdom', which allows us to intuitively understand from a contingent situation what is demanded of us, and then follow the indication from destiny without effort or struggle.

Understanding a situation and what is demanded of us is not easy. Life is exciting but it comes with many decisions, challenges and adversities for everyone. However, we should learn to remain centred and composed, free of mental blocks, and let things take their course. Only through daily meditation, training and self-renewal can we continue to maintain a position of inner-strength.

> Force of habit helps to keep order in quiet times; but in periods
> when energy is building up, everything depends on the power of the
> personality. Only a resilient man can stand up to his fate, for his inner
> security enables him to endure to the end. It is the same in life when
> destiny is at work. We should not worry and seek to shape the future by
> interfering in things before the time is ripe.

We should quietly fortify our body by consuming a wide range of healthy food, exercise our body to relieve stress, and cultivate the mind and spirit with gladness and good cheer. 'Fate comes when it will, and thus we will be ready'.[14]

The mind of the wise man is like still water, a perfect mirror

The wise man makes himself strong in every way and learns to react to whatever situation that arises around him with 'no conscious mind' by using his intuitive intelligence. He follows the principle of minimal effort and conforms to the true nature of things. Chuang Tzu said: 'The mind of the perfect man is like still water, a perfect mirror. It does not move with things, nor does it anticipate them. It responds to things, but does not retain them'.[15] In the mind of the man who is in harmony with nature, there is no violence; it is like the prow of a ship that cleaves water, and yet it leaves in its wake water unbroken. He is able to deal successfully with things, without being affected.

The spiritual man, who is in harmony with the 'Universe' and acts in conformity with the contingent situation, is absolutely free and happy, because his inner security and strength allow him to stand up to his fate. He is able to transcend all distinctions and face things exactly as they are, without any kind of self-deception or illusion. He is contented in any new situation or experience that life is offering to him, because he knows how to interpret the subtle signs that develop out of events, by which the new path takes shape and begins.

Knowledge is not experience: life, the master teacher

Nonetheless, these are only beautiful and elegant concepts that will remain so, if we are not able to live them and make them truly ours. Knowledge does not have the same value as experience. Words cannot replace the object that they attempt to describe. If we want to describe how an apple looks, we can research it in a book and by studying its biology become experts. However, if we want to know how it tastes, we will certainly not go to the library, but go to an orchard where we can pick one. If we do not know the whereabouts of an orchard, we can search for information on the Internet, which can only provide guidance on where to find apple trees. It may describe its taste, but the words have no taste. Only by biting the fruit, will we understand its real flavour. The same applies to every experience that we have in life: to learn to play the violin, to prune a tree or navigate within us. Understanding something does not automatically translate into action.

This is why it is extremely important that we fully live our life: it is our only teacher. We should also learn to allocate time wisely. The time we have in this life is limited. If we waste it to achieve unimportant things, and we work long hours to accumulate and maintain unnecessary objects and things, then we won't have enough to develop ourselves, to cultivate our inner strength and become 'free' human beings, more kind-hearted, empathic, altruistic and wise. This is crucial because, as I have already said, I firmly believe that the root of everything that happens within and around us is just the reflection of the energy emanating from our inner being. Our soul is like a magnet. The stronger its force, the larger the magnetic field. That is why it is said: 'The way to do is being'.

HAPPINESS: A PLANT TO NURTURE?

The meaning of the word 'happiness' can change from person to person, over time and in different cultural traditions. Nevertheless, in the past as nowadays, buying, for instance, a new house, a fashionable dress or a precious jewel, falling in love or enjoying a delicious meal, are conditions that many people would consider forerunners of joy. There is nothing wrong with all this, but we should be aware that these pleasures are typically transitory and short-lived.

Because of a phenomenon, called *dependence*, the same as that experienced by heroin or alcohol addicts, the pleasures procured from the senses and from the acquisition of material goods cannot last forever, and is inevitably followed by a state of dissatisfaction and unhappiness. The mind then seeks to renew the pleasure, often with a stronger stimulus, which is followed by a new state of dissatisfaction and so on in a vicious cycle. Not surprisingly many celebrities who are beautiful, wealthy and apparently happy, often end up being admitted to expensive rehabilitation clinics for drug and alcohol abuse, and depression. Not to mention the huge increase in consumption of antianxiety and antidepressant drugs in the rich capitalist societies, which has now reached epidemic proportions.[16]

For the Greek philosopher Epicurus (342–270 BCE) happiness is nothing but 'the absence of pain in the body and of disturbance in the soul', which he calls *ataraxia* or imperturbability. In contrast, for the German philosopher Friedrich Nietzsche (1844–1900) happiness and pain are inextricably linked. In a famous passage of his book *The Gay Science* he wrote:

*What if pleasure and displeasure were so tied together that whoever wanted
to have as much as possible of one must also have as much as possible of the
other – that whoever wanted to learn to 'jubilate up to the heavens' would
also have to be prepared for 'depression unto death'? ... You have the
choice: either as little displeasure as possible, painlessness in brief ... or as
much displeasure as possible as the price for the growth of an abundance of
subtle pleasures and joys that have rarely been relished yet? If you decide for
the former and desire to diminish and lower the level of human pain, you
also have to diminish and lower the level of the capacity for joy.[17]*

Who's right? Epicurus (and along with him, Aristotle, Seneca, Schopenhauer) or
Nietzsche?

I personally believe that neither one is correct, since true joy cannot be determined
by external forces, either active or passive, but a lasting source of happiness and
satisfaction can only come from within us, from the inexhaustible wellspring and
inner strength that reside deep in our soul. In the ancient *I Ching* it is written:

*True happiness must spring from within. But if one is empty within
and wholly given over to the world, idle pleasures come streaming in
from without. This is what many people welcome as diversion. Those
who lack inner stability and therefore need amusement will always
find opportunity of indulgence. They attract external pleasures by the
emptiness of their natures. Thus they lose themselves more and more,
which of course has bad results.[18]*

I agree with this idea of the wise men who, more than 2500 years ago, composed the *I
Ching*, and I think that to be truly joyful and experience a state of deep and enduring
gratification, we need to work on ourselves, on our thoughts and actions. The greater
the degree of harmony and cohesion between the mind, the body and our soul, the
deeper the sense of serenity, contentment and completeness. We cannot base our
happiness only on external factors, because youth, beauty and even our close relatives
will eventually disappear. We are young and beautiful until we are not. We look at
ourselves in the mirror until one day we realise that we are old and wrinkled. We
fight with our children and parents and one day realise that there is silence, because
they have both left our lives. And I can make many other examples of why we should
not base our happiness on external things, but, instead, on developing our 'inner
strength' and physical, mental and spiritual health and resilience.

Happiness, for the French Buddhist monk Matthieu Ricard, means:

*A deep sense of prosperity that comes from a mind that is exceptionally
healthy. This is not merely a feeling, an emotion, or a state of mind, but
an optimal state of being.*[19]

There is no doubt that in a sick and disabled body, suffering pain and dulled by drugs,
the mind can hardly concentrate and find harmony and cheerfulness.[20] But keeping
our body healthy is only one part. To foster happiness and inner peace it is also
imperative to develop a sense of tolerance, kindness and compassion towards other
human beings. We need to 'open' ourselves to others and be generous. Fear, jealousy
and distrust are negative sentiments that erode our joy and wellbeing. Instead, if
we help others, if we are kind and patient with our fellow citizens, we will foster
friendship and companionship, happiness and health.

As with all things we need to persevere to secure lasting results. We cannot
become healthy by eating nutritious food only one week a year; or aspire to win the
New York marathon by exercising a couple of days a month. To learn to play the
piano well, we must persevere for many years; even the most gifted musician needs
constant training. This constant exercise consolidates and strengthens the network
of synaptic protrusions of the brain regions, which control the fine movements of
the fingers, the perception of sounds, the vision of the notes, the creative processes
and the spatial-temporal reasoning.[21,22] Since the same concept applies to all kinds of
physical and mental activities,[23] why wouldn't it also be the case for happiness?

It takes time because life is not static. There are times when everything is calm,
and the sun is shining up in the sky, and then there are times when our lives are
tense, and a storm is fast approaching on the horizon. But we shouldn't give up in our
pursuit of freedom and ultimate happiness. As it is written in the *I Ching*:

*True serenity and happiness consists in keeping still when the time has
come to keep still, and going forward when the time has come to go
forward. In this way rest and movement are in agreement with the
demands of the time, and thus there is light in life.*[24]

SIX INTERVENTIONS TO DEVELOP AND INCREASE YOUR HAPPINESS

1. Nurture your physical, psychological and emotional health
Wise people never stop forging themselves. The purpose of discipline in conducting
our lives is not to live less, but more fully. Healthier people tend to be happier.
Therefore, it is important to consume a nourishing, balanced diet, engage in regular
physical and cognitive training, practise mindfulness and develop our emotional
health.[25]

2. Immerse yourself in nature

To cultivate happiness and wellbeing and tap into the unlimited reserve of universal energy it is important to spend as much time as possible in nature.[26] Enjoy the beauty and peace of walking around trees or in green spaces.[27] Learn to take in the energy of the forest and to bathe yourselves in the fresh, pure air. Morihei Ueshiba, Aikido's founder, said:

> *Now and again, it is necessary to seclude ourselves among deep mountains and hidden valleys to restore our link to the deep source of life. Breathe in and let yourself soar to the end of the universe; breathe out and bring the cosmos back inside. Next, breathe up all the fecundity and vibrancy of the earth. Finally, blend the breath of heaven and the breath of earth with that of your own, becoming the Breath of Life itself.[28]*

3. Find time to engage in creative activities that are truly absorbing

Where the arts flourish so does cultural tolerance, individual wellbeing and personal enlightenment.[29] 'Losing yourself' in visual arts, music, poetry or another one of the many performing disciplines can have transformative effects by influencing and focusing your inner self. Devote time to learn new artistic disciplines in order to express your creativity.

4. Develop the art of peace and compassion

Peace and compassion empower us, while anger, fear and distrust destroy our serenity. We live in a society that supports selfishness. A self-centred life promotes self-indulgence, greed, hate and all sorts of jealousies. These negative emotions decimate our own intuitive wisdom and create unhappiness.

> *The art of peace and compassion begins within us. We should work to cultivate the principle of kindness, reconciliation, cooperation and empathy as we interact with people at home, at work and in our social lives. Being altruistic, nurturing 'good' relationships and performing good acts for others, whether friends or strangers, better if anonymously, is important to foster harmony and happiness.[30] We should also learn the art of forgiveness and express gratitude for what we are. A healthy mind devoid of negativity is essential for the wellbeing of a human soul.*

5. Cultivate optimism and a spiritual life

Smile as much as you can. We should learn to look at the bright side of every situation and experience. It is key to refine our inner-being by engaging in spiritual activities, such as reading and pondering philosophical and spiritually oriented books, and by practising meditation, yoga and any other form of contemplative activities. Only a 'virtuous' soul can emanate positive vibrations that have the power to influence everything and everybody in its charismatic and constructive atmosphere.

6. Building confidence, inner-strength and a noble purpose in life

Optimism and emotional stability are strongly associated with happiness, especially when we have noble aspirations in life. Living a life that means something, working on purposeful projects brings joy.[31] The more meaningful our life feels, the more satisfaction we experience. Several studies have shown that a defining feature of a fulfilling life is creating or contributing to something that goes beyond our own ego, pursuing something that is bigger than ourselves, for example by contributing to the greater good of mankind or society. Indeed, useful and altruistic activities have been shown to generate positive emotions and profound social connections, both of which increase our satisfaction with life.

OF LIFE AND DEATH

Most people that I know are scared of dying because they are afraid they will completely cease to exist after death occurs; others because they fear that they will be eternally punished for their sins on earth. These fears have been used by many religions to subjugate billions of people in the course of history. But, if you think about it for a moment, you can accept that there is nothing to be worried about.

As Chuang-Tzu said in his book addressing those who feel too much sorrow for death:

> *This is to violate the principle of nature and to increase the emotion of man, forgetting what we have received from nature. The ancients called this suffering the penalty of violating the principle of nature. When the master Lao-Tzu came, it was because he had the occasion to be born; when he went, he simply followed the natural course.*[32]

Spinoza, one of my favourite philosophers, wrote a beautiful passage that summarises very well my thoughts on this regard:

> *In the order of Nature, our own particular lives are of no special importance. And unless we realise this, we are doomed to a miserable fate. We must understand that our mere bodies can never give ultimate fulfilment or blessedness of soul. Only by losing ourselves in Nature (or God) then, in his own insignificant particularity, the eternal and*

infinite order of Nature can be displayed. For in the finite is the infinite
expressed, and in the temporal, the eternal. It is this knowledge that
makes man free, which breaks the finite fetters from his soul enabling
him to embrace the infinite and to possess eternity.[33]

TRANSFORMING OURSELVES ONE STEP AT A TIME

The path to health, self-awareness and spiritual richness is a long one, an individual quest that lasts a lifetime. Some of you might already be worried and scared by the amount of things we need to put into practice to reduce the risk of getting sick and live a long, enjoyable, creative and fulfilling life with our loved ones and friends.

However, do not despair. We just need to arm ourselves with patience, determination and passion, and step by step make the concepts, that I have illustrated in this book, our own.

We have done it before, when for instance, we learned to read, write and solve complicated maths. Step by step, month after month we gradually acquired and mastered all the skills necessary to operate in our profession and in our lives. Remember that when we started out, learning to ride a bike or drive a car, it seemed so hard, and now without even thinking, we travel for miles in busy cities, while listening to music and talking to a friend. Nothing is impossible!

It takes time to digest new information, and transformation occurs only in steps. But important and meaningful changes can be implemented one step at a time. Start with a few small changes, and when they become habits, tackle bigger ones. In educating ourselves it is also important to eliminate our bad habits (like smoking, binge-drinking, eating fast-food, engaging in behaviour that leaves you angry, worried or stressed all of the time), but tolerate those habits that are harmless (eating some chocolate, drinking a good glass of wine). Because being too hard on ourselves has been shown to limit our ability to change.

The first step is accepting the present truth. You have to know where you are, as well as where you want to go, if you're going to get there. Making a start is the biggest step and it is amazing how new healthy habits quickly become old ones that can be built on.

The famous American educational David Kolb, who was the founder of Experience Based Learning Systems, demonstrated that people cannot learn just by paying attention. They must also experiment, practise and slowly integrate their newly acquired experiences with their existing ones by repeating them.[34]

If we want to master something new, at the beginning, it is helpful to divide the subject into multiple parts, and allow time to observe and ponder each experience, testing the new concepts and applying the new principles again and again.[35] You can start by improving your diet. Increase your consumption of vegetables, beans and whole grains. If you are just beginning to experiment with healthy food preparation, you may feel overwhelmed or intimidated, but remember that healthy cooking is like anything else: the more you practise, the better you will become. Once you have mastered a number of healthy and tasty recipes, you can move on to concentrating on improving your fitness or enrol in a yoga or Tai chi class.

According to Kolb, for a whole learning experience to take place, we must complete four learning stages:

1. concrete experience or assimilation of information

2. reflective observation or processing of knowledge

3. abstract conceptualisation or analysing and creating meaning from the experience

4. active experimentation or trying things out again and again.

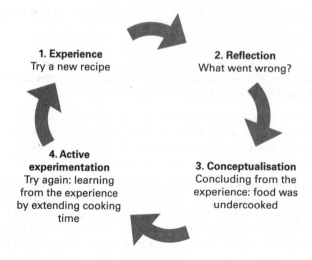

Figure 29: The four learning stages

However, this is not enough. According to Chris Argyris, an American business theorist, for people to alter their behaviour it is also necessary to change their mindset (challenge their underlying assumptions), which requires a shift in understanding, from the simple and static 'single-loop' learning method to the more comprehensive and dynamic 'double-loop' learning.[36]

Let me explain with an example. When you were a child, you were taught by your parents to eat meat and drink plenty of milk. This was considered a positive value and a behaviour to be rewarded because if you ate these foods, you would grow strong and healthy. This is largely because they were told the same thing by their parents and peers. It informed the way in which they view the world and because one thing leads to another it became a rule for how to eat. This is an example of single-loop learning.

But what do you do if you consume lots of meat and milk and you discover your blood cholesterol is markedly elevated? Do you keep eating more of these foods? Double-loop learning is when you challenge the underlying conventions and ask yourself whether meat and dairy consumption is linked with high cholesterol. To resolve your cholesterol problem you search for the best unbiased scientific information and then change your behaviour accordingly.

Argyris also believed that human beings assimilate new knowledge more effectively if they have to describe to other people how they will use what they have learned to apply it to their own situation. This is because we utilise different parts of our brain for learning and for teaching. So, I encourage you to talk with your friends and relatives about what you have learned, and what you are planning to do to improve your health and wellbeing.

There are four conditions that must be met for changing your mind-set and your behaviour:

1. Most of us will reshape our behaviours only if we have a clear understanding of why it is important to change and we approve of it. Then we just need to set our goals, pursue them and have faith in them.

2. Acquire the knowledge and skills that are required to improve your personal health and wellbeing, the health of your children, and of the environment you live in so that you can then put that knowledge into practice.

3. Key to enabling change is having the support both socially and in terms of infrastructure to make it easier. For instance, find the best markets to buy fresh, healthy and organic foods; discover parks, trails and facilities where you can practise your daily physical activity; get a bicycle if that's your chosen aerobic activity; share exercise with supportive friends and family.

4. Finally, you should establish a community of friends that help you to enthusiastically embrace your new habits. People are more prone to make changes if they become inspired by what their peers do or have achieved. When we offer people an opportunity to take a step closer to a healthier lifestyle (and we make that change feel safe), then they will pursue this change, especially if the programs are enjoyable and sociable.

Each of these conditions together tally up to a way of permanently changing your behaviour by altering attitudes about what can and should be done to improve your health and wellbeing.

PART VII

OUR WORLD

CHAPTER TWENTY-THREE

A HEALTHY SUSTAINABLE ENVIRONMENT TO LIVE IN

Writing about the care and love of our planet, Nobel-prize winning physicist Albert Einstein said:

> *Human beings are part of a whole, called by us Universe, a part limited in time and space. They experience themselves, their thoughts and feelings as something separated from the rest, a kind of optical delusion of their consciousness. This delusion is a kind of prison for us, restricting us to our personal desires and to affection for a few persons nearest to us. Our task must be to free ourselves from this prison by widening our circle of compassion to embrace all living creatures and the whole of nature in its beauty.*

Not many of us nowadays live in a pristine mountain area where the air is pure and the sun is shining above the clouds; we often live in chaotic and polluted towns and cities. Every day when we leave our home, we are immersed in noisy, congested traffic, and smoggy air. We consume foods grown in impoverished soils, sprayed with chemical fertilisers and pesticides, which seep into the deep aquifers that we collect our drinking water from.

Our detergents, and household and personal discards, very often not biodegradable, also end up in landfill and waterways that flow into rivers used for irrigation and the sea that supplies the fish we eat.[1] Industries play their own part by discarding toxic substances. Some of these pollutants can linger for months, years or centuries.

This cocktail of poisoning substances dramatically increases our risk of getting sick.[2] Modern science responds to our sicknesses with new drugs, which once taken do not magically disappear into thin air, but are eliminated via urine and faeces, which also seep into groundwater, dispersing back into the fields and the sea where the food that we eat comes from.[3] Indeed, levels of some pharmaceutical residues have increased 10 to 20 fold over the past 20 years in rivers and lakes all over the world.[4-6]

Another pressing problem, identified by scientists across the world, is that we are facing global warming, with its devastating consequences.[7] The carbon intensity of the energy system is the major culprit, but what people do not realise is that around 30 per cent of greenhouse-gas emissions are due to intensive animal farming. If cattle were their own nation, they would be the world's third-largest greenhouse-gas emitter, after the US and China.[8] And yet the consumption of meat and dairy is on the rise not only in Western countries, but also in developing countries.

By 2020, it is estimated that people in developing countries will consume 107 million metric tons (mmt) more meat and 177 mmt more milk than they did in 1996/1998. The projected increase in livestock production will require annual feed consumption of cereals to rise by nearly 300 mmt by 2020. This one dietary change will create huge environmental and health problems with potentially irreversible consequences on planetary health, for instance irreversible destruction of top soil, pollution of water and air, and global warming.[9,10]

In the long-term the trajectory is that there will be dire consequences on human and environmental health, and above all on the social and economic welfare of the entire planet.

We all know that going back to the past is not possible. Would we renounce driving our car or flying to visit Bali, the Grand Canyon in Arizona or the Sistine Chapel in Rome? Would we relinquish the convenience of being able to communicate over the internet in real time with people all over the world? Or in the event of a serious car accident would we do away with modern medicine? The answer is 'no'.

And, in fact, we don't need to give up on everything. We just need to increase our awareness, and make wise and informed choices, so that society and industry will be forced to change, and produce food, products and services that do not destroy, but enhance both human and environmental health.

For example, if we decide not to buy a product anymore, such as a certain type of food, or a polluting car, large retailers will stop ordering them from the industries that produce them, which in turn will be forced to discontinue their production, and instead create new products that meet the expectations of buyers. In this way we can build a better world for ourselves and our children, a world where innovative eco-friendly agricultural systems produce plenty of nutritious and healthy food for everybody on this planet. A world where cities are green and quiet, because our cars are powered by hybrid, electric and hydrogen engines; where buildings are energy efficient to the point that they do not require heating or air-conditioning systems, because most of the energy required can be extracted from the sun, wind and earth. We need a world where people are healthy, happy and aware, and the production model has turned towards a sustainable economy.[11]

This is not a utopia! Much of the scientific and technological knowledge needed to eliminate pollution and prevent most chronic illnesses (and their related social costs) through healthy lifestyles already exists. There is technology to build super-insulated houses which do not *consume* but *produce* energy, there is the ability to develop super-light carbon fibre cars powered by electric or hydrogen engines, and many other innovations are also already available and are being applied far beyond the development of simple prototypes.

The next step, then, will be the integrated application of all this expertise to promote human and environmental health systems that enhance and do not destroy our natural resources, our 'Natural Capital'.[12] We can collaborate to eradicate poverty, create sustainable peace and a global economic and human development plan that re-orients these unsustainable systems from an individualistic ethic of 'growth' towards an ethic of 'care' and sustainability. However, these changes will only be triggered by the choices of aware and well-informed citizens.

CHAPTER TWENTY-FOUR

POLLUTION IS MAKING US SICK

Chronic exposure to smog – a deadly cocktail of particulate matter and ozone – has been shown to reduce life expectancy by an average of 8.6 months.[1]

In particular, air pollution with fine particulate matter, PM_{10} (which has a diameter of less than 10 microns) and $PM_{2.5}$ (which has a diameter of less than 2.5 microns: one quarter of a hundredth of a millimetre), penetrates deep into our lungs, where it can cause a number of diseases, such as asthma, chronic bronchitis, heart attack, stroke and lung cancer.[2,3]

Exposure of children to fine particles has been shown to impair the development and function of their lungs, and probably also of their brains.[4] For every increase of 10 mcg per cubic metre of $PM_{2.5}$ in the air we breathe, there is an estimated 6 to 13 per cent increase in mortality.[5,6]

NO 'NORMAL' CONCENTRATIONS OF PARTICULATE MATTER EXIST

Scientific data indicate that there is no threshold below which particulate matter does not cause harm. According to a recent WHO report, globally 84 per cent of the assessed population is exposed to annual mean levels that exceed the WHO Air Quality Guidelines levels (see figure 30). The situation is particularly bad in China, India, Pakistan and the Middle East. A study found that because of the elevated $PM_{2.5}$ levels, every year approximately 1.33 million people die in China, 575,000 in India and 105,000 in Pakistan. For the European Union member states and the United States an estimated 173,000 and 52,000 people, respectively, died prematurely in 2010.[7]

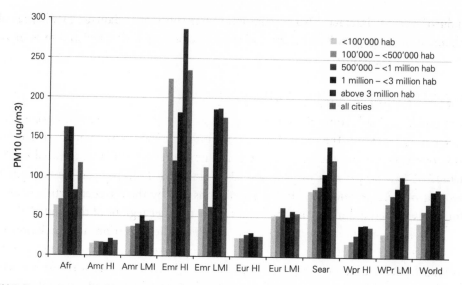

PM10: Fine particulate matter of 10 microns or less; Afr: Africa; Amr: America; Emr: Eastern Mediterranean; Eur: Europe; Sear: South-East Asia; Wpr: Western Pacific; LMI: Low- and middle-income; HI: high-income. PM10 values for the world are regional urban population-weighted.

Figure 27: PM$_{10}$ levels by region and city size, for available cities and towns latest year in the period 2008–15.[8]

WHERE DO THESE FINE PARTICLES COME FROM?

The major sources of air pollution in industrialised countries are from:

- combustion of petrol and diesel for transport by land, air and sea

- burning of coal, wood, oil and biomass for heating buildings and producing electricity for domestic and industrial use

- erosion of road surface caused by vehicular traffic and abrasion of cars' brakes and tyres

- industrial activities, such as emissions from incinerators, steel mills, refineries, construction, mining, cement industry

- intensive agriculture and industrial animal farming

- smoke from forest fires, often caused by land clearing, but also the changing climate.

So far scientific studies have failed to identify precisely what components of particulate matter are more harmful, although it seems that those resulting from the combustion of fossil fuels are the most dangerous, because they contain carcinogens and are toxic for cells.[9]

Another air pollutant is ground-level ozone, a greenhouse gas that forms when UV light, nitrogen oxides and volatile organic compounds produced by cars and industrial plants interact. Ozone pollution causes substantial damage to all types of plants, including agricultural crops and trees by oxidising leaf tissue; and to humans by entering lung tissues.

LIVESTOCK AND ENVIRONMENTAL POLLUTION

Ammonia emitted from livestock is a main precursor for forming secondary inorganic particles in the atmosphere.[10] Ammonia interacts with sunlight and other environmental factors and turns into particulate matter, which is transported by the wind.[11] About 30 per cent of PM_{10} and $PM_{2.5}$ in north Italy and the Netherlands is estimated to be produced by livestock emissions and by the nitrogen fertilisers used for industrial agriculture.[12] Similar figures apply to other regions of the world.[13,14]

But while air pollution is a serious problem, the depletion and pollution of freshwater and land resources is the most dangerous. Industrial agriculture and animal farming is responsible for 70 per cent of freshwater use, with 70 per cent of all land under tillage used to feed livestock. Chemicals, fertilisers and animal waste contaminate and degrade our soils, seep into groundwater and wash into lakes, streams and rivers, finally ending up in our seas and oceans. Worldwide figures are staggering: according to the UN Food and Agricultural Organization, approximately 56 billion animals are reared and slaughtered globally for human consumption every year with an estimated global meat output of 335 million tonnes (in carcass weight equivalent) in 2018 alone.[15] These gargantuan figures do not even include fish and other sea creatures. In the US alone, commercial slaughter in 2018 accounted for 33 million head of cattle, 124.4 million hogs, approximately 2.2 million sheep and lambs, 9.1 billion chickens, 236 million turkeys and 27.6 million ducks. In summary, total commercial red meat and poultry production in the US in 2018 was 53.6 billion kg (118.3 billion pounds), a record high.[16,17]

These creatures do not live on air, but require very large quantities of fresh water and feed. To produce the enormous supplies of corn, soybeans, grains and various herbs that are needed to feed these animals, massive quantities of nitrogen and phosphorus-based fertilisers and pesticides are dispersed annually on farmland.[18] Before World War II, most farming occurred on small family farms with limited use of chemicals, but nowadays the large corporate farms utilise massive amounts of chemical fertilisers (i.e. nitrogen, potash and phosphate) and pesticides.

In 2016, about 21 million tons of commercial fertilisers was spread on fields in the US or around 138 kg (305 lb) per hectare of arable land.[19] Corn accounts for around 40 per cent of that country's fertiliser consumption. In addition to using commercial fertilisers to increase crop yields, intensive modern agriculture uses a wide range of pesticides, herbicides, insecticides, fungicides as well as chemicals to kill birds and rodents.

In the US, about 80 per cent of the total quantity of pesticide was applied to four common crops: corn, soybeans, wheat and potatoes. Before the 1950s, only 5 to 10 per cent of corn and wheat acreage were treated with herbicides, but by 1980, herbicide was used on 90 to 99 per cent of all US corn and soybean acres planted. Notably, the four most heavily used active ingredients were: glyphosate, atrazine, acetochlor, and metolachlor.

According to the US Environmental Protection Agency, over 0.5 billion kg (1.1 billion pounds) of pesticides were used for crop production in 2012 in that country alone. Herbicides accounted for 60 per cent of total pesticide use in 2012.[20]

Where do all these substances end up? To a small extent in the actual foodstuffs, and the rest in the soil, groundwater, rivers, lakes and finally in the sea. Data from the American National Water-Quality Assessment Program show that pesticides and their degradants are present at detectable concentrations in surface waters, streams, stream sediments, aquatic biota and ground water across the United States but also in many other regions of the world.[21]

The tonnes of nitrogen and phosphorus that are released into the environment every year to grow crops, including those to be fed to animals, also gradually leaks into our rivers, lakes and seas. The ammonia and other acidic substances present in manure, in conjunction with the overabundance of nitrates and phosphates, additionally cause soil acidification and the growth of toxic algae, which in turn causes a depletion of water oxygen and leads to fish kills.[22,23] These oxygen-depleted areas are becoming more ubiquitous around the world.

The proliferation of aquatic bacteria stimulated by excess nitrogen and other chemical nutrients in the water of lakes and rivers also releases toxic substances that can affect our brains and livers. When these waters, rich in organic debris, interact with chlorine (which is used for water purification), it produces a substance called trihalomethane, which can act as a carcinogen and may trigger abortions.[24-26]

Traditional agriculture enriched the soil, by alternating crops of cereals, legumes (to fix nitrogen) and pasture. Today the intensive production of monoculture crops (e.g. the same cereal crop every season) requires the use of fertilisers and pesticides that contribute to depletion of the soil. Soil depletion associated with intensive farming in turn leads to even greater use of fossil fuels and more global warming, because more energy is need to produce more hydrocarbon-based fertilisers and pesticides in order to grow monoculture crops in topsoil increasingly depleted of nutrients. The depleted soil is also more prone to erosion.[27]

In factory farms, a range of antibiotics are also used – the same used to fight infections in humans.[28,29] The risk is that very soon, because of the disproportionate antibiotic use by farmers (and actually by many doctors as well), bacteria will develop resistance to antibiotics and we will start to die again from a simple bronchitis or for an infection contracted because of an injury.[30] The additional implications for human health of the consumption of meat, milk and eggs contaminated with traces of antibiotics are completely unknown, but potentially very harmful.[31-33]

GLOBAL HEATING

By burning fossil fuels we extract about 85 per cent of the energy that we need each day to drive cars; power trains or planes; heat, cool or power the buildings we live or work in; provide electricity for industrial activities and manufacturing, and many other applications.[34] The use of this mix of non-renewable energy sources is responsible for about 70–80 per cent of greenhouse gas emissions; the other 20 to 30 per cent is produced by intensive agriculture and animal farming.[35-38] Animal faeces, in fact, accounts for 65 per cent of global emissions of nitric oxide and 37 per cent of methane, which is a greenhouse gas 20 times more potent than carbon dioxide (CO_2).

CO_2, methane and other greenhouse gases form an invisible shield around the Earth that does not allow infrared radiation emitted by the Earth to disperse. The result is an increase in sea water temperature and energy in the atmosphere: global heating.

A dear friend of mine who works for NASA's Jet Propulsion Laboratory in Pasadena explained to me that global warming does not simply cause a general increase in temperatures, but rather greater climate variability and extreme weather events. Increasingly intense firestorms, more frequent and severe droughts and heatwaves, recurrent and more destructive hurricanes and storms, coupled with crop failures and risk of food insecurity sadly are becoming the 'norm' and will put the safety of millions of citizens at risk. Another problem will be the spread in temperate zones of tropical diseases, such as malaria, yellow fever and zika virus among other illnesses.[39]

CHAPTER TWENTY-FIVE

SECURING THE FUTURE

Most of the knowledge and technology needed to reshape our future to an environment-centred economy exists today, albeit still capable of improvement.

What is missing is the awareness that to improve human and environmental health, societal wealth and wellbeing, each of us must do something, by transforming the way we think and live. Together we can work towards a world focused on energy efficiency and resilience and the protection of our 'natural capital'.[1]

At the individual level, for instance, a conscious choice with very important repercussions for our health and our environment's health is to drastically reduce the animal products we consume and increase the variety of minimally processed organic plant foods we eat, as I tried to discuss in this book.

About 70 per cent of the planet's arable land is used to feed animals for human consumption.[2] We keep talking about hunger in the world, but few are aware that to produce a 2000-calorie meal of beef, we need 108 square metres of land, while just 3.3 square metres planted with grains and beans can provide the same amount of calories without polluting the environment, and at the same time dramatically improving our health. It takes approximately 57 calories of fossil fuel to produce a calorie of protein of lamb, 40 for a calorie of beef protein, 14 for a calorie of milk proteins, while just 2.2 calories of fossil fuel are needed to produce a calorie of protein of maize, thanks to photosynthesis.[3]

This huge cost is due to the energy required to pump an enormous quantity of water from wells to water crops and animals, to generate and sprinkle the soil with fertilisers, pesticides and herbicides, and for the transportation, slaughter, preservation, refrigeration and distribution of meat. For cereals, beans and vegetables grown with organic or biodynamic methods, the production process is much shorter, more energy-efficient and economical.[4]

It is not necessary for all of us to become vegetarians, but it certainly would be good for us and the planet to drastically change our diets. If all the world's citizens reduced their consumption of meat and milk, and consumed a diet predominantly, but not exclusively, based on plant products, the exploitation of fertile lands would be reduced by an estimated 60 to 70 per cent; there would be less deforestation; and land, water and air pollution would be substantially decreased.[5]

If people ate less food, especially less junk food (rich in empty calories and low in nutrients), and consumed more vegetables, whole grains, legumes, seeds, nuts and fruit, the prevalence of obesity, and many of the chronic diseases, as I have discussed, would decline rapidly, along with healthcare costs and global emissions. It has been estimated that approximately 4.6 per cent of carbon dioxide emissions is produced by the healthcare sector, a value that is gradually increasing across all the developed countries.[6]

Within the limits of our budget, we can all live more sustainably, using biodegradable and recyclable products (that do not need to end up in landfill, or even worse in an incinerator) and make our homes more energy-efficient, with insulation, double and triple-glazing our windows, using LED lighting and energy-efficient appliances. The lower energy needed in these houses can be generated by rooftop photovoltaic panels or geothermal heat pumps. Hot water can be produced with solar panels and other emerging technologies.

Another conscious action that we can put in place to safeguard environmental health is to move around as much as possible on foot, by using bikes (including electric), taking public transport and supporting the development of cars with low environmental impact, such as those fuelled by natural gas or electric hybrid engines.

At the community level, we also can encourage administrators, politicians and entrepreneurs to invest more financial resources in scientific research to develop:

- breakthrough materials and technologies to improve building and vehicle efficiency
- innovative technologies that better extract energy from renewable sources, like wind, sun, geothermal energy and sea currents
- chemical products with low environmental impact
- computer technology to maximise both the efficiency and resilience of our green-energy distribution networks, produced by large wind farms and large and small producers of photovoltaic energy
- the greening of our towns and cities to lower energy consumption.

All of these potential applications can also create new businesses and jobs that respect the environment.

Another vital aspect is the need to design and implement public policies that improve health literacy in order to boost preventative lifestyle interventions that will reduce the unsustainable reliance on our medical systems for conditions that should be treated with lifestyle changes. Ideally we need to put in place a system that rewards healthy behaviour, and heavily taxes products that harm human health and the environment.

Finally, we should abolish government subsidies and increase taxes for intensive, damaging agriculture, for the extraction of oil and coal and encourage, instead, companies that invest in renewable energy and sustainable farming.

Above all, we must realise that happiness and wellbeing depend not only on the acquisition of material goods and economic growth, but our physical, psychological and spiritual health, the wealth of our social relationships and the health of the environment that sustains all life on Earth, our 'natural capital'.

CHAPTER TWENTY-SIX

MY MESSAGE TO THE READER

In *The Path to Longevity* I have tried to illustrate some of the knowledge, concepts and ideas that over the years I have gained from a great variety of sources, including modern medical books, ancient philosophical texts, my scientific studies, my patients, and from working with and learning from many colleagues and friends around the world. I am still learning, we are still learning: there are so many things we don't know.

However, we already have enough knowledge to improve our chances of staying healthy, productive, empowered and independent, or to regain health, so that we can fully enjoy living in this amazing world. The road to health, happiness and self-realisation can be a long one, but it is a beautiful one. What you can achieve in this life partially depends on your current position in life. However, with enthusiasm and diligence, anything is possible.

Don't be put off by those claiming that diseases are inevitable or they are just bad luck, or bad genes. Although it is known that genetic inheritance plays a role in our risk of developing certain diseases and dying prematurely, what we do in our life turns out to be far more important and has more pervasive effects in shaping how long and well we will live. Human life is a like a magnificent jigsaw puzzle that integrates many aspects of metabolic and environmental health with our emotional, intellectual and spiritual journey into a single entity: the development of a happy, creative and fulfilling whole.

There are no magic pills, special foods or exercises that in isolation will promote longevity, health and wellbeing. So be wary of fads and snake-oil miracle cures.

What counts is our overall lifestyle, which certainly must and can be customised according to our genetic and metabolic profile, our age and individual inclinations and preferences.

We should also be mindful that ageing and the accumulation of molecular damage which leads to the decay of our body and mind, begins from conception and not when we turn 65. We can improve our situation at any age, but it is ideal to adopt a healthy lifestyle from when we are young and practise it for the rest of our life. Regardless we can learn from our mistakes and make positive changes that are life-affirming.

We can also help to spread this life-affirming knowledge with our own daily choices and by working with others who have developed their own awareness. The daily decisions of the many can affect the political, economic and financial world, changing their direction to the promotion of human and environmental health.

In conclusion, I think that the most important purpose of life should be to achieve happiness, by overcoming the suffering inflicted by physical, mental, moral and spiritual ailments. However, to achieve a real and lasting happiness it is essential to stay healthy: eating properly and practising a variety of physical, cognitive and meditative exercises that strengthen our physical endurance and our emotional, intuitive and creative intelligence. In this way, will we be able to enjoy, until late in life, together with our relatives and friends, all the wonderful experiences that life, this beautiful planet Earth, the sun, the moon and the stars present to us every day.

Life is a gift! Let's never forget that.

WHAT GETS MEASURED, GETS DONE: TRACK YOUR PROGRESS

Georg Joachim de Porris (1514–1574), a famous mathematician, astronomer and medical practitioner, the only pupil of Nicolaus Copernicus, said: 'If you can measure it, you can manage it'.

More recently this old saying has been adapted as a mantra of the most successful senior executives of the leading world's consulting firms: 'What gets measured, gets done'.

There is no doubt, in medicine as in the management of any work or life situation, being able to quantify a phenomenon, will provide the information that is necessary to make sure we actually achieve what we set out to do.

For many of us, the simple act of measuring something enhances our motivation to perform and succeed. It triggers an internal competition for improvement and reaching our objective. There is no way to know if we have improved, unless we can measure the effects of what we are doing, and as a result become more motivated to accomplish our goals. For instance, without measuring our body weight or waist circumference, it will be difficult to know if our diet and exercise program has been successful. These concrete figures will also provide an idea of what the impact of our intervention has been and, if partially successful, what we need to do differently.

Table 10 illustrates a number of parameters that we should measure with some regularity in order to assess our metabolic health and track the success of our lifestyle modifications.

THE LOWER, THE BETTER	WITHIN RANGE	THE HIGHER, THE BETTER
Waist circumference	BMI	Lean mass
LDL-cholesterol	Glucose	Insulin sensitivity (HOMA-IR)
Triglycerides	IGF-1	HDL-cholesterol
Hb1Ac	Hemoglobin	SHBG
Insulin	TSH	IGFBP-1
C-reactive protein	Leptin	IGFBP-2
AST, ALT	Vitamin D	Adiponectin
Arterial stiffness	Vitamin B12	
IMT carotid arteries	Blood pressure	VO$_2$max

Table 10: Clinical parameters to assess with regularity

MEASURING MARKERS OF SYSTEMIC HEALTH

There are a number of markers that I evaluate to assess overall health in my patients. The least invasive, as we have already discussed, is waist circumference, a very good marker of abdominal fat deposition. Unlike for body weight and BMI, the lower the circumference of our waistline the better. Ideally, we should not be able to pinch any fat with our fingers in the midsection. Remember that as your waistline improves, so does your health.[1] This is a simple but very informative measurement.

If we want to be more precise the next global indicator of health and longevity that should be measured is fasting insulin.[2] Unless, you have type 1 diabetes, the lower this marker, the better. In my clinical studies of elite athletes and people practising calorie restriction without malnutrition, the blood levels of insulin after an overnight fast were about 1.5 µU/ml (10.4 pmol/L) that is at least five times lower than the concentration of an average person.[3] Lower insulin levels have multiple anti-ageing and anticancer effects.[4]

The third universal biomarker of health is C-reactive protein, which determines the degree of systemic inflammation.[5,6] Also for this parameter, we should aim to achieve the lowest level possible. Ideally, C-reactive protein should be less than 0.7 mg/L (9.5 nmol/L).[7] In people practising calorie restriction with optimal nutrition the blood levels of C-reactive protein are so remarkably low (about 0.2 mg/L or 1.9 nmol/L) that a special highly sensitive measurement method must be employed.[8] Remember that chronic inflammation is implicated in the initiation and progression of the majority of chronic illnesses.[9]

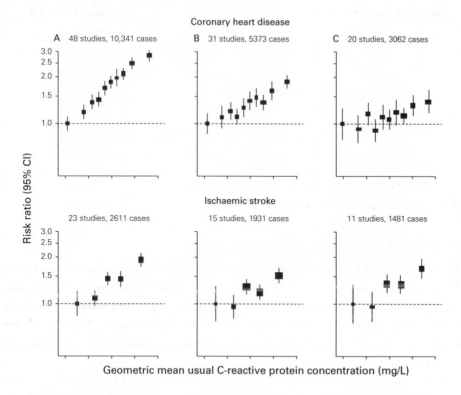

Coronary heart disease

A 48 studies, 10,341 cases   **B** 31 studies, 5373 cases   **C** 20 studies, 3062 cases

Ischaemic stroke

23 studies, 2611 cases   15 studies, 1931 cases   11 studies, 1481 cases

Risk ratio (95% CI)

Geometric mean usual C-reactive protein concentration (mg/L)

Figure 31: Relationship between C-reactive protein concentration and risk of coronary heart disease and ischaemic stroke.[10]

MEASURING MARKERS OF CARDIOVASCULAR HEALTH

There are a number of factors that we can measure to assess our risk of developing cardiometabolic diseases, the most important being total and LDL-cholesterol, HDL-cholesterol, triglycerides, blood pressure, fasting glucose and Hb1Ac. These and other risk factors, including smoking, interact and exponentially increase the risk of developing cardiovascular disease (see figure 32).[11]

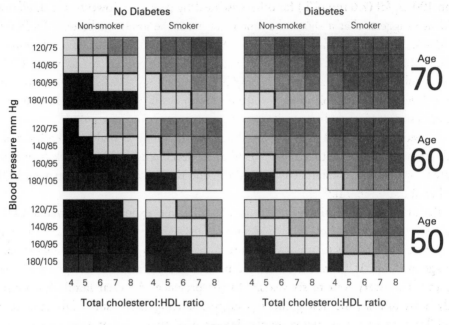

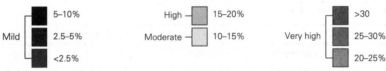

Figure 32: Framingham risk calculator

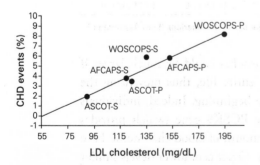

Figure 33: Coronary heart disease (CHD) event rates in primary prevention trials are directly proportional to the low-density lipoprotein (LDL) cholesterol levels.[13]

'BAD' CHOLESTEROL

There is no doubt, having abnormal high levels of LDL-cholesterol is one of the leading risk factors for developing diseases such as coronary heart disease, stroke, heart failure, vascular dementia and narrowing of the renal arteries, which can cause chronic kidney disease. Excessive LDL-cholesterol contributes to fatty build-up and hardening of the arteries, because it infiltrates the blood vessel wall where it stimulates inflammation and cell dysfunction.[12] This is why maintaining a low blood cholesterol must be on everyone's radar, starting early in life.

According to the 2018 guidelines of the American Heart Association, an optimal level is less than 100 mg/dl (2.6 mmol/L) for otherwise healthy people.[14] However, accumulating evidence suggests that it should be much less, with the lower the better.[15] Professors Goldstein and Brown, who won the 1985 Nobel prize for their studies on cholesterol biology, have postulated that we humans have been designed to maintain LDL-cholesterol levels in the range of 25 mg/dl.[16] In monkeys and human neonates the blood levels of LDL-cholesterol are usually lower than 50 mg/dl, and only in our Western society do people typically have levels higher than 100 mg/dl.[17-19]

Indeed, as illustrated in figure 33, the results of many primary prevention trials with stains have shown that the probability of developing a heart attack is linearly related with blood cholesterol concentrations, and the risk approaches zero at an LDL level of about 57 mg/dl.[20]

Because of the detrimental effects of a lifetime exposure to elevated LDL-cholesterol, screening should start as soon as possible; even in the absence of any cardiometabolic risk factors. The current recommendation is to begin testing between the age of 9 and 11 years, followed by a new screening between the ages of 17 and 21, and then every four to six years.[21] In the presence of a clear family history for early heart disease, the new guidelines suggest starting to measure LDL-cholesterol in children as young as two years old. It's essential that, even at a very young age, people follow a heart-healthy lifestyle and understand the importance of maintaining healthy cholesterol levels.

	IDEAL	NEAR IDEAL	BORDERLINE HIGH	HIGH
Total cholesterol	< 180 mg/dl <4.6 mmol/L	180-200 mg/dl 4.6-5.2 mmol/L	200-239 mg/dl 5.2-6.2 mmol/L	>240 mg/dl >6.2 mmol/L
LDL-cholesterol	<100 mg/dl <2.6 mmol/L	100-129 mg/dl 2.6-3.3 mmol/L	130-159 mg/dl 3.3-4.1 mmol/L	>160 mg/dl >4.1 mmol/L
Triglycerides	<150 mg/dl <0.17 mmol/L		150-199 mg/dl 0.17-2.25 mmol/L	>200 mg/dl >2.25 mmol/L

Table 11 – Normal and abnormal lipid values according to the 2018 guidelines of the American Heart Association[22]

We should keep in mind that the cardiovascular benefits could be much larger if plasma cholesterol was kept lower throughout our entire life, thus preventing the development of the atherosclerotic plaques from the beginning. Indeed, individuals who were born with mutations that inactivate the PCSK9 gene (which provides orders for making a protein that helps regulate the amount of blood cholesterol) have plasma LDL-cholesterol levels that are approximately 30 per cent lower (levels similar to those induced by treatment with the cholesterol lowering drugs called statins), and experience a 90 per cent reduction in heart attacks, independently of smoking, hypertension and diabetes.[23] In contrast, a similar 30 per cent reduction of serum LDL-cholesterol with statins results in only a 30 per cent lesser risk of coronary events.

These data suggest that lifelong lower levels of plasma LDL-cholesterol are much more effective than late LDL-cholesterol reductions induced by statins in preventing coronary heart disease.[24] Moreover, they suggest that the extremely low incidence of coronary heart disease observed by Ancel Keys and others in South Italy, Crete, Japan and Okinawa in the 1950s was probably due, at least in part, to the lower levels of plasma LDL-cholesterol that these populations had experienced throughout life.

'GOOD' CHOLESTEROL

Unlike for LDL-cholesterol, high-density lipoprotein (HDL) cholesterol levels should be as high as possible in people consuming a healthy diet and performing regular exercise. HDL cholesterol is also called 'good' cholesterol because it is important for removing cholesterol from the arteries.[25] In epidemiological studies, higher levels of HDL-cholesterol are strongly associated with lower risks of heart disease and ischemic stroke, independently of LDL-cholesterol concentration[26] (see figure 34).

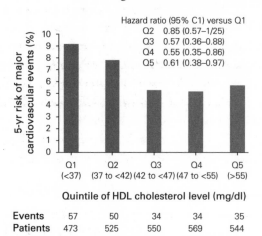

Figure 34: Relationship between major cardiovascular events and HDL-cholesterol levels stratified for LDL-cholesterol.[27]

Ideally, HDL-cholesterol levels should be higher than 60 mg/dl (1.5 mmol/L) in men and above 70 mg/dl (1.8 mmol/L) in women. However, there is one caveat because certain metabolic conditions can make HDL particles dysfunctional.

The functional capacity of HDL-cholesterol particles to remove cholesterol from arteries is influenced by several factors, the most important being inflammation. We have to think of HDL particles as airplanes transporting hundreds of cholesterol passengers from the arteries (small airports) to the liver (central hub), where excess cholesterol is excreted in the intestine as biliary acids. Although a higher number of HDL airplanes generally indicate that the system is transporting more cholesterol passengers, this is not always the case. Experimental studies have shown that high levels of inflammation drastically reduce the capacity of the HDL airplanes to embark and disembark the excess cholesterol passengers to the liver hub for excretion.[28] Therefore, the cholesterol passengers are trapped on the HDL airplanes, and might even land in the arteries. This explains why certain people with very high HDL-cholesterol levels have an increased risk of cardiovascular disease, and drugs that increase HDL-cholesterol levels (in the absence of lifestyle modifications) do not reduce the risk of developing a heart attack. It is another example of the importance of the holistic mechanism-based approach to health promotion and disease prevention.

Cholesterol:HDL ratio and non-HDL cholesterol

There are more sophisticated ways to predict our risk of developing cardiovascular disease than LDL- or HDL-cholesterol. For instance, you can calculate the **cholesterol to HDL ratio** by dividing your total cholesterol number by your HDL-cholesterol value. For example, if your total cholesterol is 180 mg/dl (4.6 mmol/L) and your HDL-c is 60 mg/dl (1.5 mmol/L), the resulting ratio is 3. This is very good because a ratio of under 4 is considered to be as a sign of healthy cholesterol levels, while a number above 6 signifies a higher risk of cardiovascular disease.[29] In general, however, the lower the ratio, the healthier your cholesterol levels are.

Another parameter that you can ask your doctor to assess is the **non-HDL cholesterol** concentration, which some studies consider to be a more precise indicator of atherogenic cholesterol and a better predictor of cardiovascular risk. Non-HDL cholesterol can be calculated by subtracting your HDL-cholesterol value from your total cholesterol number, and therefore contains not only LDL-cholesterol but also all the triglycerides-rich lipoproteins, including the very low density lipoprotein (VLDL) particles. Data from clinical trials and mendelian studies indicate that in patients with high cardiovascular risk, optimal level of non-HDL cholesterol should be less than 100 mg/dl (2.6 mmol/L).[30]

Finally, a new test that can determine how effectively your HDL particles clean up arterial cholesterol is the **cholesterol uptake capacity** method. This test can add significant information on cardiovascular risk stratification, even in patients with optimal LDL-cholesterol, independently of traditional risk factors, including HDL-cholesterol.[31]

BLOOD GLUCOSE AND OTHER MARKERS OF OPTIMAL GLUCOSE METABOLISM

Diabetes mellitus is a powerful risk factor for coronary heart disease and ischaemic stroke, independent of other conventional cardiometabolic risk factors, such as obesity or hypertension. Fasting blood glucose, in particular, is a good predictor, and is directly associated with the risk of developing cardiovascular disease and type 2 diabetes at all concentrations, including below the threshold for diabetes of 126 mg/dl (7 mmol/L).[32]

Pre-diabetes is a condition in which blood glucose levels are higher than normal (>100 mg/dl or 5.5 mmol/L), but not high enough for a diagnosis of type 2 diabetes (126 mg/dl or 7 mmol/L). Pre-diabetes has no signs or symptoms, but without lifestyle intervention one in three people will progress into type 2 diabetes, which is a major risk factor not only for cardiovascular disease, but also for diabetic nephropathy, retinopathy, neuropathy, urinary incontinence and microvascular disease, among many other complications.

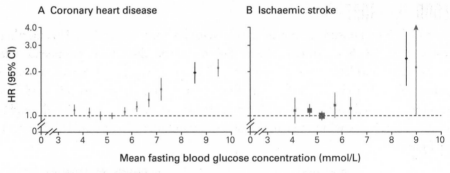

A Coronary heart disease   B Ischaemic stroke

Mean fasting blood glucose concentration (mmol/L)

- No known history of diabetes at baseline survey
- Known history of diabetes at baseline survey

Figure 35: Relationship between long-term fasting blood glucose levels and risk of coronary heart disease.[33]

The diagnosis of pre-diabetes can be done by measuring glucose levels after an overnight fast or two hours after the ingestion of a 75 g glucose load. If fasting glucose is between 100 and 125 mg/dl (5.5–7 mmol/L), the diagnosis is impaired fasting glucose, whereas a two-hour glucose between 140 and 200 mg/dl (7.7 – 11.1 mmol/L) is a sign of impaired glucose tolerance. Both conditions are associated with an increased cardiovascular risk.

It is interesting to note that, as for many other cardiometabolic risk factors, there is no threshold value below which the risk of developing complications disappears. For instance, as shown in figure 36, the risk of developing type 2 diabetes among young men starts at fasting plasma glucose levels well below what is considered the normal glucose range, especially when combined with triglyceride levels of more than 150 mg/dl.[34] Consistently, elevated fasting plasma glucose levels within the normal blood sugar level range can also predict cardio- and cerebrovascular risk in people older than 45 years.[35,36]

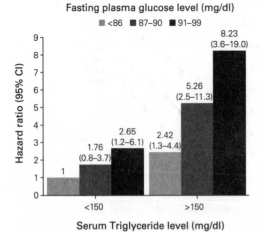

Fasting plasma glucose level (mg/dl)
■ <86 ■ 87–90 ■ 91–99

Figure 36: Relationship between blood fasting glucose and triglyceride level and risk of developing diabetes.[38]

Another test that we can use to assess glucose metabolism is HbA1c, or glycated haemoglobin, which reflects average blood glucose levels over the preceding three to four months.[37] HbA1c is regarded as the gold standard for assessing glycaemic control because it measures the amount of glucose that chemically reacts with some protein components of haemoglobin within our red blood cells. The normal range for the haemoglobin A1c level is between 4 and 5.6 per cent. People with HbA1c levels between 5.7 and 6.4 per cent have pre-diabetes and those with levels higher than 6.5 per cent have diabetes.

BLOOD PRESSURE

Abnormal blood pressure is a powerful risk factor for both ischaemic and haemorrhagic stroke, coronary heart disease, heart failure, aortic dissection, peripheral artery disease, atrial fibrillation, end-stage kidney disease and vascular dementia. Data from epidemiological studies covering 1 million people have shown that elevated blood pressure is strongly associated with heart disease and stroke mortality throughout middle and old age, without evidence of a threshold down to at least 115/75 mm Hg (see figure 37).[39]

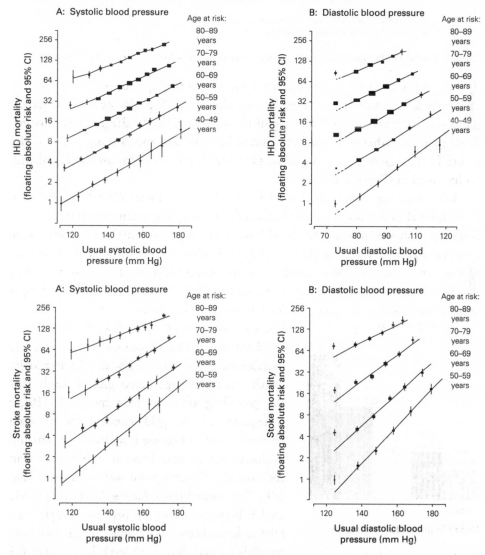

Figure 37: ischaemic heart disease (IHD) and stroke rate in each decade of age versus usual blood pressure at the start of that decade.[40]

According to the 2017 ACC–AHA Hypertension guidelines, blood pressure is considered normal when it is lower than 120/80 mm Hg, and the risk of developing cardiovascular disease doubles with each increment of 20/10 mmHg, respectively. If you have a blood pressure higher than 130/80 mm Hg, you have hypertension, while a systolic blood pressure between 120 and 129 mm Hg is considered to be prehypertension (see table 12).[41]

Blood pressure category	Definition
Normal	Systolic pressure of <120 mm Hg and diastolic pressure of <80 mm Hg
Elevated	Systolic pressure of 120–129 mm Hg and diastolic pressure of <80 mm Hg
Hypertension	
Stage 1	Systolic pressure of 130–139 mm Hg and diastolic pressure of 80–89 mm Hg
Stage 2	Systolic pressure of >140 mm Hg and diastolic pressure of >90 mm Hg

Table 12: Classification of blood pressure in adults[42]

MAXIMAL OXYGEN CONSUMPTION AND FITNESS

VO_2max, also known as maximal oxygen consumption, is the gold standard to measure our fitness or the ability to sustain work for prolonged periods. It can be used to establish our aerobic endurance capacity before and during the course of a training program. The ability to consume oxygen while exercising ultimately determines our ability for maximal work output over periods lasting greater than one minute.[43] The higher the VO_2 max, the greater the potential work rate. Aerobic fitness is related to health, and fit people are usually healthier than unfit ones.

VO_2max expressed as litres of oxygen per minute is higher in large people with more muscle mass. This is why it is preferable to correct VO_2max for body weight and express the value in millilitres of oxygen per kilogram per minute. In our studies at Washington University, endurance athletes like cyclists and runners, who rarely weigh over 80 kg, often had VO_2max values in excess of 70 ml/kg/min. In one occasion we had measured a VO_2max of 90 ml/kg/min. This is more than twice the value of the average VO_2max of a 40-year-old untrained male, which typically is around 35–40 ml/kg/min.

As shown in figure 38, VO_2max progressively diminishes with age, even in elite athletes, but aerobic training can markedly slow the decline.[44] These charts can be used to establish whether or not your fitness level is above or below the median for your age, and to monitor your progress as you improve your endurance by engaging in a regular exercise program that follows the criteria that I have described in chapter 13.

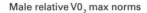
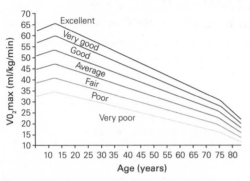
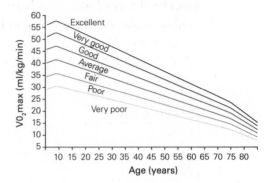

Figure 38: VO$_2$max norms charts for female and male

MONITORING PROGRESS: OTHER TESTS

There are many other elements that can be used to monitor your health progress, including IGFBP-1, IGFBP-2 and SHBG, factors that should increase if you improve your overall lifestyle. Blood IGF-1, leptin, adiponectin, TSH, vitamin D, vitamin B12 and salivary cortisol are also important parameters together with blood testosterone and oestradiol. Then, there are a number of markers of oxidative stress, plasma metabolites and instrumental tests (e.g. lean and fat mass by DXA, pulse wave velocity, augmentation index, left ventricular diastolic function, heart rate variability, intima-media thickness (IMT) of the carotid arteries, 24-hour core body temperature, polysomnography) that can be assessed with more advanced techniques, but they go beyond the scope of this book, and need highly specialised medical doctors to perform and interpret them.

> TIP: Remember that the results of these tests do not determine your future, but are very helpful to guide you in improving your health as you take the kind of action recommended in this book.

REFERENCES/BIBLIOGRAPHY

Preface

1 Centers for Disease Control and Prevention. Health and economic costs of chronic diseases. (2019). <https://www.cdc.gov/chronicdisease/about/costs/index.htm>

2 WHO. *Preventing Chronic Diseases. A Vital Investment: WHO Global Report* (2005).

3 A Publication of the American Society for Nutrition. <https://academic.oup.com/ajcn/issue-pdf/92/2/27637374/>

4 American Society for Nutrition 2019 Sustaining Partners. <https://nutrition.org/sustaining-partners/>

5 The European Food Information Council (EUFIC). Funding and governance. (2019). <https://www.eufic.org/en/who-we-are/funding-governance/>

Part I: The beginning of wisdom

Chapter 1: Are you ready to enjoy your life?

1 Benjamin, E.J., *et al.* Heart disease and stroke statistics 2018 update: a report from the American Heart Association. *Circulation,* 137, E67-E492 (2018).

2 Egan, B.M. & Stevens-Fabry, S. Prehypertension prevalence, health risks, and management strategies. *Nature Reviews: Cardiology,* 12, 289-300 (2015).

3 Ford, E.S., *et al.* C-reactive protein concentration distribution among US children and young adults: findings from the National Health and Nutrition Examination Survey, 1999-2000. *Clinical Chemistry,* 49, 1353-1357 (2003).

4 Vernon, S.T., *et al.* Increasing proportion of ST elevation myocardial infarction patients with coronary atherosclerosis poorly explained by standard modifiable risk factors. *European Journal of Preventive Cardiology,* 24, 1824-1830 (2017).

5 Breivik, G. Personality, sensation seeking and risk taking among Everest climbers. *International Journal of Sport Psychology,* 27, 308-320 (1996).

6 Reps, P. *Zen Flesh, Zen Bones: A collection of Zen and pre-Zen writings,* Tuttle Publishing. (2008).

7 *The I Ching, or, Book of Changes,* Princeton University Press; 3rd edition. (1967).

Chapter 2: Healthy centarians: the quest for healthy longevity

1 Colchero F., *et al.* The emergence of longevous populations. *Proceedings of the National Academy of Sciences of the United States of America,* 113, E7681–E7690 (2016).

2. Evert, J., Lawler, E., Bogan, H. & Perls, T. Morbidity profiles of centenarians: survivors, delayers, and escapers. *Journals of Gerontology Series A: Biological Sciences and Medical Sciences,* 58, 232-237 (2003).

3. Richmond, R.L., Law, J. & KayLambkin, F. Morbidity profiles and lifetime health of Australian centenarians. *Australasian Journal of Ageing,* 31, 227-232 (2012).

4. Baltes, P.B. & Smith, J. New frontiers in the future of aging: from successful aging of the young old to the dilemmas of the fourth age. *Gerontology,* 49, 123-135 (2003).

5. Herskind, A.M., *et al.* The heritability of human longevity: a population-based study of 2872 Danish twin pairs born 1870-1900. *Human Genetics,* 97, 319-323 (1996).

6. Lichtenstein, P., *et al.* Environmental and heritable factors in the causation of cancer analyses of cohorts of twins from Sweden, Denmark, and Finland. *The New England Journal of Medicine,* 343, 78-85 (2000).

7. Czene, K., Lichtenstein, P. & Hemminki, K. Environmental and heritable causes of cancer among 9.6 million individuals in the Swedish Family-Cancer Database. *International Journal of Cancer,* 99, 260–266 (2002).

8. Ruby, J.G., *et al.* Estimates of the heritability of human longevity are substantially inflated due to assortative mating. *Genetics,* 210, 1109–1124 (2018).

9. Sebastiani, P. & Perls, T.T. The genetics of extreme longevity: lessons from the New England centenarian study. *Frontiers in Genetics* 3, 277 (2012).

10. Willcox, B.J.; Willcox, D.C. & Suzuki, M. Demographic, phenotypic, and genetic characteristics of centenarians in Okinawa and Japan: Part 1-centenarians in Okinawa. *Mechanisms of Ageing and Development,* 165, 75–79 (2017).

11. Willcox B.J., *et al.* Caloric restriction, the traditional Okinawan diet, and healthy aging: the diet of the world's longest-lived people and its potential impact on morbidity and life span. *Annals of the New York Academy of Sciences,* 1114:434-55 (2007).

12. *Ibid.*

13. Records of the U.S. Civil Administration of the Ryukyu Islands (USCAR) 1945-72: Records of the Health, Education and Welfare Department of the Office of the Civil Administrator. Record Group 260.12.5. The U.S. National Archives and Records Administration (1949).

14. US Bureau of Agricultural Economics. Consumption of food in the United States, 1909-1948. *United States Department of Agriculture Miscellaneous Publications,* 691, (1949).

15. Kagawa, Y. Impact of westernization on the nutrition of Japanese: changes in physique, cancer, longevity and centenarians. *Preventive Medicine,* 7, 205-217 (1978).

16. *Ibid.*

17. *The I Ching, or, Book of Changes,* Princeton University Press; 3rd edition. (1967).

18. Baker, M., *et al.* Loneliness and social isolation as risk factors for mortality: a meta-analytic review. *Perspectives on Psychological Science* 10, 227-237 (2015).

19. Anjana, R., *et al.* Prevalence of diabetes and prediabetes in 15 states of India: results from the ICMR-INDIAB population-based cross-sectional study. *Lancet: Diabetes & Endocrinology,* 5, 585-596 (2017).

20. Craig, W., & Mangels, A.R. Position of the American Dietetic Association: vegetarian diets. *Journal of the American Dietetic Association,* 109, 1266-1282 (2009).

21. American Dietetic Association. Position of the American Dietetic Association and Dietitians of Canada: vegetarian diets. *Journal of the American Dietetic Association,* 64, 62-81 (2003).

22. Key, T.J.A., *et al.* Mortality in vegetarians and nonvegetarians: detailed findings from a collaborative analysis of 5 prospective studies. *American Journal of Clinical Nutrition,* 70, 516S-524S (1999).

23. Kwok, C.S., *et al.* Vegetarian diet, Seventh Day Adventists and risk of cardiovascular mortality: a systematic review and meta-analysis. *International Journal of Cardiology,* 176, 680-686 (2014).

24. Key, T.J., *et al.* Mortality in British vegetarians: results from the European Prospective Investigation into Cancer and Nutrition (EPIC-Oxford). *American Journal of Clinical Nutrition,* 89, 1613S-1619S (2009).

25. Appleby, P.N., *et al.* Mortality in vegetarians and comparable nonvegetarians in the United Kingdom. *American Journal of Clinical Nutrition,* 103, 218-230 (2016).

26. Key, T. & Davey, G. Prevalence of obesity is low in people who do not eat meat. *BMJ,* 313, 816-817 (1996).

27. Appel, L.J., *et al.* Dietary approaches to prevent and treat hypertension: a scientific statement from the American Heart Association. *Hypertension,* 47, 296-308 (2006).

28. Wang, F., *et al.* Effects of vegetarian diets on blood lipids: a systematic review and meta-analysis of randomized controlled trials. *Journal of the American Heart Association,* 4, e002408 (2015).

29. Key, T.J., *et al.* Cancer in British vegetarians: updated analyses of 4998 incident cancers in a cohort of 32,491 meat eaters, 8612 fish eaters, 18,298 vegetarians, and 2246 vegans. *The American Journal of Clinical Nutrition,* 100 (Suppl. 1), 378S-385S (2014).

30. Penniecook-Sawyers, J.A., *et al.* Vegetarian dietary patterns and the risk of breast cancer in a low-risk population. *The British Journal of Nutrition,* 115, 1790-1797 (2016).

31. Tantamango-Bartley, Y., *et al.* Are strict vegetarians protected against prostate cancer? *The American Journal of Clinical Nutrition,* 103, 153-160 (2016).

32. Heaney, R.P., *et al.* Dietary changes favorably affect bone remodeling in older adults. *Journal of the American Dietetic Association,* 99, 1228-1233 (1999).

33. Orlich, M.J., *et al.* Vegetarian dietary patterns and mortality in Adventist Health Study 2. *Journal of the American Medical Association: Internal Medicine,* 173, 1230-1238 (2013).

34. *Ibid.*

35. Orlich, M.J., *et al.* Vegetarian dietary patterns and the risk of colorectal cancers. *Journal of the American Medical Association: Internal Medicine,* 175, 767-776 (2015).

36. Orlich, M.J. & Fraser, G.E. Vegetarian diets in the Adventist Health Study 2: a review of initial published findings. *The American Journal of Clinical Nutrition,* 100 (Suppl. 1), 353S-358S (2014).

37. Antero-Jacquemin Jda, S., *et al.* Learning From Leaders: Life-span Trends in Olympians and Supercentenarians. *The Journals of Gerontology. Series A, Biological Sciences and Medical Sciences,* 70, 944-949 (2015).

38. Holloszy, J.O. Mortality rate and longevity of food-restricted exercising male rats: a reevaluation. *Journal of Applied Physiology,* 82, 399-403 (1997).

39. *Ibid.*

40. Owora, A.H., *et al.* A systematic review of etiological risk factors associated with early mortality among National Football League players. *Orthopaedic Journal of Sports Medicine,* 6, 2325967118813312 (2018).

41. Lindqvist, A.S., *et al.* Increased mortality rate and suicide in Swedish former elite male athletes in power sports. *Scandinavian Journal of Medicine & Science in Sports,* 24, 1000-1005 (2014).

Chapter 3: Healthspan and the mechanisms of ageing

1. Lopez-Otin, C., *et al.* The hallmarks of aging. *Cell,* 153, 1194-1217 (2013).

2. Evert, J., *et al.* Morbidity profiles of centenarians: survivors, delayers, and escapers. *The Journals of Gerontology. Series A, Biological Sciences and Medical Sciences,* 58, 232-237 (2003).

3. Fontana, L., Partridge, L. & Longo, V.D. Extending healthy life span – from yeast to humans. *Science,* 328, 321-326 (2010).

4. Fontana, L. & Partridge, L. Promoting health and longevity through diet: from model organisms to humans. *Cell,* 161, 106-118 (2015).

5. Fontana L, *et al.* Medical research: treat ageing. *Nature,* 511:405-7 (2014).

6. Shimokawa, I., *et al.* Diet and the suitability of the male Fischer 344 rat as a model for aging research. *Journal of Gerontology,* 48, B27-32 (1993).

7. Ikeno, Y., *et al.* Delayed occurrence of fatal neoplastic diseases in Ames dwarf mice: correlation to extended longevity. *The Journals of Gerontology. Series A, Biological Sciences and Medical Sciences,* 58, 291-296 (2003).

8. Ikeno, Y., *et al.* Do long-lived mutant and calorie-restricted mice share common anti-aging mechanisms? A pathological point of view. *Age,* 28, 163-171 (2006).

9. Vergara, M., *et al.* Hormone-treated Snell dwarf mice regain fertility but remain long lived and disease resistant. *The Journals of Gerontology. Series A, Biological Sciences and Medical Sciences,* 59, 1244-1250 (2004).

10. Eijkelenboom, A. & Burgering, B.M. FOXOs: signalling integrators for homeostasis maintenance. *Nature Reviews: Molecular Cell Biology,* 14, 83-97 (2013).

11. Hotamisligil, G.S. Inflammation, metaflammation and immunometabolic disorders. *Nature,* 542, 177-185 (2017).

12. Bertozzi, B., Tosti, V. & Fontana, L. Beyond calories: an integrated approach to promote health, longevity, and well-being. *Gerontology,* 63, 13-19 (2017).

13. Fontana, L. Interventions to promote cardiometabolic health and slow cardiovascular ageing. *Nature Reviews: Cardiology,* 15, 566-577 (2018).

14. *Ibid.*

15. Pencina M.J., *et al.* Predicting the 30-year risk of cardiovascular disease: the framingham heart study. *Circulation,* 119:3078-84 (2009).

16. Joseph, A., *et al.* Manifestations of coronary atherosclerosis in young trauma victims – an autopsy study. *Journal of the American College of Cardiology,* 22, 459-467 (1993).

17. Lloyd-Jones, D.M., *et al.* Prediction of lifetime risk for cardiovascular disease by risk factor burden at 50 years of age. *Circulation,* 113, 791-798 (2006).

18. O'Keefe, J.H., Cordain, L., Harris, W.H., Moe, R.M. & Vogel, R. Optimal low-density lipoprotein is 50 to 70 mg/dl – lower is better and physiologically normal. *Journal of the American College of Cardiology,* 43, 2142-2146 (2004).

19. Coutinho, M., *et al.* The relationship between glucose and incident cardiovascular events. *Diabetes Care,* 22, 233-240 (1999).

20. Vidal-Petiot, E., *et al.* The 2018 ESC-ESH guidelines for the management of arterial hypertension leave clinicians facing a dilemma in half of the patients. *European Heart Journal,* 39, 4040-4041 (2018).

21. Ridker, P.M., *et al.* C-reactive protein and other markers of inflammation in the prediction of cardiovascular disease in women. *New England Journal of Medicine,* 342, 836-843 (2000).

22. Calle, E.E. & Kaaks, R. Overweight, obesity and cancer: epidemiological evidence and proposed mechanisms. *Nature Reviews: Cancer,* 4, 579-591 (2004).

23. Wood, L.D., *et al.* The genomic landscapes of human breast and colorectal cancers. *Science,* 318, 1108-1113 (2007).

24. Umar, A., Dunn, B.K. & Greenwald, P. Future directions in cancer prevention. *Nature Reviews: Cancer,* 12, 835-848 (2012).

25. Longo, V.D. & Fontana, L. Calorie restriction and cancer prevention: metabolic and molecular mechanisms. *Trends in Pharmacological Sciences,* 31, 89-98 (2010).

26. Seyfried, T.N. & Huysentruyt, L.C. On the origin of cancer metastasis. *Critical Reviews in Oncogenesis,* 18, 43-73 (2013).

27. Fidler, I.J. The pathogenesis of cancer metastasis: the 'seed and soil' hypothesis revisited. *Nature Reviews: Cancer,* 3, 453-458 (2003).

28. Pollak, M. The insulin and insulin-like growth factor receptor family in neoplasia: an update. *Nature Reviews: Cancer,* 12, 159-169 (2012).

29. Liu, P., Cheng, H., Roberts, T.M. & Zhao, J.J. Targeting the phosphoinositide 3-kinase pathway in cancer. *Nature Reviews: Drug discovery,* 8, 627-644 (2009).

30. Pugeat, M., *et al.* Pathophysiology of sex hormone binding globulin (SHBG): relation to insulin. *The Journal of steroid biochemistry and molecular biology,* 40, 841-849 (1991).

31. Powell, D.R., *et al.* Insulin inhibits transcription of the human gene for insulin-like growth factor-binding protein-1. *The Journal of biological chemistry,* 266, 18868-18876 (1991).

32. Yu, H., *et al.* Joint effect of insulin-like growth factors and sex steroids on breast cancer risk. *Cancer Epidemiology, Biomarkers & Prevention,* 12, 1067-1073 (2003).

33. Michelet, X., *et al.* Metabolic reprogramming of natural killer cells in obesity limits antitumor responses. *Nature Immunology,* 19, 1330-1340 (2018).

Part II: Nourishing your body

Chapter 4: The science of healthy nutrition

1. Hippocrates. *The Aphorisms of Hippocrates,* (Andesite Press, 2015).

2. Fang, B.J.Q.J.Y. *Prescriptions Worth a Thousand in Gold for Every Emergency Vol. II-IV,* The Chinese Medicine Database: Bilingual Edition, 2008.

3. Enqin, Z. *Health Preservation and Rehabilitation,* Publishing House of Shanghai College of Traditional Chinese Medicine, 1988.

4. Fontana, L. & Partridge, L. Promoting health and longevity through diet: from model organisms to humans. *Cell,* 161, 106-118 (2015).

5. Subramanian, S., *et al.* Cultivating healthy growth and nutrition through the gut microbiota. *Cell,* 161, 36-48 (2015).

6. Mattson, M.P., *et al.* Meal frequency and timing in health and disease. *Proceedings of the National Academy of Sciences,* 111, 16647-16653 (2014).

7. Carpenter, K.J. A short history of nutritional science: part 1 (1785-1885). *The Journal of Nutrition,* 133, 638-645 (2003).

8. Scheja, L. & Heeren, J. The endocrine function of adipose tissues in health and cardiometabolic disease. *Nature Reviews: Endocrinology,* 15, 507-524 (2019).

9. Colditz, G.A., *et al.* Weight gain as a risk factor for clinical diabetes mellitus in women. *Annals of Internal Medicine,* 122, 481-486 (1995).

10. Flegal, K.M., *et al.* Trends in Obesity Among Adults in the United States, 2005 to 2014. *Journal of the American Medical Association,* 315, 2284-2291 (2016).

11. Jaacks, L.M., *et al.* The obesity transition: stages of the global epidemic. *Lancet: Diabetes & Endocrinology,* 7, 231-240 (2019).

12. Chan, J.M., *et al.* Obesity, fat distribution, and weight gain as risk factors for clinical diabetes in men. *Diabetes Care,* 17, 961-969 (1994).

13. National Institutes of Health. Clinical guidelines on the identification, evaluation, and treatment of overweight and obesity in adults – the evidence report. *Obesity Research,* 6 (Suppl. 2), 51S-209S (1998).

14. Shaper, A.G., Wannamethee, S.G. & Walker, M. Body weight: implications for the prevention of coronary heart disease, stroke, and diabetes mellitus in a cohort study of middle aged men. *BMJ,* 314, 1311-1317 (1997).

15. Walker, S.P., *et al.* Body size and fat distribution as predictors of stroke among US men. *American Journal of Epidemiology,* 144, 1143-1150 (1996).

16. Rexrode, K.M., *et al.* A prospective study of body mass index, weight change, and risk of stroke in women. *Journal of the American Medical Association,* 277, 1539-1545 (1997).

17. Haslam, D.W. & James, W.P. Obesity. *Lancet,* 366, 1197-1209 (2005).

18. Rinella, M.E. Nonalcoholic fatty liver disease: a systematic review. *Journal of the American Medical Association,* 313, 2263-2273 (2015).

19. Bell, C.L., *et al.* Late-life factors associated with healthy aging in older men. *Journal of the American Geriatrics Society,* 62, 880-888 (2014).

20. Kalkhoff, R. & Ferrou, C. Metabolic differences between obese overweight and muscular overweight men. *The New England Journal of Medicine,* 284, 1236-1239 (1971).

21. Veronese, N., *et al.* Combined associations of body weight and lifestyle factors with all cause and cause specific mortality in men and women: prospective cohort study. *BMJ,* 355, i5855 (2016).

22. *Ibid.*

23. Willett, W.C., Dietz, W.H. & Colditz, G.A. Guidelines for healthy weight. *The New England Journal of Medicine,* 341, 427-434 (1999).

24. Willcox, B.J., *et al.* Midlife risk factors and healthy survival in men. *Journal of the American Medical Association,* 296, 2343-2350 (2006).

25. Sun, Q., *et al.* Adiposity and weight change in mid-life in relation to healthy survival after age 70 in women: prospective cohort study. *BMJ,* 339, b3796 (2009).

26. *Ibid.*

27. Hall, K.D., *et al.* Quantification of the effect of energy imbalance on bodyweight. *Lancet,* 378, 826-837 (2011).

28. Tracy, R.P. Is visceral adiposity the "enemy within"? *Arteriosclerosis, Thrombosis, and Vascular Biology,* 21, 881-883 (2001).

29. Karpe, F. & Pinnick, K.E. Biology of upper-body and lower-body adipose tissue – link to whole-body phenotypes. *Nature Reviews: Endocrinology,* 11, 90-100 (2015).

30. Zhang, C., *et al.* Abdominal obesity and the risk of all-cause, cardiovascular, and cancer mortality: sixteen years of follow-up in US women. *Circulation,* 117, 1658-1667 (2008).

31. Pischon, T., *et al.* General and abdominal adiposity and risk of death in Europe. *The New England Journal of Medicine,* 359, 2105-2120 (2008).

32. Fang H., *et al.* How to best assess abdominal obesity. *Current Opinion in Clincal Nutrition and Metabolic Care,* 21:360-365 (2018).

33. Alberti, K.G., Zimmet, P. & Shaw, J. Metabolic syndrome – a new world-wide definition. A consensus statement from the International Diabetes Federation. *Diabetic Medicine,* 23, 469-480 (2006).

34. Sun, Q., *et al.* Adiposity and weight change. *BMJ* (2009).

35. Goldstein, D.J. Beneficial health effects of modest weight loss. *International Journal of Obesity and Related Metabolic Disorders,* 16, 397-415 (1992).

36. Racette, S.B., *et al.* One year of caloric restriction in humans: feasibility and effects on body composition and abdominal adipose tissue. *The Journals of Gerontology Series A: Biological Sciences and Medical Sciences,* 61, 943-950 (2006).

37. Fontana, L., *et al.* Calorie restriction or exercise: effects on coronary heart disease risk factors. A randomized, controlled trial. *American Journal of Physiology-Endocrinology and Metabolism,* 293, E197-E202 (2007).

38. Weiss, E.P. & Holloszy, J.O. Improvements in body composition, glucose tolerance, and insulin action induced by increasing energy expenditure or decreasing energy intake. *The Journal of Nutrition,* 137, 1087-1090 (2007).

39. Riordan, M.M., *et al.* The effects of caloric restriction-and exercise-induced weight loss on left ventricular diastolic function. *American Journal of Physiology-Heart and Circulatory Physiology* 294, H1174-H1182 (2008).

40. Racette, S.B., *et al.* One year of caloric restriction in humans. *The Journals of Gerontology Series A,* 61, 943-950 (2006).

41. Lean, M.E.J., *et al.* Durability of a primary care-led weight-management intervention for remission of type 2 diabetes: 2-year results of the DiRECT open-label, cluster-randomised trial. *Lancet: Diabetes & Endocrinology,* 7, 344-355 (2019).

42 Vilar-Gomez E, *et al.* Weight loss through lifestyle modification significantly reduces features of nonalcoholic steatohepatitis. *Gastroenterology,* 149, 367-378 (2015).

43. Fontana, L., *et al.* Effects of 2-year calorie restriction on circulating levels of IGF-1, IGF-binding proteins and cortisol in nonobese men and women: a randomized clinical trial. *Aging Cell,* 15, 22-27 (2016).

44. Fontana, L., *et al.* Effect of long-term calorie restriction with adequate protein and micronutrients on thyroid hormones. *The Journal of Clinical Endocrinology & Metabolism,* 91, 3232-3235 (2006).

45. Weiss, E.P., *et al.* Caloric restriction but not exercise-induced reductions in fat mass decrease plasma triiodothyronine concentrations: a randomized controlled trial. *Rejuvenation Research,* 11, 605-609 (2008).

46. Griffin, N.W., *et al.* Prior dietary practices and connections to a human gut microbial metacommunity alter responses to diet interventions. *Cell Host & Microbe,* 21, 84-96 (2017).

Chapter 5: Longevity effects of restricting calories and fasting

1. Weindruch, R. & Walford, R.L. Dietary restriction in mice beginning at 1 year of age: effect on life-span and spontaneous cancer incidence. *Science,* 215, 1415-1418 (1982).

2. McCay, C.M., Crowell, M.F. & Maynard, L.A. The effect of retarded growth upon the length of life span and upon the ultimate body size. 1935. *Nutrition,* 5, 155-171 (1989).

3. Ingram, D.K. & de Cabo, R. Calorie restriction in rodents: Caveats to consider. *Ageing Research Reviews,* 39:15-28 (2017).

4. Fontana, L. & Klein, S. Aging, adiposity, and calorie restriction. *Journal of the American Medical Association,* 297, 986-994 (2007).

5. Albanes, D. Total calories, body weight, and tumor incidence in mice. *Cancer Research,* 47, 1987-1992 (1987).

6. Weindruch, R. & Sohal, R.S. Seminars in medicine. Caloric intake and aging. *The New England Journal of Medicine,* 337, 986-994 (1997).

7. Shimokawa, I., *et al.* Diet and the suitability of the male Fischer 344 rat as a model for aging research. *Journal of Gerontology,* 48, B27-32 (1993).

8. Vermeij, W.P., *et al.* Restricted diet delays accelerated ageing and genomic stress in DNA-repair-deficient mice. *Nature,* 537, 427-431 (2016).

9. Fontana, L., *et al.* Calorie restriction in non-human and human primates. *Handbook of the Biology of Aging,* Elsevier; 7th ed. (2011).

10. Colman, R.J., *et al.* Caloric restriction delays disease onset and mortality in rhesus monkeys. *Science,* 325, 201-204 (2009).

11. Colman, R.J., *et al.* Caloric restriction reduces age-related and all-cause mortality in rhesus monkeys. *Nature Communications,* 5:3557 (2014).

12. Mattison, J.A., *et al.* Caloric restriction improves health and survival of rhesus monkeys. *Nature Communications,* 8, 14063 (2017).

13. McKiernan, S.H., *et al.* Caloric restriction delays aging-induced cellular phenotypes in rhesus monkey skeletal muscle. *Experimental Gerontology,* 46, 23-29 (2011).

14. Someya, S., Tanokura, M., Weindruch, R., Prolla, T.A. & Yamasoba, T. Effects of caloric restriction on age-related hearing loss in rodents and rhesus monkeys. *Current Aging Science,* 3, 20-25 (2010).

15. Yamada, Y., *et al.* Caloric restriction and healthy life span: frail phenotype of nonhuman primates in the Wisconsin National Primate Research Center caloric restriction study. *The journals of gerontology. Series A, Biological Sciences and Medical Sciences,* 73, 273-278 (2018).

16. Enqin, Z. *Health Preservation and Rehabilitation,* Publishing House of Shanghai College of Traditional Chinese Medicine. (1988).

17. Most, J., *et al.* Calorie restriction in humans: an update. *Ageing Research Reviews,* 39, 36-45 (2017).

18. Spelta, F., *et al.* Calorie restriction, endothelial function and blood pressure homeostasis. *Vascular Pharmacology,* 65, 1 (2015).

19. Fontana, L., *et al.* Long-term calorie restriction is highly effective in reducing the risk for atherosclerosis in humans. *Proceedings of the National Academy of Sciences,* 101, 6659-6663 (2004).

20. Barzilai, N., *et al.* Offspring of centenarians have a favorable lipid profile. *Journal of the American Geriatrics Society,* 49, 76-79 (2001).

21. Meyer, T.E., *et al.* Long-term caloric restriction ameliorates the decline in diastolic function in humans. *Journal of the American College of Cardiology,* 47, 398-402 (2006).

22. Lloyd-Jones, D.M., *et al.* Prediction of lifetime risk for cardiovascular disease by risk factor burden at 50 years of age. *Circulation,* 113, 791-798 (2006).

23. Kraus, W.E., *et al.* 2 years of calorie restriction and cardiometabolic risk (CALERIE): exploratory outcomes of a multicentre, phase 2, randomised controlled trial. *Lancet: Diabetes & Endocrinology,* 7, 673-683 (2019).

24. Riordan, M.M., *et al.* The Effects of Caloric Restriction- and Exercise-Induced Weight Loss on Left Ventricular Diastolic Function. *American Journal of Physiology: Heart and Circulatory Physiology,* 294:H1174-82 (2008).

25. Meyer, T.E., *et al.* Long-term caloric restriction. *American College of Cardiology* (2006).

26. Stein, P.K., *et al.* Caloric restriction may reverse age-related autonomic decline in humans. *Aging Cell,* 11, 644-650 (2012).

27. Fontana, L., *et al.* Effects of 2-year calorie restriction on circulating levels of IGF-1, IGF-binding proteins and cortisol in nonobese men and women: a randomized clinical trial. *Aging Cell,* 15, 22-27 (2016).

28. Cangemi, R., *et al.* Long-term effects of calorie restriction on serum sex-hormone concentrations in men. *Aging Cell,* 9, 236-242 (2010).

29. Fontana, L., Klein, S. & Holloszy, J.O. Effects of long-term calorie restriction and endurance exercise on glucose tolerance, insulin action, and adipokine production. *Age,* 32, 97-108 (2010).

30. Hofer, T., *et al.* Long-term effects of caloric restriction or exercise on DNA and RNA oxidation levels in white blood cells and urine in humans. *Rejuvenation Research,* 11, 793-799 (2008).

31. Il'yasova, D., *et al.* Effects of 2 years of caloric restriction on oxidative status assessed by urinary F2-isoprostanes: The CALERIE 2 randomized clinical trial. *Aging Cell,* 17, e12719 (2018).

32. Meydani, S.N., *et al.* Long-term moderate calorie restriction inhibits inflammation without impairing cell-mediated immunity: a randomized controlled trial in non-obese humans. *Aging,* 8, 1416 (2016).

33. Yang, L., *et al.* Long-term calorie restriction enhances cellular quality-control processes in human skeletal muscle. *Cell Reports* 14, 422-428 (2016).

34. *Ibid.*

35. Omodei, D., *et al.* Serum from humans on long-term calorie restriction enhances stress resistance in cell culture. *Aging,* 5, 599 (2013).

36. Mercken, E.M., *et al.* Calorie restriction in humans inhibits the PI 3 K/AKT pathway and induces a younger transcription profile. *Aging Cell,* 12, 645-651 (2013).

37. *Ibid.*

38. Fontana, L., *et al.* The effects of graded caloric restriction: XII. Comparison of mouse to human impact on cellular senescence in the colon. *Aging Cell,* 17, e12746 (2018).

39. Mitchell, S.J., *et al.* Effects of sex, strain, and energy intake on hallmarks of aging in Mice. *Cell Metabolism,* 23, 1093-1112 (2016).

40. Mozaffarian, D., *et al.* Changes in diet and lifestyle and long-term weight gain in women and men. *The New England Journal of Medicine,* 364, 2392-2404 (2011).

41. Berrino, F., *et al.* Reducing bioavailable sex hormones through a comprehensive change in diet: the diet and androgens (DIANA) randomized trial. *Cancer Epidemiology, Biomarkers & Prevention,* 10, 25-33 (2001).

42. Enqin, Z. *Health Preservation and Rehabilitation,* Publishing House of Shanghai College of Traditional Chinese Medicine. (1988).

43. *Ibid.*

44. Mattson, M.P., *et al.* Meal frequency and timing in health and disease. *Proceedings of the National Academy of Sciences,* 111, 16647-16653 (2014).

45. Baugh, L.R. To grow or not to grow: nutritional control of development during Caenorhabditis elegans L1 arrest. *Genetics,* 194, 539-555 (2013).

46. Fontana, L., Partridge, L. & Longo, V.D. Extending healthy life span – from yeast to humans. *Science,* 328, 321-326 (2010).

47. Renehan, A.G., *et al.* Insulin-like growth factor (IGF)-I, IGF binding protein-3, and cancer risk: systematic review and meta-regression analysis. *Lancet,* 363, 1346-1353 (2004).

48. de Cabo, R. & Mattson, M.P. Effects of Intermittent Fasting on Health, Aging, and Disease. *New England Journal of Medicine,* 381:2541-2551 (2019).

49. Yang, L., *et al.* Long-term calorie restriction enhances cellular quality-control processes in human skeletal muscle. *Cell reports* 14, 422-428 (2016).

50. Kozumbo, W.J. & Calabrese, E.J. Two decades (1998-2018) of research Progress on Hormesis: advancing biological understanding and enabling novel applications. *Journal of Cell Communication and Signaling,* 13, 273-275 (2019).

51. Chaix, A., *et al.* Time-restricted feeding is a preventative and therapeutic intervention against diverse nutritional challenges. *Cell Metabolism,* 20, 991-1005 (2014).

52. Enqin, Z. *Health Preservation,* Shanghai College of Traditional Chinese Medicine. (1988).

53. Jakubowicz, D., *et al.* Effects of caloric intake timing on insulin resistance and hyperandrogenism in lean women with polycystic ovary syndrome. *Clinical Science,* 125, 423-432 (2013).

54. Eijkelenboom, A. & Burgering, B.M. FOXOs: signalling integrators for homeostasis maintenance. *Nature Reviews: Molecular Cell Biology,* 14, 83-97 (2013).

55. Dixit, V.D., *et al.* Ghrelin inhibits leptin- and activation-induced proinflammatory cytokine expression by human monocytes and T cells. *The Journal of Clinical Investigation,* 114, 57-66 (2004).

56. Alberti, K.G., Zimmet, P. & Shaw, J. Metabolic syndrome – a new world-wide definition. A consensus statement from the International Diabetes Federation. *Diabetic Medicine,* 23, 469-480 (2006).

57. Yamaji, T., *et al.* Slow down, you eat too fast: fast eating associated with obesity and future prevalence of metabolic syndrome. *Circulation,* 136, 2 (2017).

Chapter 6: Healthy Children

1. Lane, M., Robker, R.L. & Robertson, S.A. Parenting from before conception. *Science (New York, N.Y.),* 345, 756-760 (2014).

2. Sinclair, K.D. & Watkins, A.J. Parental diet, pregnancy outcomes and offspring health: metabolic determinants in developing oocytes and embryos. *Reproduction, Fertility, and Development,* 26, 99-114 (2013).

3. Stephenson, J., *et al.* Before the beginning: nutrition and lifestyle in the preconception period and its importance for future health. *Lancet,* 391, 1830-1841 (2018).

4. Fleming, T.P., *et al.* Origins of lifetime health around the time of conception: causes and consequences. *Lancet,* 391, 1842-1852 (2018).

5. Sinclair, K.D. & Watkins, A.J. Parental diet. *Reproduction, Fertility, and Development* (2013).

6. Jones, P.A. Functions of DNA methylation: islands, start sites, gene bodies and beyond. *Nature Reviews: Genetics,* 13, 484-492 (2012).

7. Benayoun, B.A., *et al.* Epigenetic regulation of ageing: linking environmental inputs to genomic stability. Nat *Nature Reviews: Molecular Cell Biology,* 16:593-610 (2015).

8. Rando, O.J. Daddy issues: paternal effects on phenotype. *Cell,* 151, 702-708 (2012).

9. Rechavi, O., *et al,* Starvation-induced transgenerational inheritance of small RNAs in C. elegans. *Cell,* 158, 277-287 (2014).

10. Sinclair, K.D. & Watkins, A.J. Parental diet. *Reproduction, Fertility, and Development* (2013).

11. Pembrey, M., Saffery, R. & Bygren, L.O. Human transgenerational responses to early-life experience: potential impact on development, health and biomedical research. *Journal of Medical Genetics,* 51, 563-572 (2014).

12. De-Regil, L.M., *et al.* Effects and safety of periconceptional oral folate supplementation for preventing birth defects. *The Cochrane Database of Systematic Reviews,* 10, CD007950 (2015).

13. Mastroiacovo, P. & Leoncini, E. More folic acid, the five questions: why, who, when, how much, and how. *BioFactors,* 37, 272-279 (2011).

14. Gao, Y., *et al.* New perspective on impact of folic acid supplementation during pregnancy on neurodevelopment/ autism in the offspring children – a systematic review. *PLOS One,* 11, e0165626 (2016).

15. He Y., *et al.* Folic acid supplementation, birth defects, and adverse pregnancy outcomes in Chinese women: a population-based mega-cohort study. *Lancet,* 388, 91 (2016).

16. Bath, S.C., *et al.* Effect of inadequate iodine status in UK pregnant women on cognitive outcomes in their children: results from the Avon Longitudinal Study of Parents and Children (ALSPAC). *Lancet,* 382, 331-337 (2013).

17. Barker, D.J., *et al.* Resource allocation in utero and health in later life. *Placenta,* 33 (Suppl. 2), e30-34 (2012).

18. Been, J.V., *et al.* Effect of smoke-free legislation on perinatal and child health: a systematic review and meta-analysis. *Lancet,* 383, 1549-1560 (2014).

19. Caputo, C., Wood, E. & Jabbour, L. Impact of fetal alcohol exposure on body systems: A systematic review. *Birth Defects Research. Part C, Embryo Today: Reviews,* 108, 174-180 (2016).

20. Papadopoulou, E., *et al.* Maternal caffeine intake during pregnancy and childhood growth and overweight: results from a large Norwegian prospective observational cohort study. *BMJ Open,* 8, e018895 (2018).

21. Hales, C.N. & Barker, D.J. The thrifty phenotype hypothesis. *British Medical Bulletin,* 60, 5-20 (2001).

22. Gluckman, P.D. & Hanson, M.A. The developmental origins of the metabolic syndrome. *Trends in Endocrinology and Metabolism: TEM,* 15, 183-187 (2004).

23. Mackenzie, H.S. & Brenner, B.M. Fewer nephrons at birth: a missing link in the etiology of essential hypertension? *American Journal of Kidney Diseases,* 26, 91-98 (1995).

24. Keller, G., *et al.* Nephron number in patients with primary hypertension. *The New England Journal of Medicine,* 348, 101-108 (2003).

25. Widiker, S., *et al.* High-fat diet leads to a decreased methylation of the Mc4r gene in the obese BFMI and the lean B6 mouse lines. *Journal of Applied Genetics,* 51, 193-197 (2010).

26. Brait, M., *et al.* Association between lifestyle factors and CpG island methylation in a cancer-free population. *Cancer Epidemiology, Biomarkers & Prevention,* 18, 2984-2991 (2009).

27. Tarry-Adkins, J.L. & Ozanne, S.E. Nutrition in early life and age-associated diseases. *Ageing Research Reviews,* 39, 96-105 (2017).

28. Ozanne, S.E. & Hales, C.N. Lifespan: catch-up growth and obesity in male mice. *Nature,* 427, 411-412 (2004).

29. Ozanne, S.E. & Nicholas Hales, C. Poor fetal growth followed by rapid postnatal catch-up growth leads to premature death. *Mechanisms of Ageing and Development,* 126, 852-854 (2005).

30. Mangano, K.M., *et al.* Dietary protein is associated with musculoskeletal health independently of dietary pattern: the Framingham Third Generation Study. *The American Journal of Clinical Nutrition,* 105, 714-722 (2017).

31. Maslova, E., *et al.* Maternal protein intake during pregnancy and offspring overweight 20 y later. *The American Journal of Clinical Nutrition,* 100, 1139-1148 (2014).

32. Silva Idos, S., De Stavola, B. & McCormack, V. Birth size and breast cancer risk: re-analysis of individual participant data from 32 studies. *PLOS Medicine,* 5, e193 (2008).

33. McCormack, V.A., *et al.* Fetal growth and subsequent risk of breast cancer: results from long term follow up of Swedish cohort. *BMJ,* 326, 248 (2003).

34. Tibblin, G., *et al.* High birthweight as a predictor of prostate cancer risk. *Epidemiology,* 6, 423-424 (1995).

35. Sandhu, M.S., *et al.* Self-reported birth weight and subsequent risk of colorectal cancer. *Cancer Epidemiology, Biomarkers & Prevention,* 11, 935-938 (2002).

36. Dipietro, L., *et al.* Benefits of physical activity during pregnancy and postpartum: an umbrella review. *Medicine and Science in Sports and Exercise,* 51, 1292-1302 (2019).

37. Subramanian, S., *et al.* Cultivating healthy growth and nutrition through the gut microbiota. *Cell,* 161, 36-48 (2015).

38. Goyal, M.S., *et al.* Feeding the brain and nurturing the mind: Linking nutrition and the gut microbiota to brain development. *Proceedings of the National Academy of Sciences of the United States of America,* 112, 14105-14112 (2015).

39. Keski-Nisula, L., *et al.* Maternal intrapartum antibiotics and decreased vertical transmission of Lactobacillus to neonates during birth. *Acta Paediatrica,* 102, 480-485 (2013).

40. Martin, R., *et al.* Isolation of bifidobacteria from breast milk and assessment of the bifidobacterial population by PCR-denaturing gradient gel electrophoresis and quantitative real-time PCR. *Applied and Environmental Microbiology,* 75, 965-969 (2009).

41. Turroni, F., *et al.* Ability of Bifidobacterium breve to grow on different types of milk: exploring the metabolism of milk through genome analysis. *Applied and Environmental Microbiology,* 77, 7408-7417 (2011).

42. Bjerke, G.A., *et al.* Mother-to-child transmission of and multiple-strain colonization by Bacteroides fragilis in a cohort of mothers and their children. *Applied and Environmental Microbiology,* 77, 8318-8324 (2011).

43. David, L.A., *et al.* Diet rapidly and reproducibly alters the human gut microbiome. *Nature,* 505, 559-563 (2014).

44. Clemente, J.C., *et al,* The impact of the gut microbiota on human health: an integrative view. *Cell,* 148, 1258-1270 (2012).

45. Thorburn, A.N., Macia, L. & Mackay, C.R. Diet, metabolites, and "Western-lifestyle" inflammatory diseases. *Immunity,* 40, 833-842 (2014).

46. Zimmermann, M., *et al.* Mapping human microbiome drug metabolism by gut bacteria and their genes. *Nature,* 570, 462-467 (2019).

47. Victora, C.G., *et al.* Breastfeeding in the 21st century: epidemiology, mechanisms, and lifelong effect. *Lancet,* 387, 475-490 (2016).

48. Djuric, Z., *et al.* Effects of high fruit-vegetable and/or low-fat intervention on breast nipple aspirate fluid micronutrient levels. *Cancer Epidemiology, Biomarkers & Prevention,* 16, 1393-1399 (2007).

49. Mennella, J.A., *et al.* The timing and duration of a sensitive period in human flavor learning: a randomized trial. *The American Journal of Clinical Nutrition,* 93, 1019-1024 (2011).

50. Cowardin, C.A., *et al.* Mechanisms by which sialylated milk oligosaccharides impact bone biology in a gnotobiotic mouse model of infant undernutrition. *Proceedings of the National Academy of Sciences,* 116, 11988-11996 (2019).

51. World Health Organization. Early initiation of breastfeeding to promote exclusive breastfeeding. (2019).<http://www.who.int/elena/titles/early_breastfeeding/en/>

52. Holt, P.G. & Jones, C.A. The development of the immune system during pregnancy and early life. *Allergy,* 55, 688-697 (2000).

53. Quigley, M.A., Kelly, Y.J. & Sacker, A. Breastfeeding and hospitalization for diarrheal and respiratory infection in the United Kingdom Millennium Cohort Study. *Pediatrics,* 119, e837-842 (2007).

54. Wilson, A.C., *et al.* Relation of infant diet to childhood health: seven year follow up of cohort of children in Dundee infant feeding study. *BMJ,* 316, 21-25 (1998).

55. Belfort, M.B., *et al.* Infant feeding and childhood cognition at ages 3 and 7 years: Effects of breastfeeding duration and exclusivity. *Journal of the American Medical Association Pediatrics,* 167, 836-844 (2013).

56. Horwood, L.J. & Fergusson, D.M. Breastfeeding and later cognitive and academic outcomes. *Pediatrics,* 101, E9 (1998).

57. Ziegler, A.G., *et al.* Early infant feeding and risk of developing type 1 diabetes-associated autoantibodies. *Journal of the American Medical Association,* 290, 1721-1728 (2003).

58. Horta, B.L., Loret de Mola, C. & Victora, C.G. Long-term consequences of breastfeeding on cholesterol, obesity, systolic blood pressure and type 2 diabetes: a systematic review and meta-analysis. *Acta Paediatrica,* 104, 30-37 (2015).

59. Owen, C.G., *et al.* Effect of infant feeding on the risk of obesity across the life course: a quantitative review of published evidence. *Pediatrics,* 115, 1367-1377 (2005).

60. Singhal, A., *et al.* Nutrition in infancy and long-term risk of obesity: evidence from 2 randomized controlled trials. *The American Journal of Clinical Nutrition,* 92, 1133-1144 (2010).

61. Weber, M., *et al.* Lower protein content in infant formula reduces BMI and obesity risk at school age: follow-up of a randomized trial. *The American Journal of Clinical Nutrition,* 99, 1041-1051 (2014).

62. Socha, P., *et al.* Endocrine and metabolic biomarkers predicting early childhood obesity risk. *Nestle Nutrition Institute Workshop Series,* 85, 81-88 (2016).

63. Labbok, M.H. Effects of breastfeeding on the mother. *Pediatric Clinics of North America,* 48, 143-158 (2001).

64. Dewey, K.G., Heinig, M.J. & Nommsen, L.A. Maternal weight-loss patterns during prolonged lactation. *The American Journal of Clinical Nutrition,* 58, 162-166 (1993).

65. Stuebe, A.M., *et al.* Duration of lactation and incidence of type 2 diabetes. *Journal of the American Medical Association,* 294, 2601-2610 (2005).

66. Collaborative Group on Hormonal Factors in Breast Cancer. Breast cancer and breastfeeding: collaborative reanalysis of individual data from 47 epidemiological studies in 30 countries, including 50302 women with breast cancer and 96973 women without the disease. *Lancet,* 360, 187-195 (2002).

67. Luan, N.N., *et al.* Breastfeeding and ovarian cancer risk: a meta-analysis of epidemiologic studies. *The American Journal of Clinical Nutrition,* 98, 1020-1031 (2013).

68. Michels, K.B. & Willett, W.C. Breast cancer – early life matters. *The New England Journal of Medicine,* 351, 1679-1681 (2004).

69. Gunnell, D., Rogers, J. & Dieppe, P. Height and health: predicting longevity from bone length in archaeological remains. *Journal of Epidemiology and Community Health,* 55, 505-507 (2001).

70. Micozzi, M.S. Functional consequences from varying patterns of growth and maturation during adolescence. *Hormone Research,* 39 (Suppl. 3), 49-58 (1993).

71. Michels, K.B. & Willett, W.C. Breast cancer – early life matters. *The New England Journal of Medicine,* 351, 1679-1681 (2004).

72. Maclure, M., *et al.* A prospective cohort study of nutrient intake and age at menarche. *The American Journal of Clinical Nutrition,* 54, 649-656 (1991).

73. Cho, G.J., *et al.* Age at menarche in a Korean population: secular trends and influencing factors. *European Journal of Pediatrics,* 169, 89-94 (2010).

74. Russo, J., Tay, L.K. & Russo, I.H. Differentiation of the mammary gland and susceptibility to carcinogenesis. *Breast Cancer Research and Treatment,* 2, 5-73 (1982).

75. Clifton, K.H. & Crowley, J.J. Effects of radiation type and dose and the role of glucocorticoids, gonadectomy, and thyroidectomy in mammary tumor induction in mammotropin-secreting pituitary tumor-grafted rats. *Cancer Research,* 38, 1507-1513 (1978).

76. Land, C.E. Studies of cancer and radiation dose among atomic bomb survivors. The example of breast cancer. *Journal of the American Medical Association,* 274, 402-407 (1995).

77. Ahlgren, M., *et al.* Growth patterns and the risk of breast cancer in women. *The New England Journal of Medicine,* 351, 1619-1626 (2004).

78. Stefan, N., *et al.* Divergent associations of height with cardiometabolic disease and cancer: epidemiology, pathophysiology, and global implications. *Lancet: Diabetes & Endocrinology,* 4, 457-467 (2016).

Chapter 7: Diet Quality Matters

1. Partridge, L. & Fontana, L. Promoting health and longevity through diet: from model organisms to humans. *Cell,* 161, 106-118 (2015).

2. Maeda, H., *et al.* Nutritional influences on aging of Fischer 344 rats: II. Pathology. *Journal of Gerontology,* 40, 671-688 (1985).

3. Solon-Biet, S.M., *et al.* The ratio of macronutrients, not caloric intake, dictates cardiometabolic health, aging, and longevity in ad libitum-fed mice. *Cell Metabolism,* 19, 418-430 (2014).

4. Mittendorfer, B., Klein, S. & Fontana L. A word of caution against excessive protein intake. *Nature Reviews: Endocrinology,* 16, 59-66 (2019).

5. Leidy, H.J., *et al.* The role of protein in weight loss and maintenance. *The American Journal of Clinical Nutrition,* 101, 1320s-1329s (2015).

6. Vergnaud, A.C., *et al.* Macronutrient composition of the diet and prospective weight change in participants of the EPIC-PANACEA study. *PLOS One,* 8, e57300 (2013).

7. Kim, J.E., *et al.* Effects of dietary protein intake on body composition changes after weight loss in older adults: a systematic review and meta-analysis. *Nutrition Reviews,* 74, 210-224 (2016).

8. Foster, G.D., *et al.* Weight and metabolic outcomes after 2 years on a low-carbohydrate versus low-fat diet: a randomized trial. *Annals of Internal Medicine,* 153, 147-157 (2010).

9. Gardner, C.D., *et al.* Effect of low-fat vs low-carbohydrate diet on 12-month weight loss in overweight adults and the association with genotype pattern or insulin secretion: the DIETFITS randomized clinical trial. *Journal of the American Medical Association,* 319, 667-679 (2018).

10. Kim, J.E., *et al.* Effects of dietary protein intake. *Nutrition Reviews* (2016).

11. Smith, G.I., *et al.* Effect of protein supplementation during diet-induced weight loss on muscle mass and strength: a randomized controlled study. *Obesity (Silver Spring, Md.),* 26, 854-861 (2018).

12. Mangano, K.M., *et al.* Dietary protein is associated with musculoskeletal health independently of dietary pattern: the Framingham Third Generation Study. *The American Journal of Clinical Nutrition,* 105, 714-722 (2017).

13. Baer, D.J., *et al.* Whey protein but not soy protein supplementation alters body weight and composition in free-living overweight and obese adults. *The Journal of Nutrition,* 141, 1489-1494 (2011).

14. Zhu, K., *et al.* Two-year whey protein supplementation did not enhance muscle mass and physical function in well-nourished healthy older postmenopausal women. *The Journal of Nutrition,* 145, 2520-2526 (2015).

15. Reidy, P.T., *et al.* Protein supplementation has minimal effects on muscle adaptations during resistance exercise training in young men: a double-blind randomized clinical trial. *The Journal of Nutrition,* 146, 1660-1669 (2016).

16. Reidy, P.T., *et al.* Protein supplementation does not affect myogenic adaptations to resistance training. *Medicine and Science in Sports and Exercise,* 49, 1197-1208 (2017).

17. Chale, A., *et al.* Efficacy of whey protein supplementation on resistance exercise-induced changes in lean mass, muscle strength, and physical function in mobility-limited older adults. *The Journals of Gerontology. Series A, Biological Sciences and Medical Sciences,* 68, 682-690 (2013).

18. Bray, G.A., *et al.* Effect of dietary protein content on weight gain, energy expenditure, and body composition during overeating: a randomized controlled trial. *Journal of the American Medical Association,* 307, 47-55 (2012).

19. Rand, W.M., Pellett, P.L. & Young, V.R. Meta-analysis of nitrogen balance studies for estimating protein requirements in healthy adults. *The American Journal of Clinical Nutrition,* 77, 109-127 (2003).

20. World Health Organization. Protein and Amino Acid Requirements in Human Nutrition. *WHO Press,* Report Series 935, 1–265 (2007).

21. Mittendorfer, B., Klein, S. & Fontana L. A word of caution against excessive protein intake. *Nature Reviews: Endocrinology,* 16, 59-66 (2019).

22. Finger, D., *et al.* Effects of protein supplementation in older adults undergoing resistance training: a systematic review and meta-analysis. *Sports Medicine,* 45, 245-255 (2015).

23. Morton, R.W., *et al.* A systematic review, meta-analysis and meta-regression of the effect of protein supplementation on resistance training-induced gains in muscle mass and strength in healthy adults. *British Journal of Sports Medicine,* 52, 376-384 (2018).

24. Reidy, P.T. & Rasmussen, B.B. Role of ingested amino acids and protein in the promotion of resistance exercise-induced muscle protein anabolism. *The Journal of Nutrition,* 146, 155-183 (2016).

25. Holm, L. & Nordsborg, N.B. Supplementing a normal diet with protein yields a moderate improvement in the robust gains in muscle mass and strength induced by resistance training in older individuals. *The American Journal of Clinical Nutrition,* 106, 971-972 (2017).

26. Liao, C.D., *et al.* Effects of protein supplementation combined with resistance exercise on body composition and physical function in older adults: a systematic review and meta-analysis. *The American Journal of Clinical Nutrition,* 106, 1078-1091 (2017).

27. Moore, D.R., *et al.* Protein ingestion to stimulate myofibrillar protein synthesis requires greater relative protein intakes in healthy older versus younger men. *The Journals of Gerontology. Series A, Biological Sciences and Medical Sciences,* 70, 57-62 (2015).

28. Murphy, C.H., Oikawa, S.Y. & Phillips, S.M. Dietary protein to maintain muscle mass in aging: a case for per-meal protein recommendations. *The Journal of Frailty & Aging,* 5, 49-58 (2016).

29. Moore, D.R., *et al.* Ingested protein dose response of muscle and albumin protein synthesis after resistance exercise in young men. *The American Journal of Clinical Nutrition,* 89, 161-168 (2009).

30. Malik, V.S., *et al.* Dietary protein intake and risk of type 2 diabetes in US men and women. *American Journal of Epidemiology,* 183, 715-728 (2016).

31. Shang, X., *et al.* Dietary protein intake and risk of type 2 diabetes: results from the Melbourne Collaborative Cohort Study and a meta-analysis of prospective studies. *The American Journal of Clinical Nutrition,* 104, 1352-1365 (2016).

32. Wang, E.T., de Koning, L. & Kanaya, A.M. Higher protein intake is associated with diabetes risk in South Asian Indians: the Metabolic Syndrome and Atherosclerosis in South Asians Living in America (MASALA) study. *The Journal of American College of Nutrition,* 29, 130-135 (2010).

33. Simila, M.E., *et al.* Carbohydrate substitution for fat or protein and risk of type 2 diabetes in male smokers. *European Journal of Clinical Nutrition,* 66, 716-721 (2012).

34. Lagiou, P., *et al.* Low carbohydrate-high protein diet and mortality in a cohort of Swedish women. *Journal of Internal Medicine,* 261, 366-374 (2007).

35. Wang, E.T. Higher protein intake is associated with diabetes risk. *The Journal of American College of Nutrition* (2010).

36. Tinker, L.F., *et al.* Biomarker-calibrated dietary energy and protein intake associations with diabetes risk among postmenopausal women from the Women's Health Initiative. *The American Journal of Clinical Nutrition,* 94, 1600-1606 (2011).

37. Sluijs, I., *et al.* Dietary intake of total, animal, and vegetable protein and risk of type 2 diabetes in the European Prospective Investigation into Cancer and Nutrition (EPIC)-NL study. *Diabetes Care,* 33, 43-48 (2010).

38. Rand, W.M., Pellett, P.L. & Young, V.R. Meta-analysis of nitrogen balance studies. *The American Journal of Clinical Nutrition,* (2003).

39. Fontana, L., *et al.* Decreased consumption of branched-chain amino acids improves metabolic health. *Cell Reports,* 16, 520-530 (2016).

40. Zhang, Y., *et al.* The starvation hormone, fibroblast growth factor-21, extends lifespan in mice. *eLife,* 1, e00065 (2012).

41. Fontana, L., *et al.* Decreased consumption of branched-chain amino acids. *Cell Reports,* (2016).

42. Smith, G.I., *et al.* High-protein intake during weight loss therapy eliminates the weight-loss-induced improvement in insulin action in obese postmenopausal women. *Cell Reports,* 17, 849-861 (2016).

43. Levine, M.E., *et al.* Low protein intake is associated with a major reduction in IGF-1, cancer, and overall mortality in the 65 and younger but not older population. *Cell Metabolism,* 19, 407-417 (2014).

44. Simpson, S.J., *et al.* Dietary protein, aging and nutritional geometry. *Ageing Research Reviews,* 39, 78-86 (2017).

45. Solon-Biet, S.M., *et al.* The ratio of macronutrients, not caloric intake. *Cell Metabolism,* (2014).

46. Mensink, R. Effects of saturated fatty acids on serum lipids and lipoproteins: a systematic review and regression analysis. *World Health Organization,* (2016).

47. Tang, W.H., *et al.* Intestinal microbial metabolism of phosphatidylcholine and cardiovascular risk. *The New England Journal of Medicine,* 368, 1575-1584 (2013).

48. Bastide, N.M., Pierre, F.H. & Corpet, D.E. Heme iron from meat and risk of colorectal cancer: a meta-analysis and a review of the mechanisms involved. *Cancer Prevention Research,* 4, 177-184 (2011).

49. Efeyan, A., Zoncu, R. & Sabatini, D.M. Amino acids and mTORC1: from lysosomes to disease. *Trends in Molecular Medicine,* 18, 524-533 (2012).

50. Weickert, M.O., *et al.* Effects of supplemented isoenergetic diets differing in cereal fiber and protein content on insulin sensitivity in overweight humans. *The American Journal of Clinical Nutrition,* 94, 459-471 (2011).

51. Hattersley, J.G., *et al.* Modulation of amino acid metabolic signatures by supplemented isoenergetic diets differing in protein and cereal fiber content. *The Journal*

of Clinical Endocrinology and Metabolism, 99, E2599-2609 (2014).

52. Sargrad, K.R., *et al.* Effect of high protein vs high carbohydrate intake on insulin sensitivity, body weight, hemoglobin A1c, and blood pressure in patients with type 2 diabetes mellitus. *Journal of the American Dietetic Association,* 105, 573-580 (2005).

53. Malik, V.S., *et al.* Dietary protein intake. *American Journal of Epidemiology,* (2016).

54. Sluijs, I., *et al.* Dietary intake of total, animal, and vegetable protein and risk of type 2 diabetes. *Diabetes Care,* (2010).

55. Fontana, L., *et al.* Decreased consumption of branched-chain amino acids. *Cell Reports,* (2016).

56. Smith, G.I., *et al.* Protein ingestion induces muscle insulin resistance independent of leucine-mediated mTOR activation. *Diabetes,* 64, 1555-1563 (2015).

57. Ericksen, R.E., *et al.* Loss of BCAA catabolism during carcinogenesis enhances mTORC1 activity and promotes tumor development and progression. *Cell Metabolism,* 29, 1151-1165.e1156 (2019).

58. Fontana, L., *et al.* Dietary protein restriction inhibits tumor growth in human xenograft models of prostate and breast cancer. *Oncotarget,* 4, 2451 (2013).

59. Levine, M.E., *et al.* Low protein intake is associated with a major reduction in IGF-1, cancer. *Cell Metabolism,* (2014).

60. Song, M., *et al.* Association of animal and plant protein intake with all-cause and cause-specific mortality. *Journal of the American Medical Association: Internal Medicine,* 176, 1453-1463 (2016).

61. Ables, G.P., *et al.* The first international mini-symposium on methionine restriction and lifespan. *Frontiers in Genetics,* 5, 122 (2014).

62. Miller, R.A., *et al.* Methionine-deficient diet extends mouse lifespan, slows immune and lens aging, alters glucose, T4, IGF-I and insulin levels, and increases hepatocyte MIF levels and stress resistance. *Aging Cell,* 4, 119-125 (2005).

63. Mensink, R.P., *et al.* Effects of dietary fatty acids and carbohydrates on the ratio of serum total to HDL cholesterol and on serum lipids and apolipoproteins: a meta-analysis of 60 controlled trials. *The American Journal of Clinical Nutrition,* 77, 1146-1155 (2003).

64. *Ibid.*

65. Mozaffarian, D., *et al.* Trans fatty acids and cardiovascular disease. *The New England Journal of Medicine,* 354, 1601-1613 (2006).

66. Kris-Etherton, P.M. AHA Science Advisory. Monounsaturated fatty acids and risk of cardiovascular disease. American Heart Association Nutrition Committee. *Circulation,* 100, 1253-1258 (1999).

67. Mensink, R.P., *et al.* Effects of dietary fatty acids. *The American Journal of Clinical Nutrition* (2003).

68. Garg, A., Grundy, S.M. & Koffler, M. Effect of high carbohydrate intake on hyperglycemia, islet function, and plasma lipoproteins in NIDDM. *Diabetes Care,* 15, 1572-1580 (1992).

69. Guasch-Ferre, M., *et al.* Associations of monounsaturated fatty acids from plant and animal sources with total and cause-specific mortality in two US prospective cohort studies. *Circulation Research,* 124, 1266-1275 (2019).

70. Innes, J.K. & Calder, P.C. Omega-6 fatty acids and inflammation. *Prostaglandins, Leukotrienes, and Essential Fatty Acids,* 132, 41-48 (2018).

71. Welsch, C.W. Relationship between dietary fat and experimental mammary tumorigenesis: a review and critique. *Cancer Research,* 52, 2040s-2048s (1992).

72. Russo, G.L. Dietary n-6 and n-3 polyunsaturated fatty acids: from biochemistry to clinical implications in cardiovascular prevention. *Biochemical Pharmacology,* 77, 937-946 (2009).

73. Visioli, F., *et al.* An overview of the pharmacology of olive oil and its active ingredients. *British Journal of Pharmacology* (2019).

74. Heaton, K.W., *et al.* Particle size of wheat, maize, and oat test meals: effects on plasma glucose and insulin responses and on the rate of starch digestion in vitro. *The American Journal of Clinical Nutrition,* 47, 675-682 (1988).

75. Bjorck, I. & Elmstahl, H.L. The glycaemic index: importance of dietary fibre and other food properties. *The Proceedings of the Nutrition Society,* 62, 201-206 (2003).

76. Haber, G.B., *et al.* Depletion and disruption of dietary fibre. Effects on satiety, plasma-glucose, and serum-insulin. *Lancet,* 2, 679-682 (1977).

77. Brand-Miller, J.C., *et al.* Glycemic index and obesity. *The American Journal of Clinical Nutrition,* 76, 281s-285s (2002).

78. Huang, T., *et al.* Consumption of whole grains and cereal fiber and total and cause-specific mortality: prospective analysis of 367,442 individuals. *BMC Medicine,* 13, 59 (2015).

79. Hajishafiee, M., *et al.* Cereal fibre intake and risk of mortality from all causes, CVD, cancer and inflammatory diseases: a systematic review and meta-analysis of prospective cohort studies. *The British Journal of Nutrition,* 116, 343-352 (2016).

80. Xu, M., *et al.* Ready-to-eat cereal consumption with total and cause-specific mortality: prospective analysis of 367,442 individuals. *The Journal of American College of Nutrition,* 35, 217-223 (2016).

81. Colonna, P., Leloup, V. & Buleon, A. Limiting factors of starch hydrolysis. *European Journal of Clinical Nutrition,* 46 (Suppl. 2), S17-32 (1992).

82. Thomsen, C., *et al.* The glycemic index of spaghetti and gastric emptying in non-insulin-dependent diabetic patients. *European Journal of Clinical Nutrition,* 48, 776-780 (1994).

83. Englyst, K.N., *et al.* Rapidly available glucose in foods: an in vitro measurement that reflects the glycemic response. *The American Journal of Clinical Nutrition,* 69, 448-454 (1999).

84. Collier, G., McLean, A. & O'Dea, K. Effect of co-ingestion of fat on the metabolic responses to slowly and

rapidly absorbed carbohydrates. *Diabetologia, 26,* 50-54 (1984).

85. Chuang, S.C., *et al.* Fiber intake and total and cause-specific mortality in the European Prospective Investigation into Cancer and Nutrition cohort. *The American Journal of Cinical Nutrition, 96,* 164-174 (2012).

86. Reynolds, A., *et al.* Carbohydrate quality and human health: a series of systematic reviews and meta-analyses. *Lancet, 393,* 434-445 (2019).

87. Yang, Y., *et al.* Association between dietary fiber and lower risk of all-cause mortality: a meta-analysis of cohort studies. *American Journal of Epidemiology, 181,* 83-91 (2015).

88. Bingham, S.A., *et al.* Dietary fibre in food and protection against colorectal cancer in the European Prospective Investigation into Cancer and Nutrition (EPIC): an observational study. *Lancet, 361,* 1496-1501 (2003).

89. Reynolds, A., *et al.* Carbohydrate quality and human health. *Lancet* (2019).

90. Huang, T., *et al.* Consumption of whole grains. *BMC Medicine* (2015).

91. Bingham, S.A. Mechanisms and experimental and epidemiological evidence relating dietary fibre (non-starch polysaccharides) and starch to protection against large bowel cancer. *The Proceedings of the Nutrition Society, 49,* 153-171 (1990).

92. Cummings, J.H. Fermentation in the human large intestine: evidence and implications for health. *Lancet, 1,* 1206-1209 (1983).

93. Bingham, S.A. Mechanisms and experimental. *The Proceedings of the Nutrition Society* (1990).

94. Muegge, B.D., *et al.* Diet drives convergence in gut microbiome functions across mammalian phylogeny and within humans. *Science, 332,* 970-974 (2011).

95. Stephen, A.M. & Cummings, J.H. Mechanism of action of dietary fibre in the human colon. *Nature, 284,* 283-284 (1980).

96. Bonithon-Kopp, C., *et al.* Calcium and fibre supplementation in prevention of colorectal adenoma recurrence: a randomised intervention trial. European Cancer Prevention Organisation Study Group. *Lancet, 356,* 1300-1306 (2000).

97. Donaldson, M.S. Metabolic vitamin B12 status on a mostly raw vegan diet with follow-up using tablets, nutritional yeast, or probiotic supplements. *Annals of Nutrition & Metabolism, 44,* 229-234 (2000).

98. *Ibid.*

99. Herrmann, W. & Geisel, J. Vegetarian lifestyle and monitoring of vitamin B-12 status. *Clinica Chimica Acta: International Journal of Clinical Chemistry, 326,* 47-59 (2002).

100. Savva, S.C. & Kafatos, A. Is red meat required for the prevention of iron deficiency among children and adolescents? *Current Pediatric Reviews, 10,* 177-183 (2014).

101. Hallberg, L. & Hulthen, L. Prediction of dietary iron absorption: an algorithm for calculating absorption and bioavailability of dietary iron. *The American Journal of Clinical Nutrition, 71,* 1147-1160 (2000).

102. Fleming, D.J., *et al.* Dietary factors associated with the risk of high iron stores in the elderly Framingham Heart Study cohort. *The American Journal of Clinical Nutrition, 76,* 1375-1384 (2002).

103. Gillooly, M., *et al.* The effects of organic acids, phytates and polyphenols on the absorption of iron from vegetables. *The British Journal of Nutrition, 49,* 331-342 (1983).

104. Manary, M.J., *et al.* Community-based dietary phytate reduction and its effect on iron status in Malawian children. *Annals of Tropical Paediatrics, 22,* 133-136 (2002).

105. Bhatia, A. & Khetarpaul, N. Development, acceptability and nutritional evaluation of 'Doli Ki Roti'--an indigenously fermented bread. *Nutrition and Health, 15,* 113-120 (2001).

106. Hurrell, R.F., Reddy, M. & Cook, J.D. Inhibition of non-haem iron absorption in man by polyphenolic-containing beverages. *The British Journal of Nutrition, 81,* 289-295 (1999).

107. Weaver, C.M. & Plawecki, K.L. Dietary calcium: adequacy of a vegetarian diet. *The American Journal of Clinical Nutrition, 59,* 1238s-1241s (1994).

108. Weaver, C.M., Proulx, W.R. & Heaney, R. Choices for achieving adequate dietary calcium with a vegetarian diet. *The American Journal of Clinical Nutrition, 70,* 543s-548s (1999).

109. Tesar, R., *et al.* Axial and peripheral bone density and nutrient intakes of postmenopausal vegetarian and omnivorous women. *The American Journal of Clinical Nutrition, 56,* 699-704 (1992).

110. Fontana, L., *et al.* Low bone mass in subjects on a long-term raw vegetarian diet. *Archives of Internal Medicine, 165,* 684-689 (2005).

111. Satija, A., *et al.* Healthful and unhealthful plant-based diets and the risk of coronary heart disease in U.S. adults. *Journal of the American College of Cardiology, 70,* 411-422 (2017).

112. Satija, A., *et al.* Plant-Based Dietary Patterns and Incidence of Type 2 Diabetes in US Men and Women: Results from Three Prospective Cohort Studies. *PLoS medicine 13,* e1002039 (2016).

113. Micha, R. & Mozaffarian, D. Trans fatty acids: effects on metabolic syndrome, heart disease and diabetes. *Nature Reviews: Endocrinology 5,* 335-344 (2009).

Part III: From the Mediterranean to the modern healthy longevity diet

Chapter 8: The Mediterranean diet

1. Keys, A. From Naples to seven countries – a sentimental journey. *Progress in Biochemical Pharmacology, 19,* 1-30 (1983).

2. *Ibid.*

3. Keys, A., *et al.* Studies on serum cholesterol and other characteristics of clinically healthy men in Naples. *JAMA Internal Medicine*, 93, 328-336 (1954).

4. Taylor, H.L., *et al.* Coronary heart disease in seven countries. XI. Five years of follow-up of railroad men in Italy. *Circulation*, 41, I113-122 (1970).

5. Keys, A., *et al.* The diet and 15-year death rate in the seven countries study. *American Journal of Epidemiology*, 124, 903-915 (1986).

6. *Ibid.*

7. Tosti, V., Bertozzi, B. & Fontana, L. Health benefits of the mediterranean diet: metabolic and molecular mechanisms. *The Journals of Gerontology: Series A*, 73, 318-326 (2017).

8. de Lorgeril, M., *et al.* Mediterranean diet, traditional risk factors, and the rate of cardiovascular complications after myocardial infarction: final report of the Lyon Diet Heart Study. *Circulation*, 99, 779-785 (1999).

9. Singh, R.B., *et al.* Effect of an Indo-Mediterranean diet on progression of coronary artery disease in high risk patients (Indo-Mediterranean Diet Heart Study): a randomised single-blind trial. *Lancet*, 360, 1455-1461 (2002).

10. Estruch, R., *et al.* Primary prevention of cardiovascular disease with a mediterranean diet supplemented with extra-virgin olive oil or nuts. *The New England Journal of Medicine*, 378, e34 (2018).

11. Salas-Salvado, J., *et al.* Reduction in the incidence of type 2 diabetes with the Mediterranean diet: results of the PREDIMED-Reus nutrition intervention randomized trial. *Diabetes Care*, 34, 14-19 (2011).

12. Toledo, E., *et al.* Mediterranean Diet and Invasive Breast Cancer Risk Among Women at High Cardiovascular Risk in the PREDIMED Trial: A Randomized Clinical Trial. *Journal of the American Medical Association: Internal Medicine*, 175, 1752-1760 (2015).

13. Martinez-Gonzalez, M.A., *et al.* Extravirgin olive oil consumption reduces risk of atrial fibrillation: the PREDIMED trial. *Circulation*, 130, 18-26 (2014).

14. Li, Y., *et al.* Saturated fats compared with unsaturated fats and sources of carbohydrates in relation to risk of coronary heart disease: a prospective cohort study. *Journal of the American College of Cardiology*, 66, 1538-1548 (2015).

15. Sacks, F.M., *et al.* Dietary fats and cardiovascular disease: a presidential advisory from the American Heart Association. *Circulation*, 136, e1-e23 (2017).

16. Abumweis, S.S., Barake, R. & Jones, P.J. Plant sterols/stanols as cholesterol lowering agents: a meta-analysis of randomized controlled trials. *Food & Nutrition Research*, 52 (2008).

17. Jenkins, D.J., *et al.* Effect of a dietary portfolio of cholesterol-lowering foods given at 2 levels of intensity of dietary advice on serum lipids in hyperlipidemia: a randomized controlled trial. *Journal of the American Medical Association*, 306, 831-839 (2011).

18. Hu, F.B. & Stampfer, M.J. Nut consumption and risk of coronary heart disease: a review of epidemiologic evidence. *Current Atherosclerosis Reports*, 1, 204-209 (1999).

19. Stender, S. In equal amounts, the major ruminant trans fatty acid is as bad for LDL cholesterol as industrially produced trans fatty acids, but the latter are easier to remove from foods. *The American Journal of Clinical Nutrition*, 102, 1301-1302 (2015).

20. Theuwissen, E. & Mensink, R.P. Water-soluble dietary fibers and cardiovascular disease. *Physiology & Behavior*, 94, 285-292 (2008).

21. Salas-Salvado, J., *et al.* Effect of two doses of a mixture of soluble fibres on body weight and metabolic variables in overweight or obese patients: a randomised trial. *The British Journal of Nutrition*, 99, 1380-1387 (2008).

22. Yusuf, S., *et al.* Effect of potentially modifiable risk factors associated with myocardial infarction in 52 countries (the INTERHEART study): case-control study. *Lancet*, 364, 937-952 (2004).

23. Lim, C.C., *et al.* Mediterranean Diet and the Association Between Air Pollution and Cardiovascular Disease Mortality Risk. *Circulation*, 139, 1766-1775 (2019).

24. Meisinger, C., *et al.* Plasma oxidized low-density lipoprotein, a strong predictor for acute coronary heart disease events in apparently healthy, middle-aged men from the general population. *Circulation*, 112, 651-657 (2005).

25. Fito, M., *et al.* Effect of a traditional Mediterranean diet on lipoprotein oxidation: a randomized controlled trial. *Archives of Internal Medicine*, 167, 1195-1203 (2007).

26. Calder, P.C., *et al.* Dietary factors and low-grade inflammation in relation to overweight and obesity. *The British Journal of Nutrition*, 106 (Suppl. 3), S5-78 (2011).

27. *Ibid.*

28. Oh, D.Y., *et al.* GPR120 is an omega-3 fatty acid receptor mediating potent anti-inflammatory and insulin-sensitizing effects. *Cell*, 142, 687-698 (2010).

29. Yan, Y., *et al.* Omega-3 fatty acids prevent inflammation and metabolic disorder through inhibition of NLRP3 inflammasome activation. *Immunity*, 38, 1154-1163 (2013).

30. Visioli, F., *et al.* An overview of the pharmacology of olive oil and its active ingredients. *British Journal of Pharmacology* (2019).

31. Muegge, B.D., *et al.* Diet drives convergence in gut microbiome functions across mammalian phylogeny and within humans. *Science*, 332, 970-974 (2011).

32. Haro, C., *et al.* Consumption of two healthy dietary patterns restored microbiota dysbiosis in obese patients with metabolic dysfunction. *Molecular Nutrition & Food Research*, 61 (2017).

33. De Filippis, F., *et al.* High-level adherence to a Mediterranean diet beneficially impacts the gut microbiota and associated metabolome. *Gut*, 65, 1812-1821 (2016).

34. Mazmanian, S.K., *et al.* An immunomodulatory molecule of symbiotic bacteria directs maturation of the host immune system. *Cell,* 122, 107-118 (2005).

35. Round, J.L. & Mazmanian, S.K. Inducible Foxp3+ regulatory T-cell development by a commensal bacterium of the intestinal microbiota. *Proceedings of the National Academy of Sciences of the United States of America,* 107, 12204-12209 (2010).

36. Arpaia, N., *et al.* Metabolites produced by commensal bacteria promote peripheral regulatory T-cell generation. *Nature,* 504, 451-455 (2013).

37. Thorburn, A.N., Macia, L. & Mackay, C.R. Diet, metabolites, and "Western-lifestyle" inflammatory diseases. *Immunity,* 40, 833-842 (2014).

38. Llewellyn, S.R., *et al.* Interactions between diet and the intestinal microbiota alter intestinal permeability and colitis severity in mice. *Gastroenterology,* 154, 1037-1046.e1032 (2018).

39. Jowett, S.L., *et al.* Influence of dietary factors on the clinical course of ulcerative colitis: a prospective cohort study. *Gut,* 53, 1479-1484 (2004).

40. Ananthakrishnan, A.N., *et al.* High school diet and risk of Crohn's disease and ulcerative colitis. *Inflammatory Bowel Diseases,* 21, 2311-2319 (2015).

41. Brotherton, C.S., *et al.* Avoidance of fiber is associated with greater risk of Crohn's disease flare in a 6-month period. *Clinical Gastroenterology and Hepatology,* 14, 1130-1136 (2016).

42. Hallert, C., *et al.* Ispaghula husk may relieve gastrointestinal symptoms in ulcerative colitis in remission. *Scandinavian Journal of Gastroenterology,* 26, 747-750, (1991).

43. Tang, W.H., *et al.* Intestinal microbial metabolism of phosphatidylcholine and cardiovascular risk. *The New England Journal of Medicine,* 368, 1575-1584 (2013).

44. Griffin, N.W., *et al.* Prior dietary practices and connections to a human gut microbial metacommunity alter responses to diet interventions. *Cell Host & Microbe,* 21, 84-96 (2017).

45. Sonnenburg, E.D., *et al.* Diet-induced extinctions in the gut microbiota compound over generations. *Nature,* 529, 212-215 (2016).

46. Barratt, M.J., *et al.* The Gut Microbiota, Food Science, and Human Nutrition: A Timely Marriage. *Cell Host Microbe,* 22:134-141 (2017).

Chapter 9: Move to the modern healthy longevity diet

1. Fontana, L. & Partridge, L. Promoting health and longevity through diet: from model organisms to humans. *Cell,* 161, 106-118 (2015).

2. Abete, I., *et al.* Obesity and metabolic syndrome: potential benefit from specific nutritional components. *Nutrition, Metabolism and Cardiovascular Disease,* 10, 1016 (2011).

3. Speakman, J.R., & Mitchell, S.E., Caloric restriction. *Molecular Aspects of Medicine,* 32, 159-221 (2011).

4. Liu, R.H. Potential synergy of phytochemicals in cancer prevention: mechanism of action. *The Journal of Nutrition,* 134, 3479s-3485s (2004).

5. Velmurugan, B., Mani, A. & Nagini, S. Combination of S-allylcysteine and lycopene induces apoptosis by modulating Bcl-2, Bax, Bim and caspases during experimental gastric carcinogenesis. *European Journal of Cancer Prevention,* 14, 387-393 (2005).

6. Swami, S., *et al.* Genistein potentiates the growth inhibitory effects of 1,25-dihydroxyvitamin D3 in DU145 human prostate cancer cells: role of the direct inhibition of CYP24 enzyme activity. *Molecular and Cellular Endocrinology,* 241, 49-61 (2005).

7. Li, W., *et al.* Emerging senolytic agents derived from natural products. *Mechanisms of Ageing and Development,* 181, 1-6 (2019).

8. de Oliveira Otto, M.C., *et al.* Dietary Diversity: Implications for Obesity Prevention in Adult Populations: A Science Advisory From the American Heart Association. *Circulation,* 138, e160-e168 (2018).

9. Zimmermann, M.B., Jooste, P.L. & Pandav, C.S. Iodine-deficiency disorders. *Lancet,* 372, 1251-1262 (2008).

10. Liu, R.H. Health benefits of fruit and vegetables are from additive and synergistic combinations of phytochemicals. *The American Journal of Clinical Nutrition,* 78, 517s-520s (2003).

11. Kris-Etherton, P.M., *et al.* Bioactive compounds in foods: their role in the prevention of cardiovascular disease and cancer. *The American Journal of Medicine,* 113 (Suppl. 9B), 71s-88s (2002).

12. Howitz, K.T. & Sinclair, D.A. Xenohormesis: Sensing the chemical cues of other species. *Cell,* 133, 387-391 (2008).

13. Collett, N.P., *et al.* Cancer prevention with natural compounds. *Seminars in Oncology,* 37, 258-281 (2010).

14. Aune, D., *et al.* Fruit and vegetable intake and the risk of cardiovascular disease, total cancer and all-cause mortality-a systematic review and dose-response meta-analysis of prospective studies. *International Journal of Epidemiology,* 46, 1029-1056 (2017).

15. Leenders, M., *et al.* Fruit and vegetable intake and cause-specific mortality in the EPIC study. *European Journal of Epidemiology,* 29, 639-652 (2014).

16. Hung, H.C., *et al.* Fruit and vegetable intake and risk of major chronic disease. *Journal of the National Cancer Institute,* 96, 1577-1584 (2004).

17. Bhupathiraju, S.N., *et al.* Quantity and variety in fruit and vegetable intake and risk of coronary heart disease. *The American Journal of Clinical Nutrition,* 98, 1514-1523 (2013).

18. Sacks, F.M., *et al.* Effects on blood pressure of reduced dietary sodium and the Dietary Approaches to Stop Hypertension (DASH) diet. DASH-Sodium Collaborative Research Group. *The New England Journal of Medicine,* 344, 3-10 (2001).

19. de Kok, T.M., *et al.* Antioxidative and antigenotoxic properties of vegetables and dietary phytochemicals: the value of genomics biomarkers in molecular epidemiology. *Molecular Nutrition & Food Research,* 54, 208-217 (2010).

20. Jung, S., *et al.* Fruit and vegetable intake and risk of breast cancer by hormone receptor status. *Journal of the National Cancer Institute,* 105, 219-236 (2013).

21. Lee, J.E., *et al.* Intakes of fruits, vegetables, vitamins A, C, and E, and carotenoids and risk of renal cell cancer. *Cancer Epidemiology, Biomarkers & Prevention,* 15, 2445-2452 (2006).

22. Linseisen, J., *et al.* Fruit and vegetable consumption and lung cancer risk: updated information from the European Prospective Investigation into Cancer and Nutrition (EPIC). *International Journal of Cancer,* 121, 1103-1114 (2007).

23. Boeing, H., *et al.* Intake of fruits and vegetables and risk of cancer of the upper aero-digestive tract: the prospective EPIC-study. *Cancer Causes & Control: CCC,* 17, 957-969 (2006).

24. Guo, W., *et al.* A nested case-control study of oesophageal and stomach cancers in the Linxian nutrition intervention trial. *International Journal of Epidemiology,* 23, 444-450 (1994).

25. Jeurnink, S.M., *et al.* Variety in vegetable and fruit consumption and the risk of gastric and esophageal cancer in the European Prospective Investigation into Cancer and Nutrition. *International Journal of Cancer,* 131, E963-973 (2012).

26. Aune, D., *et al.* Dietary compared with blood concentrations of carotenoids and breast cancer risk: a systematic review and meta-analysis of prospective studies. *The American Journal of Clinical Nutrition,* 96, 356-373 (2012).

27. Bertoia, M.L., *et al.* Changes in intake of fruits and vegetables and weight change in United States men and women followed for up to 24 years: analysis from three prospective cohort studies. *PLOS Medicine,* 12, e1001878 (2015).

28. Berrino, F., *et al.* Reducing bioavailable sex hormones through a comprehensive change in diet: the diet and androgens (DIANA) randomized trial. *Cancer Epidemiology, Biomarkers & Prevention,* 10, 25-33 (2001).

29. DiMeglio, L.A., Evans-Molina, C. & Oram, R.A. Type 1 diabetes. *Lancet,* 391, 2449-2462 (2018).

30. de la Cuesta-Zuluaga, J., *et al.* Age- and Sex-Dependent Patterns of Gut Microbial Diversity in Human Adults. *mSystems,* 4, e00261-e00319 (2019).

31. Cooper, A.J., *et al.* A prospective study of the association between quantity and variety of fruit and vegetable intake and incident type 2 diabetes. *Diabetes Care,* 35, 1293-1300 (2012).

32. Jeurnink, S.M., *et al.* Variety in vegetable and fruit consumption and the risk of gastric and esophageal cancer in the European Prospective Investigation into Cancer and Nutrition. *International Journal of Cancer,* 131, E963-973 (2012).

33. Jansen, M.C., *et al.* Quantity and variety of fruit and vegetable consumption and cancer risk. *Nutrition and Cancer,* 48, 142-148 (2004).

34. Buchner, F.L., *et al.* Variety in fruit and vegetable consumption and the risk of lung cancer in the European prospective investigation into cancer and nutrition. *Cancer Epidemiology, Biomarkers & Prevention,* 19, 2278-2286 (2010).

35. Buchner, F.L., *et al.* Variety in vegetable and fruit consumption and risk of bladder cancer in the European Prospective Investigation into Cancer and Nutrition. *International Journal of Cancer,* 128, 2971-2979 (2011).

36. Almeida-de-Souza, J., *et al.* Associations between fruit and vegetable variety and low-grade inflammation in Portuguese adolescents from LabMed Physical Activity Study. *European Journal of Nutrition,* 57, 2055-2068 (2018).

37. Jaszewski, R., *et al.* Folic acid supplementation inhibits recurrence of colorectal adenomas: a randomized chemoprevention trial. *World Journal of Gastroenterology,* 14, 4492-4498 (2008).

38. Krinsky, N.I., Landrum, J.T. & Bone, R.A. Biologic mechanisms of the protective role of lutein and zeaxanthin in the eye. *Annual Review of Nutrition,* 23, 171-201 (2003).

39. Petropoulos, S., *et al.* Chemical composition and yield of six genotypes of common purslane (Portulaca oleracea l.): an alternative source of omega-3 fatty acids. *Plant Foods for Human Nutrition,* 70, 420-426 (2015).

40. Verkerk, R., *et al.* Glucosinolates in Brassica vegetables: the influence of the food supply chain on intake, bioavailability and human health. *Molecular Nutrition & Food Research,* 53 (Suppl. 2), S219 (2009).

41. *Ibid.*

42. Formica, J.V. & Regelson, W. Review of the biology of quercetin and related bioflavonoids. *Food and Chemical Toxicology,* 33, 1061-1080 (1995).

43. Mackraj, I., Govender, T. & Ramesar, S. The antihypertensive effects of quercetin in a salt-sensitive model of hypertension. *Journal of Cardiovascular Pharmacology,* 51, 239-245 (2008).

44. Rivera, L., *et al.* Quercetin ameliorates metabolic syndrome and improves the inflammatory status in obese Zucker rats. *Obesity,* 16, 2081-2087 (2008).

45. Talalay, P. & Fahey, J.W. Phytochemicals from cruciferous plants protect against cancer by modulating carcinogen metabolism. *The Journal of Nutrition,* 131, 3027s-3033s (2001).

46. Fahey, J.W., Zhang, Y. & Talalay, P. Broccoli sprouts: an exceptionally rich source of inducers of enzymes that protect against chemical carcinogens. *Proceedings of the National Academy of Sciences of the United States of America,* 94, 10367-10372 (1997).

47. Axelsson, A.S., *et al.* Sulforaphane reduces hepatic glucose production and improves glucose control in patients with type 2 diabetes. *Science Translational Medicine,* 9 (2017).

48. Singh, K., *et al.* Sulforaphane treatment of autism spectrum disorder (ASD). *Proceedings of the National Academy of Sciences of the United States of America,* 111, 15550-15555 (2014).

49. Abdull Razis, A.F. & Noor, N.M. Cruciferous vegetables: dietary phytochemicals for cancer prevention. *Asian Pacific Journal of Cancer Prevention: APJCP,* 14, 1565-1570 (2013).

50. Gupta, P., *et al.* Molecular targets of isothiocyanates in cancer: Recent advances. *Molecular Nutrition & Food Research,* 58, 1685-1707 (2014).

51. Lee, Y.R., *et al.* Reactivation of PTEN tumor suppressor for cancer treatment through inhibition of a MYC-WWP1 inhibitory pathway. *Science,* 364 (2019).

52. Ortega-Molina, A., *et al.* Pten positively regulates brown adipose function, energy expenditure, and longevity. *Cell Metabolism,* 15, 382-394 (2012).

53. Rock, C.L., *et al.* Bioavailability of beta-carotene is lower in raw than in processed carrots and spinach in women. *The Journal of Nutrition,* 128, 913-916 (1998).

54. Christensen, L.P. & Brandt, K. Bioactive polyacetylenes in food plants of the Apiaceae family: occurrence, bioactivity and analysis. *Journal of Pharmaceutical and Biomedical Analysis,* 41, 683-693 (2006).

55. Paetau, I., *et al.* Interactions in the postprandial appearance of beta-carotene and canthaxanthin in plasma triacylglycerol-rich lipoproteins in humans. *The American Journal of Clinical Nutrition,* 66, 1133-1143 (1997).

56. Giovannucci, E. Tomatoes, tomato-based products, lycopene, and cancer: review of the epidemiologic literature. *Journal of the National Cancer Institute,* 91, 317-331 (1999).

57. Kucuk, O., *et al.* Phase II randomized clinical trial of lycopene supplementation before radical prostatectomy. *Cancer Epidemiology, Biomarkers & Prevention,* 10, 861-868 (2001).

58. Vrieling, A., *et al.* Lycopene supplementation elevates circulating insulin-like growth factor binding protein-1 and -2 concentrations in persons at greater risk of colorectal cancer. *The American Journal of Clinical Nutrition,* 86, 1456-1462 (2007).

59. van het Hof, K.H., *et al.* Carotenoid bioavailability in humans from tomatoes processed in different ways determined from the carotenoid response in the triglyceride-rich lipoprotein fraction of plasma after a single consumption and in plasma after four days of consumption. *The Journal of Nutrition,* 130, 1189-1196 (2000).

60. Block, E. The chemistry of garlic and onions. *Scientific American* 252, 114-119 (1985).

61. Song, K. & Milner, J.A. The influence of heating on the anticancer properties of garlic. *The Journal of Nutrition,* 131, 1054s-1057s (2001).

62. Dong, Y., Lisk, D., Block, E. & Ip, C. Characterization of the biological activity of gamma-glutamyl-Se-methylselenocysteine: a novel, naturally occurring anticancer agent from garlic. *Cancer Research,* 61, 2923-2928 (2001).

63. Wargovich, M.J. Diallyl sulfide, a flavor component of garlic (Allium sativum), inhibits dimethylhydrazine-induced colon cancer. *Carcinogenesis,* 8, 487-489 (1987).

64. Breithaupt-Grogler, K., *et al.* Protective effect of chronic garlic intake on elastic properties of aorta in the elderly. *Circulation,* 96, 2649-2655 (1997).

65. Milner, J.A. A historical perspective on garlic and cancer. *The Journal of Nutrition,* 131, 1027s-1031s (2001).

66. Knowles, L.M. & Milner, J.A. Possible mechanism by which allyl sulfides suppress neoplastic cell proliferation. *The Journal of Nutrition,* 131, 1061s-1066s (2001).

67. Dorant, E., *et al.* Consumption of onions and a reduced risk of stomach carcinoma. *Gastroenterology,* 110, 12-20 (1996).

68. Brusselmans, K., *et al.* Induction of cancer cell apoptosis by flavonoids is associated with their ability to inhibit fatty acid synthase activity. *The Journal of Biological Chemistry,* 280, 5636-5645 (2005).

69. Muraki, I., *et al.* Potato consumption and risk of type 2 diabetes: results from three prospective cohort studies. *Diabetes Care,* 39, 376-384 (2016).

70. Borgi, L., *et al.* Potato intake and incidence of hypertension: results from three prospective US cohort studies. *BMJ,* 353, i2351 (2016).

71. Veronese, N., *et al.* Fried potato consumption is associated with elevated mortality: an 8-y longitudinal cohort study. *The American Journal of Clinical Nutrition,* 106, 162-167 (2017).

72. Ceccanti, C., *et al.* Mediterranean wild edible plants: weeds or "new functional crops"? *Molecules (Basel, Switzerland),* 23, 2299 (2018).

73. van der Walt, A.M., *et al.* Linolenic acid and folate in wild-growing African dark leafy vegetables (morogo). *Public Health Nutrition,* 12, 525-530 (2009).

74. Perez-Jimenez, J., *et al.* Identification of the 100 richest dietary sources of polyphenols: an application of the Phenol-Explorer database. *European Journal of Clinical Nutrition,* 64 (Suppl. 3), S112-120 (2010).

75. Caterina, M.J., *et al.* The capsaicin receptor: a heat-activated ion channel in the pain pathway. *Nature,* 389, 816-824 (1997).

76. Zhang, L.L., *et al.* Activation of transient receptor potential vanilloid type-1 channel prevents adipogenesis and obesity. *Circulation Research,* 100, 1063-1070 (2007).

77. Kang, J.H., *et al.* Dietary capsaicin reduces obesity-induced insulin resistance and hepatic steatosis in obese mice fed a high-fat diet. *Obesity,* 18, 780-787 (2010).

78. Snitker, S., *et al.* Effects of novel capsinoid treatment on fatness and energy metabolism in humans: possible pharmacogenetic implications. *The American Journal of Clinical Nutrition,* 89, 45-50 (2009).

79. Yoneshiro, T., *et al.* Recruited brown adipose tissue as an antiobesity agent in humans. *The Journal of clinical investigation* 123, 3404-3408 (2013).

80. Luo, X.J., Peng, J. & Li, Y.J. Recent advances in the study on capsaicinoids and capsinoids. *European Journal of Pharmacology,* 650, 1-7 (2011).

81. Ruby, A.J., *et al.* Anti-tumour and antioxidant activity of natural curcuminoids. *Cancer Letters,* 94, 79-83 (1995).

82. Aggarwal, B.B., Kumar, A. & Bharti, A.C. Anticancer potential of curcumin: preclinical and clinical studies. *Anticancer Research*, 23, 363-398 (2003).

83. Kuttan, G., *et al*. Antitumour, anti-invasion, and antimetastatic effects of curcumin. *Advances in Experimental Medicine and Biology*, 595, 173-184 (2007).

84. Li, M., *et al*. Curcumin, a dietary component, has anticancer, chemosensitization and radiosensitization effects on down-regulating the MDM2 oncogene through the P13K/mTOR/ETS2 pathway. *Cancer Research*, 10.1158/0008-5472.CAN-06-3066 (2007).

85. Cruz-Correa, M., *et al*. Combination treatment with curcumin and quercetin of adenomas in familial adenomatous polyposis. *Clinical Gastroenterology and Hepatology*, Vol 4, Issue 8, 1035-1038 (2006).

86. Yang, F., *et al*. Curcumin inhibits formation of amyloid beta oligomers and fibrils, binds plaques, and reduces amyloid in vivo. *The Journal of Biological Chemistry*, 280, 5892-5901 (2005).

87. Aggarwal, B.B. & Sung, B. Pharmacological basis for the role of curcumin in chronic diseases: an age-old spice with modern targets. *Trends in Pharmacological Sciences*, 30, 85-94 (2009).

88. Anand, P., *et al*. Bioavailability of curcumin: problems and promises. *Molecular Pharmaceutics*, 4, 807-818 (2007).

89. Arun, K.B., *et al*. Nutraceutical properties of cumin residue generated from Ayurvedic industries using cell line models. *Journal of Food Science and Technology*, 53, 3814-3824 (2016).

90. Lee, S.H., *et al*. Inhibitory effect of 2'-hydroxycinnamaldehyde on nitric oxide production through inhibition of NF-kappa B activation in RAW 264.7 cells. *Biochemical Pharmacology*, 69, 791-799 (2005).

91. Dugoua, J.J., *et al*. From type 2 diabetes to antioxidant activity: a systematic review of the safety and efficacy of common and cassia cinnamon bark. *Canadian Journal of Physiology and Pharmacology*, 85, 837-847 (2007).

92. Blevins, S.M., *et al*. Effect of cinnamon on glucose and lipid levels in non insulin-dependent type 2 diabetes. *Diabetes Care*, 30, 2236-2237 (2007).

93. Khan, A., *et al*. Cinnamon improves glucose and lipids of people with type 2 diabetes. *Diabetes Care*, 26, 3215-3218 (2003).

94. Qin, B., *et al*. Cinnamon extract prevents the insulin resistance induced by a high-fructose diet. *Hormone and metabolic research = Hormon- und Stoffwechselforschung = Hormones et metabolisme* 36, 119-125 (2004).

95. Mang, B., *et al*. Effects of a cinnamon extract on plasma glucose, HbA, and serum lipids in diabetes mellitus type 2. *European Journal of Clinical Investigation*, 36, 340-344 (2006).

96. Lee, S.H., Cekanova, M. & Baek, S.J. Multiple mechanisms are involved in 6-gingerol-induced cell growth arrest and apoptosis in human colorectal cancer cells. *Molecular Carcinogenesis*, 47, 197-208 (2008).

97. Zeng, G.F., *et al*. Protective effects of ginger root extract on Alzheimer disease-induced behavioral dysfunction in rats. *Rejuvenation Research*, 16, 124-133 (2013).

98. Mansour, M.S., *et al*. Ginger consumption enhances the thermic effect of food and promotes feelings of satiety without affecting metabolic and hormonal parameters in overweight men: a pilot study. *Metabolism*, 61, 1347-1352 (2012).

99. Wu, K.L., *et al*. Effects of ginger on gastric emptying and motility in healthy humans. *European Journal of Gastroenterology & Hepatology*, 20, 436-440 (2008).

100. Marx, W.M., *et al*. Ginger (Zingiber officinale) and chemotherapy-induced nausea and vomiting: a systematic literature review. *Nutrition Reviews*, 71, 245-254 (2013).

101. Larkin, M. Surgery patients at risk for herb-anaesthesia interactions. *Lancet*, 354, 1362 (1999).

102. Perez-Jimenez, J., *et al*. Identification of the 100 richest dietary sources of polyphenols. *European Journal of Clinical Nutrition*. (2010).

103. Jiang, T.A. Health Benefits of Culinary Herbs and Spices. *Journal of AOAC International*, 102, 395-411 (2019).

104. Shukla, S. & Gupta, S. Apigenin: a promising molecule for cancer prevention. *Pharmaceutical Research*, 27, 962-978 (2010).

105. Jayasinghe, C., *et al*. Phenolics composition and antioxidant activity of sweet basil (Ocimum basilicum L.). *Journal of Agricultural and Food Chemistry*, 51, 4442-4449 (2003).

106. Elufioye, T.O. & Habtemariam, S. Hepatoprotective effects of rosmarinic acid: insight into its mechanisms of action. *Biomedicine & Pharmacotherapy = Biomedecine & Pharmacotherapie*, 112, 108600 (2019).

107. Habtemariam, S. The therapeutic potential of rosemary (Rosmarinus officinalis) diterpenes for Alzheimer's disease. *Evidence-based Complementary and Alternative Medicine: eCAM*, 2016, 2680409 (2016).

108. Lopresti, A.L. Salvia (sage): a review of its potential cognitive-enhancing and protective effects. *Drugs in R&D*, 17, 53-64 (2017).

109. Losch, S., *et al*. Stable isotope and trace element studies on gladiators and contemporary Romans from Ephesus (Turkey, 2nd and 3rd Ct. AD) – implications for differences in diet. *PLOS One*, 9, e110489 (2014).

110. Kushi, L.H., Meyer, K.A. & Jacobs, D.R., Jr. Cereals, legumes, and chronic disease risk reduction: evidence from epidemiologic studies. *The American Journal of Clinical Nutrition*, 70, 451s-458s (1999).

111. Higgins, J.A. Whole grains, legumes, and the subsequent meal effect: implications for blood glucose control and the role of fermentation. *Journal of Nutrition and Metabolism*, 2012, 829238 (2012).

112. Hajishafiee, M., *et al*. Cereal fibre intake and risk of mortality from all causes, CVD, cancer and inflammatory diseases: a systematic review and meta-analysis of prospective cohort studies. *The British Journal of Nutrition*, 116, 343-352 (2016).

113. Reddy, B.S., *et al.* Preventive potential of wheat bran fractions against experimental colon carcinogenesis: implications for human colon cancer prevention. *Cancer Research,* 60, 4792-4797 (2000).

114. Yang, C.S., *et al.* Inhibition of carcinogenesis by dietary polyphenolic compounds. *Annual Review of Nutrition,* 21, 381-406 (2001).

115. Ghosh, S., *et al.* New insights into the ameliorative effects of ferulic acid in pathophysiological conditions. *Food and Chemical Toxicology,* 103, 41-55 (2017).

116. Eisenberg, T., *et al.* Cardioprotection and lifespan extension by the natural polyamine spermidine. *Nature Medicine,* 22, 1428-1438 (2016).

117. Gaesser, G.A. Carbohydrate quantity and quality in relation to body mass index. *Journal of the American Dietetic Association,* 107, 1768-1780 (2007).

118. McKeown, N.M., *et al.* Whole-grain intake is favorably associated with metabolic risk factors for type 2 diabetes and cardiovascular disease in the Framingham Offspring Study. *The American Journal of Clinical Nutrition,* 76, 390-398 (2002).

119. Flight, I. & Clifton, P. Cereal grains and legumes in the prevention of coronary heart disease and stroke: a review of the literature. *European Journal of Clinical Nutrition,* 60, 1145-1159 (2006).

120. Randi, G., *et al.* Dietary patterns and the risk of colorectal cancer and adenomas. *Nutrition Reviews,* 68, 389-408 (2010).

121. Huang, T., *et al.* Consumption of whole grains and cereal fiber and total and cause-specific mortality: prospective analysis of 367,442 individuals. *BMC Medicine,* 13, 59 (2015).

122. de Munter, J.S., *et al.* Whole grain, bran, and germ intake and risk of type 2 diabetes: a prospective cohort study and systematic review. *PLOS Medicine,* 4, e261 (2007).

123. Ye, E.Q., *et al.* Greater whole-grain intake is associated with lower risk of type 2 diabetes, cardiovascular disease, and weight gain. *The Journal of Nutrition,* 142, 1304-1313 (2012).

124. Flint, A.J., *et al.* Whole grains and incident hypertension in men. *The American Journal of Clinical Nutrition,* 90, 493-498 (2009).

125. Aune, D., *et al.* Dietary fibre, whole grains, and risk of colorectal cancer: systematic review and dose-response meta-analysis of prospective studies. *BMJ,* 343, d6617 (2011).

126. Farvid, M.S., *et al.* Lifetime grain consumption and breast cancer risk. *Breast Cancer Research and Treatment,* 159, 335-345 (2016).

127. *Ibid.*

128. Khanam, A. & Platel, K. Bioavailability and bioactivity of selenium from wheat (Triticum aestivum), maize (Zea mays), and pearl millet (Pennisetum glaucum), in selenium-deficient rats. *Journal of Agricultural and Food Chemistry,* 67, 6366-6376 (2019).

129. Alminger, M. & Eklund-Jonsson, C. Whole-grain cereal products based on a high-fibre barley or oat genotype lower post-prandial glucose and insulin responses in healthy humans. *European Journal of Nutrition,* 47, 294-300 (2008).

130. Delaney, B., *et al.* Beta-glucan fractions from barley and oats are similarly antiatherogenic in hypercholesterolemic Syrian golden hamsters. *The Journal of Nutrition,* 133, 468-475 (2003).

131. O'Keefe, J.H., Gheewala, N.M. & O'Keefe, J.O. Dietary strategies for improving post-prandial glucose, lipids, inflammation, and cardiovascular health. *Journal of the American College of Cardiology,* 51, 249-255 (2008).

132. Gaitan, E., *et al.* Antithyroid and goitrogenic effects of millet: role of C-glycosylflavones. *The Journal of Clinical Endocrinology and Metabolism,* 68, 707-714 (1989).

133. Dias-Martins, *et al.* Potential use of pearl millet (Pennisetum glaucum (L.) R. Br.) in Brazil: Food security, processing, health benefits and nutritional products. *Food Research International,* 109, 175-186 (2018).

134. Khanam, A. & Platel, K. Bioavailability and bioactivity of selenium. *Journal of Agricultural and Food Chemistry* (2019).

135. Lasztity, R. The chemistry of oats. *Cereal Chemistry.* Akademiai Kiado. (1999).

136. Naumann, E., *et al.* Beta-glucan incorporated into a fruit drink effectively lowers serum LDL-cholesterol concentrations. *The American Journal of Clinical Nutrition,* 83, 601-605 (2006).

137. Kreft, M. Buckwheat phenolic metabolites in health and disease. *Nutrition Research Reviews,* 29, 30-39 (2016).

138. Darmadi-Blackberry, I., *et al.* Legumes: the most important dietary predictor of survival in older people of different ethnicities. *Asia Pacific Journal of Clinical Nutrition,* 13, 217-220 (2004).

139. Chang, W.C., *et al.* A bean-free diet increases the risk of all-cause mortality among Taiwanese women: the role of the metabolic syndrome. *Public Health Nutrition,* 15, 663-672 (2012).

140. Mollard, R.C., *et al.* First and second meal effects of pulses on blood glucose, appetite, and food intake at a later meal. *Applied Physiology, Nutrition, and Metabolism,* 36, 634-642 (2011).

141. Jenkins, D.J., *et al.* Effect of legumes as part of a low glycemic index diet on glycemic control and cardiovascular risk factors in type 2 diabetes mellitus: a randomized controlled trial. *Archives of Internal Medicine,* 172, 1653-1660 (2012).

142. Hosseinpour-Niazi, S., *et al.* Substitution of red meat with legumes in the therapeutic lifestyle change diet based on dietary advice improves cardiometabolic risk factors in overweight type 2 diabetes patients: a cross-over randomized clinical trial. *European Journal of Clinical Nutrition,* 69, 592-597 (2015).

143. Bazzano, L.A., *et al.* Non-soy legume consumption lowers cholesterol levels: a meta-analysis of randomized controlled trials. *Nutrition, Metabolism, and Cardiovascular Diseases: NMCD,* 21, 94-103 (2011).

144. Abumweis, S.S., Barake, R. & Jones, P.J. Plant sterols/stanols as cholesterol lowering agents: a meta-analysis of randomized controlled trials. *Food & Nutrition Research,* 52 (2008).

145. Papanikolaou, Y. & Fulgoni, V.L., 3rd bean consumption is associated with greater nutrient intake, reduced systolic blood pressure, lower body weight, and a smaller waist circumference in adults: results from the National Health and Nutrition Examination Survey 1999-2002. *The Journal of American College of Nutrition,* 27, 569-576 (2008).

146. Venn, B.J., *et al.* The effect of increasing consumption of pulses and wholegrains in obese people: a randomized controlled trial. *The Journal of American College of Nutrition,* 29, 365-372 (2010).

147. Jayalath, V.H., *et al.* Effect of dietary pulses on blood pressure: a systematic review and meta-analysis of controlled feeding trials. *American Journal of Hypertension,* 27, 56-64 (2014).

148. Hosseinpour-Niazi, S., *et al.* Non-soya legume-based therapeutic lifestyle change diet reduces inflammatory status in diabetic patients: a randomised cross-over clinical trial. *The British Journal of Nutrition,* 114, 213-219 (2015).

149. Whelton, P.K., *et al.* Effects of oral potassium on blood pressure. Meta-analysis of randomized controlled clinical trials. *Journal of the American Medical Association,* 277, 1624-1632 (1997).

150. Deng, G., *et al.* Phytoestrogens: science, evidence, and advice for breast cancer patients. *Journal of the Society for Integrative Oncology,* 8, 20-30 (2010).

151. Xu, B. & Chang, S.K. Phenolic substance characterization and chemical and cell-based antioxidant activities of 11 lentils grown in the northern United States. *Journal of Agricultural and Food Chemistry,* 58, 1509-1517 (2010).

152. Xu, B.J., Yuan, S.H. & Chang, S.K. Comparative analyses of phenolic composition, antioxidant capacity, and color of cool season legumes and other selected food legumes. *Journal of Food Science,* 72, S167-177 (2007).

153. Duane, W.C. Effects of legume consumption on serum cholesterol, biliary lipids, and sterol metabolism in humans. *Journal of Lipid Research,* 38, 1120-1128 (1997).

154. Luzzatto, L. & Arese, P. Favism and glucose-6-phosphate dehydrogenase deficiency. *The New England Journal of Medicine,* 378, 60-71 (2018).

155. Hughes, G.J., *et al.* Protein digestibility-corrected amino acid scores (PDCAAS) for soy protein isolates and concentrate: criteria for evaluation. *Journal of Agricultural and Food Chemistry,* 59, 12707-12712 (2011).

156. Welty, F.K., *et al.* Effect of soy nuts on blood pressure and lipid levels in hypertensive, prehypertensive, and normotensive postmenopausal women. *Archives of Internal Medicine,* 167, 1060-1067 (2007).

157. Pawlowski, J.W., *et al.* Impact of equol-producing capacity and soy-isoflavone profiles of supplements on bone calcium retention in postmenopausal women: a randomized crossover trial. *The American Journal of Clinical Nutrition,* 102, 695-703 (2015).

158. Eakin, A., Kelsberg, G. & Safranek, S. Clinical inquiry: does high dietary soy intake affect a woman's risk of primary or recurrent breast cancer? *The Journal of Family Practice,* 64, 660-662 (2015).

159. Taku, K., *et al.* Extracted or synthesized soybean isoflavones reduce menopausal hot flash frequency and severity: systematic review and meta-analysis of randomized controlled trials. *Menopause,* 19, 776-790 (2012).

160. Bazzano, L.A., *et al.* Legume consumption and risk of coronary heart disease in US men and women: NHANES I Epidemiologic Follow-up Study. *Archives of Internal Medicine,* 161, 2573-2578 (2001).

161. Jenkins, D.J., *et al.* Effect of legumes. *Archives of Internal Medicine* (2012).

162. Sievenpiper, J.L., *et al.* Effect of non-oil-seed pulses on glycaemic control: a systematic review and meta-analysis of randomised controlled experimental trials in people with and without diabetes. *Diabetologia,* 52, 1479-1495 (2009).

163. Ha, V., *et al.* Effect of dietary pulse intake on established therapeutic lipid targets for cardiovascular risk reduction: a systematic review and meta-analysis of randomized controlled trials. *CMAJ: Canadian Medical Association Journal,* 186, E252-262 (2014).

164. Afshin, A., *et al.* Consumption of nuts and legumes and risk of incident ischemic heart disease, stroke, and diabetes: a systematic review and meta-analysis. *The American Journal of Clinical Nutrition,* 100, 278-288 (2014).

165. Sanchez-Chino, X., *et al.* Nutrient and nonnutrient components of legumes, and its chemopreventive activity: a review. *Nutrition and Cancer,* 67, 401-410 (2015).

166. Campos-Vega, R., *et al.* Common Beans and Their Non-Digestible Fraction: Cancer Inhibitory Activity-An Overview. *Foods,* 2, 374-392 (2013).

167. Douglas, C.C., Johnson, S.A. & Arjmandi, B.H. Soy and its isoflavones: the truth behind the science in breast cancer. *Anti-cancer Agents in Medicinal Chemistry,* 13, 1178-1187 (2013).

168. Yang, W.S., *et al.* Soy intake is associated with lower lung cancer risk: results from a meta-analysis of epidemiologic studies. *The American Journal of Clinical Nutrition,* 94, 1575-1583 (2011).

169. Farvid, M.S., *et al.* Lifetime grain consumption and breast cancer risk. *Breast Cancer Research and Treatment* (2016).

170. Deng, G., *et al.* Phytoestrogens. *Journal of the Society for Integrative Oncology* (2010).

171. Urbano, G., *et al.* The role of phytic acid in legumes: antinutrient or beneficial function? *Journal of Physiology and Biochemistry,* 56, 283-294 (2000).

172. Hu, F.B. & Stampfer, M.J. Nut consumption and risk of coronary heart disease: a review of epidemiologic

evidence. *Current Atherosclerosis Reports,* 1, 204-209 (1999).

173. Hou, Y.Y., *et al.* A randomized controlled trial to compare the effect of peanuts and almonds on the cardio-metabolic and inflammatory parameters in patients with type 2 diabetes mellitus. *Nutrients,* 10, E1565 (2018).

174. Sabate, J., Oda, K. & Ros, E. Nut consumption and blood lipid levels: a pooled analysis of 25 intervention trials. *Archives of Internal Medicine,* 170, 821-827 (2010).

175. Jenkins, D.J., *et al.* Effect of a dietary portfolio of cholesterol-lowering foods given at 2 levels of intensity of dietary advice on serum lipids in hyperlipidemia: a randomized controlled trial. *Journal of the American Medical Association,* 306, 831-839 (2011).

176 US Department of Agriculture, Agricultural Research Service, quoted by Peanut Company of Australia (http://pca.com.au/index.php

177. Anderson, K.J., *et al.* Walnut polyphenolics inhibit in vitro human plasma and LDL oxidation. *The Journal of Nutrition,* 131, 2837-2842 (2001).

178. Maguire, L.S., *et al.* Fatty acid profile, tocopherol, squalene and phytosterol content of walnuts, almonds, peanuts, hazelnuts and the macadamia nut. *International Journal of Food Sciences and Nutrition,* 55, 171-178 (2004).

179. Pan, A., *et al.* Walnut consumption is associated with lower risk of type 2 diabetes in women. *The Journal of Nutrition,* 143, 512-518 (2013).

180. Yu, Z., *et al.* Associations between nut consumption and inflammatory biomarkers. *The American Journal of Clinical Nutrition,* 104, 722-728 (2016).

181. Bolling, B.W., *et al.* Tree nut phytochemicals: composition, antioxidant capacity, bioactivity, impact factors. A systematic review of almonds, Brazils, cashews, hazelnuts, macadamias, pecans, pine nuts, pistachios and walnuts. *Nutrition Research Reviews,* 24, 244-275 (2011).

182. Blade, C., Arola, L. & Salvado, M.J. Hypolipidemic effects of proanthocyanidins and their underlying biochemical and molecular mechanisms. *Molecular Nutrition & Food Research,* 54, 37-59 (2010).

183. Serafini, M., *et al.* Plasma antioxidants from chocolate. *Nature,* 424, 1013 (2003).

184. Bolling, B.W., *et al.* Tree nut phytochemicals. *Nutrition Research Reviews,* 24, 244-275 (2011).

185. Kendall, C.W., Josse, A.R., Esfahani, A. & Jenkins, D.J. The impact of pistachio intake alone or in combination with high-carbohydrate foods on post-prandial glycemia. *European Journal of Clinical Nutrition,* 65, 696-702 (2011).

186. Bryan, J., *et al.* Nutrients for cognitive development in school-aged children. *Nutrition Reviews,* 62, 295-306 (2004).

187. Hirata, F., *et al.* Hypocholesterolemic effect of sesame lignan in humans. *Atherosclerosis,* 122, 135-136 (1996).

188. Francois, C.A., *et al.* Supplementing lactating women with flaxseed oil does not increase docosahexaenoic acid in their milk. *The American Journal of Clinical Nutrition,* 77, 226-233 (2003).

189. Pan, A., *et al.* Meta-analysis of the effects of flaxseed interventions on blood lipids. *The American Journal of Clinical Nutrition,* 90, 288-297 (2009).

190. Adlercreutz, H., Lignans and human health. *Critical Reviews in Clinical Laboratory Sciences,* 44, 483-525 (2007).

191. de Souza Ferreira, C., *et al.* Effect of chia seed (Salvia hispanica l.) consumption on cardiovascular risk factors in humans: a systematic review. *Nutricion Hospitalaria,* 32, 1909-1918 (2015).

192. Nieman, D.C., *et al.* Chia seed does not promote weight loss or alter disease risk factors in overweight adults. *Nutrition Research,* 29, 414-418 (2009).

193. Zhang, Y., *et al.* A major inducer of anticarcinogenic protective enzymes from broccoli: isolation and elucidation of structure. *Proceedings of the National Academy of Sciences of the United States of America,* 89, 2399-2403 (1992).

194. Talalay, P. & Fahey, J.W. Phytochemicals from cruciferous plants. *The Journal of Nutrition,* (2001).

195. Cornblatt, B.S., *et al.* Preclinical and clinical evaluation of sulforaphane for chemoprevention in the breast. *Carcinogenesis,* 28, 1485-1490 (2007).

196. Juturu, V., Bowman, J.P. & Deshpande, J. Overall skin tone and skin-lightening-improving effects with oral supplementation of lutein and zeaxanthin isomers: a double-blind, placebo-controlled clinical trial. *Clinical, Cosmetic and Investigational Dermatology,* 9, 325-332 (2016).

197. Sommerburg, O., *et al.* Fruits and vegetables that are sources for lutein and zeaxanthin: the macular pigment in human eyes. *The British Journal of Ophthalmology,* 82, 907-910 (1998).

198. Ridaura, V.K., *et al.* Gut microbiota from twins discordant for obesity modulate metabolism in mice. *Science,* 341, 1241214 (2013).

199. Henning, S.M., *et al.* Health benefit of vegetable/fruit juice-based diet: role of microbiome. *Scientific Reports,* 7, 2167 (2017).

200. Scott, K.J., *et al.* The correlation between the intake of lutein, lycopene and beta-carotene from vegetables and fruits, and blood plasma concentrations in a group of women aged 50-65 years in the UK. *The British Journal of Nutrition,* 75, 409-418 (1996).

201. Black, H.S. & Rhodes, L.E. Potential benefits of omega-3 fatty acids in non-melanoma skin cancer. *Journal of Clinical Medicine,* 5, E23 (2016).

202. Katiyar, S.K., *et al.* Green tea polyphenol (-)-epigallocatechin-3-gallate treatment of human skin inhibits ultraviolet radiation-induced oxidative stress. *Carcinogenesis,* 22, 287-294 (2001).

203. Carpenter, K.J. A short history of nutritional science: part 1 (1785-1885). *The Journal of Nutrition,* 133, 638-645 (2003).

204. Farvid, M.S., *et al.* Dairy consumption in adolescence and early adulthood and risk of breast cancer. *Cancer Epidemiology, Biomarkers & Prevention,* 27, 575-584 (2018).

205. Liu, R.H. Health-promoting components of fruits and vegetables in the diet. *Advances in Nutrition,* 4, 384s-392s (2013).

206. Lampe, J.W. Health effects of vegetables and fruit: assessing mechanisms of action in human experimental studies. *The American Journal of Clinical Nutrition,* 70, 475s-490s (1999).

207. Liu, R.H. Health benefits of fruit and vegetables. *The American Journal of Clinical Nutrition,* (2003).

208. Dalgard, C., *et al.* Supplementation with orange and blackcurrant juice, but not vitamin E, improves inflammatory markers in patients with peripheral arterial disease. *The British Journal of Nutrition,* 101, 263-269 (2009).

209. Kang, I., *et al.* Raspberry seed flour attenuates high-sucrose diet-mediated hepatic stress and adipose tissue inflammation. *The Journal of Nutritional Biochemistry,* 32, 64-72 (2016).

210. Gil, M.I., *et al.* Antioxidant activity of pomegranate juice and its relationship with phenolic composition and processing. *Journal of Agricultural and Food Chemistry,* 48, 4581-4589 (2000).

211. Aviram, M., *et al.* Pomegranate juice consumption reduces oxidative stress, atherogenic modifications to LDL, and platelet aggregation: studies in humans and in atherosclerotic apolipoprotein E-deficient mice. *The American Journal of Clinical Nutrition,* 71, 1062-1076 (2000).

212. Aviram, M. & Dornfeld, L. Pomegranate juice consumption inhibits serum angiotensin converting enzyme activity and reduces systolic blood pressure. *Atherosclerosis,* 158, 195-198 (2001).

213. Pantuck, A.J., *et al.* Phase II study of pomegranate juice for men with rising prostate-specific antigen following surgery or radiation for prostate cancer. *Clinical Cancer Research,* 12, 4018-4026 (2006).

214. Paller, C.J., *et al.* A randomized phase II study of pomegranate extract for men with rising PSA following initial therapy for localized prostate cancer. *Prostate Cancer and Prostatic Diseases,* 16, 50-55 (2013).

215. Pantuck, A.J., *et al.* A randomized, double-blind, placebo-controlled study of the effects of pomegranate extract on rising PSA levels in men following primary therapy for prostate cancer. *Prostate Cancer and Prostatic Diseases,* 18, 242-248 (2015).

216. Dewailly, E., *et al.* N-3 Fatty acids and cardiovascular disease risk factors among the Inuit of Nunavik. *The American Journal of Clinical Nutrition,* 74, 464-473 (2001).

217. Kromhout, D., Bosschieter, E.B. & de Lezenne Coulander, C. The inverse relation between fish consumption and 20-year mortality from coronary heart disease. *The New England Journal of Medicine,* 312, 1205-1209 (1985).

218. Leung Yinko, S.S., *et al.* Fish consumption and acute coronary syndrome: a meta-analysis. *The American Journal of Medicine,* 127, 848-857.e842 (2014).

219. Rimm, E.B., *et al.* Seafood long-chain n-3 polyunsaturated fatty acids and cardiovascular disease: a science advisory from the American Heart Association. *Circulation,* 138, e35-e47 (2018).

220. Mozaffarian, D., *et al.* Cardiac benefits of fish consumption may depend on the type of fish meal consumed: the Cardiovascular Health Study. *Circulation,* 107, 1372-1377 (2003).

221. He, K., *et al.* Fish consumption and risk of stroke in men. *Journal of the American Medical Association,* 288, 3130-3136 (2002).

222. US Department of Agriculture and US Department of Health and Human Services. *Dietary Guidelines for Americans,* US Government Printing Office; 7th ed. (2010).

223. Leaf, A., *et al.* Clinical prevention of sudden cardiac death by n-3 polyunsaturated fatty acids and mechanism of prevention of arrhythmias by n-3 fish oils. *Circulation,* 107, 2646-2652 (2003).

224. Leaf, A. , *et al.* Prevention of fatal arrhythmias in high-risk subjects by fish oil n-3 fatty acid intake. *Circulation,* 112, 2762-2768 (2005).

225. Rimm, E.B., *et al.* Seafood long-chain n-3 polyunsaturated fatty acids and cardiovascular disease: a science advisory from the American Heart Association. *Circulation,* 138, e35-e47 (2018).

226. Norat, T., *et al.* Meat, fish, and colorectal cancer risk: the European Prospective Investigation into cancer and nutrition. *Journal of the National Cancer Institute,* 97, 906-916 (2005).

227. Visioli, F., *et al.* An overview of the pharmacology of olive oil and its active ingredients. *British Journal of Pharmacology* (2019).

228. Covas, M.I., *et al.* The effect of polyphenols in olive oil on heart disease risk factors: a randomized trial. *Annals of Internal Medicine,* 145, 333-341 (2006).

229. Lopez-Miranda, J., *et al.* Olive oil and health: summary of the II international conference on olive oil and health consensus report, Jaen and Cordoba (Spain) 2008. *Nutrition, Metabolism, and Cardiovascular Diseases: NMCD,* 20, 284-294 (2010).

230. Fito, M., *et al.* Anti-inflammatory effect of virgin olive oil in stable coronary disease patients: a randomized, crossover, controlled trial. *European Journal of Clinical Nutrition,* 62, 570-574 (2008).

231. Beauchamp, G.K., *et al.* Phytochemistry: ibuprofen-like activity in extra-virgin olive oil. *Nature,* 437, 45-46 (2005).

232. Patrono, C. & Baigent, C. Role of aspirin in primary prevention of cardiovascular disease. *Nature Reviews: Cardiology,* 16, 675-686 (2019).

233. Steinbach, G., *et al.* The effect of celecoxib, a cyclooxygenase-2 inhibitor, in familial adenomatous polyposis. *The New England Journal of Medicine,* 342, 1946-1952 (2000).

234. Zhou, Y., *et al.* Nonsteroidal anti-inflammatory drugs can lower amyloidogenic Abeta42 by inhibiting Rho. *Science,* 302, 1215-1217 (2003).

235. Vallee, A., Lecarpentier, Y. & Vallee, J.N. Targeting the canonical WNT/beta-catenin pathway in cancer treatment using non-steroidal anti-inflammatory drugs. *Cells,* 8, E726 (2019).

236. Poole, R., *et al.* Coffee consumption and health: umbrella review of meta-analyses of multiple health outcomes. *BMJ,* 359, j5024 (2017).

237. Kim, H.S., Quon, M.J. & Kim, J.A. New insights into the mechanisms of polyphenols beyond antioxidant properties; lessons from the green tea polyphenol, epigallocatechin 3-gallate. *Redox Biology,* 2, 187-195 (2014).

238. Higdon, J.V. & Frei, B. Tea catechins and polyphenols: health effects, metabolism, and antioxidant functions. *Critical Reviews in Food Science and Nutrition,* 43, 89-143 (2003).

239. Graham, H.N. Green tea composition, consumption, and polyphenol chemistry. *Preventive Medicine,* 21, 334-350 (1992).

240. Yang, C.S., *et al.* Cancer prevention by tea: animal studies, molecular mechanisms and human relevance. *Nature Reviews: Cancer,* 9, 429-439 (2009).

241. Aneja, R., *et al.* Theaflavin, a black tea extract, is a novel anti-inflammatory compound. *Critical Care Medicine,* 32, 2097-2103 (2004).

242. Khan, N., *et al.* Targeting multiple signaling pathways by green tea polyphenol (-)-epigallocatechin-3-gallate. *Cancer Research,* 66, 2500-2505 (2006).

243. Baliga, M.S., Meleth, S. & Katiyar, S.K. Growth inhibitory and antimetastatic effect of green tea polyphenols on metastasis-specific mouse mammary carcinoma 4T1 cells in vitro and in vivo systems. *Clinical Cancer Research,* 11, 1918-1927 (2005).

244. Bettuzzi, S., *et al.* Chemoprevention of human prostate cancer by oral administration of green tea catechins in volunteers with high-grade prostate intraepithelial neoplasia: a preliminary report from a one-year proof-of-principle study. *Cancer Research,* 66, 1234-1240 (2006).

245. Duffy, S.J., *et al.* Short- and long-term black tea consumption reverses endothelial dysfunction in patients with coronary artery disease. *Circulation,* 104, 151-156 (2001).

246. Nagaya, N., *et al.* Green tea reverses endothelial dysfunction in healthy smokers. *Heart,* 90, 1485-1486 (2004).

247. Amsterdam, J.D., *et al.* A randomized, double-blind, placebo-controlled trial of oral Matricaria recutita (chamomile) extract therapy for generalized anxiety disorder. *Journal of Clinical Psychopharmacology,* 29, 378-382 (2009).

248. Zick, S.M., *et al.* Preliminary examination of the efficacy and safety of a standardized chamomile extract for chronic primary insomnia: a randomized placebo-controlled pilot study. *BMC Complementary and Alternative Medicine,* 11, 78 (2011).

249. Adib-Hajbaghery, M. & Mousavi, S.N. The effects of chamomile extract on sleep quality among elderly people: a clinical trial. *Complementary Therapies in Medicine,* 35, 109-114 (2017).

250. Saker, P., *et al.* Influence of anterior midcingulate cortex on drinking behavior during thirst and following satiation. *Proceedings of the National Academy of Sciences of the United States of America,* 115, 786-791 (2018).

Chapter 10: Foods to eliminated or drastically reduce

1. Rico-Campa, A., *et al.* Association between consumption of ultra-processed foods and all cause mortality: SUN prospective cohort study. *BMJ,* 365, l1949 (2019).

2. Srour, B., *et al.* Ultra-processed food intake and risk of cardiovascular disease: prospective cohort study (NutriNet-Sante). *BMJ,* 365, l1451 (2019).

3. Fiolet, T., *et al.* Consumption of ultra-processed foods and cancer risk: results from NutriNet-Sante prospective cohort. *BMJ,* 360, k322 (2018).

4. Panel on Contaminants in the Food Chain. Acrylamide in Food. *EFSA Journal,* 13:4104doi:10.2903/j.efsa (2015).

5. IARC. Carbon black, titanium dioxide, and talc. *IARC Monographs on the Evaluation of Carcinogenic Risks to Humans,* 93, 1-413 (2010).

6. Muncke, J. Endocrine disrupting chemicals and other substances of concern in food contact materials: an updated review of exposure, effect and risk assessment. *The Journal of Steroid Biochemistry and Molecular Biology,* 127, 118-127 (2011).

7. Hall, K.D., *et al.* Ultra-processed diets cause excess calorie intake and weight gain: an inpatient randomized controlled trial of ad libitum food intake. *Cell Metabolism,* 30, 67-77.e63 (2019).

8. Vos, M.B., *et al.* Added sugars and cardiovascular disease risk in children: a scientific statement from the American Heart Association. *Circulation,* 135, e1017-e1034 (2017).

9. Malik, V.S., *et al.* Long-term consumption of sugar-sweetened and artificially sweetened beverages and risk of mortality in US adults. *Circulation,* 139, 2113-2125 (2019).

10. Vos, M.B., *et al.* Added sugars and cardiovascular disease risk in children. *Circulation,* (2017).

11. Malik, V.S., *et al.* Sugar-sweetened beverages and weight gain in children and adults: a systematic review and meta-analysis. *The American Journal of Clinical Nutrition,* 98, 1084-1102 (2013).

12. Pollock, N.K., *et al.* Greater fructose consumption is associated with cardiometabolic risk markers and visceral adiposity in adolescents. *The Journal of Nutrition,* 142, 251-257 (2012).

13. Ludwig, D.S., Peterson, K.E. & Gortmaker, S.L. Relation between consumption of sugar-sweetened drinks and childhood obesity: a prospective, observational analysis. *Lancet,* 357, 505-508 (2001).

14. Hu, F.B. Resolved: there is sufficient scientific evidence that decreasing sugar-sweetened beverage consumption will reduce the prevalence of obesity and obesity-related diseases. *Obesity Reviews: An Official Journal of the International Association for the Study of Obesity,* 14, 606-619 (2013).

15. Shi, L. & van Meijgaard, J. Substantial decline in sugar-sweetened beverage consumption among California's children and adolescents. *International Journal of General Medicine,* 3, 221-224 (2010).

16. Pollock, N.K., *et al.* Greater fructose consumption is associated with cardiometabolic risk markers. *The Journal of Nutrition,* (2012).

17. Lustig, R.H., *et al.* Isocaloric fructose restriction and metabolic improvement in children with obesity and metabolic syndrome. *Obesity,* 24, 453-460 (2016).

18. Lin, W.T., *et al.* Fructose-rich beverage intake and central adiposity, uric acid, and pediatric insulin resistance. *The Journal of Pediatrics,* 171, 90-96.e91 (2016).

19. Romero-Gomez, M., Zelber-Sagi, S. & Trenell, M. Treatment of NAFLD with diet, physical activity and exercise. *Journal of Hepatology,* 67, 829-846 (2017).

20. de Koning, L., *et al.* Sweetened beverage consumption, incident coronary heart disease, and biomarkers of risk in men. *Circulation,* 125, 1735-1741, s1731 (2012).

21. Mueller, N.T., *et al.* Soft drink and juice consumption and risk of pancreatic cancer: the Singapore Chinese Health Study. *Cancer Epidemiology, Biomarkers & Prevention,* 19, 447-455 (2010).

22. Hodge, A.M., *et al.* Consumption of sugar-sweetened and artificially sweetened soft drinks and risk of obesity-related cancers. *Public Health Nutrition,* 21, 1618-1626 (2018).

23. Goncalves, M., *et al.* High-fructose corn syrup enhances intestinal tumor growth in mice. *Science,* 363, 1345-1349 (2019).

24. Wang, Q.P., *et al.* Sucralose promotes food intake through NPY and a neuronal fasting response. *Cell Metabolism,* 24, 75-90 (2016).

25. The Australian Government National Health and Medical Research Council. Nutrient Reference Values for Australia and New Zealand: Including Recommended Dietary Intakes. *NHMRC Publications,* 1.2 (2017).

26. He, F.J., Li, J. & Macgregor, G.A. Effect of longer term modest salt reduction on blood pressure: Cochrane systematic review and meta-analysis of randomised trials. *BMJ,* 346, f1325 (2013).

27. Elliott, P., *et al.* Intersalt revisited: further analyses of 24 hour sodium excretion and blood pressure within and across populations. Intersalt Cooperative Research Group. *BMJ,* 312, 1249-1253 (1996).

28. Sacks, F.M., *et al.* Effects on blood pressure of reduced dietary sodium and the Dietary Approaches to Stop Hypertension (DASH) diet. DASH-Sodium Collaborative Research Group. *The New England Journal of Medicine,* 344, 3-10 (2001).

29. He, F.J., Li, J. & Macgregor, G.A. Effect of longer term modest salt reduction on blood pressure. *BMJ,* 346, f1326 (2013).

30. Aburto, N.J., *et al.* Effect of lower sodium intake on health: systematic review and meta-analyses. *BMJ,* 346, f1326 (2013).

31. Wenstedt EF, *et al.* Salt increases monocyte CCR2 expression and inflammatory responses in humans. *JCI Insight,* 4, 130508 (2019).

32. Cook, N.R., Appel, L.J. & Whelton, P.K. Sodium intake and all-cause mortality over 20 years in the trials of hypertension prevention. *Journal of the American College of Cardiology,* 68, 1609-1617 (2016).

33. Aburto, N.J., *et al.* Effect of lower sodium intake on health: systematic review and meta-analyses. *BMJ,* 346, f1326 (2013).

34. Opie, L.H. & Seedat, Y.K. Hypertension in sub-Saharan African populations. *Circulation,* 112, 3562-3568 (2005).

35. Fontana, L., *et al.* Long-term calorie restriction is highly effective in reducing the risk for atherosclerosis in humans. *Proceedings of the National Academy of Sciences,* 101, 6659-6663 (2004).

36. Kraus, W.E., *et al.* 2 years of calorie restriction and cardiometabolic risk (CALERIE): exploratory outcomes of a multicentre, phase 2, randomised controlled trial. *The Lancet: Diabetes & Endocrinology,* 7, 673-683 (2019).

37. Australian Population Development Principal Committee. The prevalence and severity of iodine deficiency in Australia. (2007)

38. de Escobar, G.M., Obregon, M.J. & del Rey, F.E. Iodine deficiency and brain development in the first half of pregnancy. *Public Health Nutrition,* 10, 1554-1570 (2007).

39. Aghini Lombardi, F.A., *et al.* Mild iodine deficiency during fetal/ neonatal life and neuropsychological impairment in Tuscany. *Journal of Endocrinological Investigation,* 18, 57-62 (1995).

40. Vermiglio, F., *et al.* Attention deficit and hyperactivity disorders in the offspring of mothers exposed to mild-moderate iodine deficiency: a possible novel iodine deficiency disorder in developed countries. *The Journal of Clinical Endocrinology and Metabolism,* 89, 6054-6060 (2004).

41. OECD-FAO Agricultural Outlook ECD and Food and Agriculture Organization of the United Nations. *OECD-FAO Agricultural Outlook 2019-2028,* OECD Publishing (2019).

41. Armstrong, B., Doll, R., Environmental factors and cancer incidence and mortality in different countries, with specific reference to dietary practices. *International Journal of Cancer,* 15, 617-631 (1975).

42. World Cancer Research Fund. Continuous Update Project Expert Report 2018. (2018). <https://www.wcrf.org/dietandcancer/about>

43. IARC Working Group on the Evaluation of Carcinogenic Risk to Humans. Red meat and

processed meat. *IARC Monographs on the Evaluation of Carcinogenic Risks to Humans*, 114, (2018).

44. Norat, T., *et al.* Meat, fish, and colorectal cancer risk: the European Prospective Investigation into cancer and nutrition. *Journal of the National Cancer Institute*, 97, 906-916 (2005).

45. Sandhu, M.S., White, I.R. & McPherson, K. Systematic review of the prospective cohort studies on meat consumption and colorectal cancer risk: a meta-analytical approach. *Cancer Epidemiology, Biomarkers & Prevention*, 10, 439-446 (2001).

46. Chan, D.S., *et al.* Red and processed meat and colorectal cancer incidence: meta-analysis of prospective studies. *PLOS One*, 6, e20456 (2011).

47. *Ibid.*

48. Bouvard, V., *et al.* Carcinogenicity of consumption of red and processed meat. *The Lancet: Oncology*, 16, 1599-1600 (2015).

49. IARC Working Group. Red meat. *IARC Monographs*, (2018).

50. Mozaffarian, D., *et al.* Changes in diet and lifestyle and long-term weight gain in women and men. *The New England Journal of Medicine*, 364, 2392-2404 (2011).

51. Rohrmann, S., *et al.* Meat consumption and mortality-results from the European Prospective Investigation into Cancer and Nutrition. *BMC Medicine*, 11, 63 (2013).

52. Micha, R., Michas, G. & Mozaffarian, D. Unprocessed red and processed meats and risk of coronary artery disease and type 2 diabetes – an updated review of the evidence. *Current Atherosclerosis Reports*, 14, 515-524 (2012).

53. Pan, A., *et al.* Red meat consumption and risk of type 2 diabetes: 3 cohorts of US adults and an updated meta-analysis. *The American Journal of Clinical Nutrition*, 94, 1088-1096 (2011).

54. Zheng, Y., *et al.* Association of changes in red meat consumption with total and cause specific mortality among US women and men: two prospective cohort studies. *BMJ*, 365, l2110 (2019).

55. van den Bogaard, A.E. & Stobberingh, E.E. Epidemiology of resistance to antibiotics. Links between animals and humans. *International Journal of Antimicrobial Agents*, 14, 327-335 (2000).

56. Martinez, J.L. Environmental pollution by antibiotics and by antibiotic resistance determinants. *Environmental Pollution*, 157, 2893-2902 (2009).

57. Sapkota, A.R., *et al.* What do we feed to food-production animals? A review of animal feed ingredients and their potential impacts on human health. *Environmental Health Perspectives*, 115, 663-670 (2007).

58. Fernandes, A.R., *et al.* The assimilation of dioxins and PCBs in conventionally reared farm animals: occurrence and biotransfer factors. *Chemosphere*, 83, 815-822 (2011).

59. Bauman, D.E. Bovine somatotropin: review of an emerging animal technology. *Journal of Dairy Science*, 75, 3432-3451 (1992).

60. Goldstein, J.L. & Brown, M.S. A century of cholesterol and coronaries: from plaques to genes to statins. *Cell*, 161, 161-172 (2015).

61. Zhu, W., *et al.* Gut microbial metabolite TMAO enhances platelet hyperreactivity and thrombosis risk. *Cell*, 165, 111-124 (2016).

62. Bastide, N.M., Pierre, F.H. & Corpet, D.E. Heme iron from meat and risk of colorectal cancer: a meta-analysis and a review of the mechanisms involved. *Cancer Prevention Research*, 4, 177-184 (2011).

63. Samraj, A.N., *et al.* A red meat-derived glycan promotes inflammation and cancer progression. *Proceedings of the National Academy of Sciences of the United States of America*, 112, 542-547 (2015).

64. Office of Chemical Safety, Australian Government Department of Health and Ageing. National Dioxins Program Technical. *Australian Government Department of the Environment and Heritage*, 12, (2005).

65. Weber, R., *et al.* Reviewing the relevance of dioxin and PCB sources for food from animal origin and the need for their inventory, control and management. *Environmental Sciences Europe*, 30, 42 (2018).

66. Assessment of the health risk of dioxins: re-evaluation of the tolerable daily intake (TDI). Geneva, Switzerland. *Food Additives and Contaminants*, 17, 223-369 (2000).

67. Shimada, T., *et al.* Activation of chemically diverse procarcinogens by human cytochrome P-450 1B1. *Cancer Research*, 56, 2979-2984 (1996).

68. Steenland, K., *et al.* Dioxin revisited: developments since the 1997 IARC classification of dioxin as a human carcinogen. *Environmental Health Perspectives*, 112, 1265-1268 (2004).

69. Fernandez-Salguero, P., *et al.* Immune system impairment and hepatic fibrosis in mice lacking the dioxin-binding Ah receptor. *Science*, 268, 722-726 (1995).

70. Sugimura, T. Carcinogenicity of mutagenic heterocyclic amines formed during the cooking process. *Mutation Research*, 150, 33-41 (1985).

71. Turesky, R.J. & Le Marchand, L. Metabolism and biomarkers of heterocyclic aromatic amines in molecular epidemiology studies: lessons learned from aromatic amines. *Chemical Research in Toxicology*, 24, 1169-1214 (2011).

72. Loh, Y.H., *et al.* N-Nitroso compounds and cancer incidence: the European Prospective Investigation into Cancer and Nutrition (EPIC)-Norfolk Study. *The American Journal of Clinical Nutrition*, 93, 1053-1061 (2011).

73. Mirvish, S.S. Role of N-nitroso compounds (NOC) and N-nitrosation in etiology of gastric, esophageal, nasopharyngeal and bladder cancer and contribution to cancer of known exposures to NOC. *Cancer Letters*, 93, 17-48 (1995).

74. Pili, R. & Fontana, L. Low-protein diet in cancer: ready for prime time? *Nature Reviews: Endocrinology*, 14, 384-386 (2018).

75. Orillion, A., *et al.* Dietary protein restriction reprograms tumor-associated macrophages and enhances immunotherapy. *Clinical Cancer Research*, 24, 6383-6395 (2018).

76. Gao, X., *et al.* Dietary methionine influences therapy in mouse cancer models and alters human metabolism. *Nature*, 572, 397-401 (2019).

77. Adelaiye, R.M., *et al.* Tumor growth inhibition and epigenetic changes following protein diet restriction in a human prostate cancer model. *American Association for Cancer Research*, 73, 4859 (2013).

78. Lamming, D.W., *et al.* Restriction of dietary protein decreases mTORC1 in tumors and somatic tissues of a tumor-bearing mouse xenograft model. *Oncotarget*, 6, 31233 (2015).

79. Orillion, A., *et al.* Dietary protein restriction. *Clinical Cancer Research* (2018).

80. Rubio-Patino, C., *et al.* Low-protein diet induces IRE1α-dependent anticancer immunosurveillance. *Cell Metabolism*, 27, 828-842.e827 (2018).

81. Orillion, A.R., *et al.* Methionine restriction increases macrophage tumoricidal activity and significantly inhibits prostate cancer growth. *American Association for Cancer Research*, 77, 250 (2017).

82. Fortmann, S.P., *et al.* Vitamin and mineral supplements in the primary prevention of cardiovascular disease and cancer: an updated systematic evidence review for the US Preventive Services Task Force. *Annals of Internal Medicine*, 159, 824-834 (2013).

83. Bjelakovic, G., *et al.* Antioxidant supplements for prevention of mortality in healthy participants and patients with various diseases. *The Cochrane Database of Systematic Reviews*, 3, CD007176 (2012).

84. Rautiainen, S., *et al.* Dietary supplements and disease prevention – a global overview. *Nature Reviews: Endocrinology*, 12, 407-420 (2016).

85. Griffin, N.W., *et al.* Prior dietary practices and connections to a human gut microbial metacommunity alter responses to diet interventions. *Cell Host & Microbe*, 21, 84-96 (2017).

86. Dey, N., *et al.* Regulators of gut motility revealed by a gnotobiotic model of diet-microbiome interactions related to travel. *Cell*, 163, 95-107 (2015).

Part IV: Physical exercise as a daily medicine

Chapter 11: Maximising health through physical exercise

1. Eijsvogels, T.M., *et al.* Exercise at the Extremes: The Amount of Exercise to Reduce Cardiovascular Events. *Journal of the American College of Cardiology*, 67, 316-329 (2016).

2. Pate, R.R., *et al.* Physical activity and public health. A recommendation from the Centers for Disease Control and Prevention and the American College of Sports Medicine. *Journal of the American Medical Association*, 273, 402-407 (1995).

3. Hupin, D., *et al.* Even a low-dose of moderate-to-vigorous physical activity reduces mortality by 22% in adults aged >/=60 years: a systematic review and meta-analysis. *British Journal of Sports Medicine*, 49, 1262-1267 (2015).

4. Eijsvogels, T.M., *et al.* Exercise at the Extremes. *Journal of the American College of Cardiology*. (2016).

5. Wen, C.P., *et al.* Minimum amount of physical activity for reduced mortality and extended life expectancy: a prospective cohort study. *Lancet*, 378, 1244-1253 (2011).

6. Biswas, A., *et al.* Sedentary time and its association with risk for disease incidence, mortality, and hospitalization in adults: a systematic review and meta-analysis. *Annals of Internal Medicine*, 162, 123-132 (2015).

7. Nguyen, L.H., *et al.* Sedentary behaviors, TV viewing time, and risk of young-onset colorectal cancer. *JNCI Cancer Spectrum*, 2, pky073 (2018).

8. Healy, G.N., *et al.* Breaks in sedentary time: beneficial associations with metabolic risk. *Diabetes Care*, 31, 661-666 (2008).

9. Dunstan, D.W., *et al.* Breaking up prolonged sitting reduces postprandial glucose and insulin responses. *Diabetes Care*, 35, 976-983 (2012).

10. Matthews, C.E., *et al.* Mortality benefits for replacing sitting time with different physical activities. *Medicine and Science in Sports and Exercise*, 47, 1833-1840 (2015).

11. Lee, D.C., *et al.* Leisure-time running reduces all-cause and cardiovascular mortality risk. *Journal of the American College of Cardiology*, 64, 472-481 (2014).

12. Arem, H., *et al.* Leisure time physical activity and mortality: a detailed pooled analysis of the dose-response relationship. *Journal of the American Medical Association: Internal Medicine*, 175, 959-967 (2015).

13. Piercy, K.L., *et al.* The physical activity guidelines for Americans. *Journal of the American Medical Association*, 320, 2020-2028 (2018).

14. *Ibid.*

15. Bhishagratna, K. L. *An English translation of the Sushruta Samhita*. Chowkhamba Sanskrit Series Office; 2nd ed. (1963).

16. Wong, K.C. & Wu, L. *History of Chinese Medicine*. National Quarantine Service; 2nd ed. (1936).

17. Vogel, C.J. *Pythagoras and early pythagoreanism*. Royal Van Gorcum & Company. (1966).

18. Hippocrates. *Hippocrates, translated by Jones WHS*. William Heinemann; vol. 1. (1923).

19. Hagberg, J.M., *et al.* The historical context and scientific legacy of John O. Holloszy. *Journal of Applied Physiology*, 127, 277-305 (2019).

Chapter 12: Beneficial effects of aerobic exercise

1. Holloszy, J.O. Biochemical adaptations in muscle. Effects of exercise on mitochondrial oxygen uptake and respiratory enzyme activity in skeletal muscle. *The Journal of Biological Chemistry*, 242, 2278-2282 (1967).

2. Spina, R.J., *et al.* Mitochondrial enzymes increase in muscle in response to 7-10 days of cycle exercise. *Journal of Applied Physiology*, 80, 2250-2254 (1996).

3. Coggan, A.R., *et al*. Skeletal muscle adaptations to endurance training in 60- to 70-yr-old men and women. *Journal of Applied Physiology, 72*, 1780-1786 (1992).

4. Weiss, E. Washington University School of Medicine CAERIE Group. *American Journal Clinical Nutrition* (2006).

5. Bourey, R.E., *et al*. Effect of exercise on glucose disposal: response to a maximal insulin stimulus. *Journal of Applied Physiology, 69*, 1689-1694 (1990).

6. King, D.S., *et al*. Effects of exercise and lack of exercise on insulin sensitivity and responsiveness. *Journal of Applied Physiology, 64*, 1942-1946 (1988).

7. Stephenson, E.J., Smiles, W. & Hawley, J.A. The relationship between exercise, nutrition and type 2 diabetes. *Medicine and Sport Science, 60*, 1-10 (2014).

8. Holloszy, J.O. Regulation of mitochondrial biogenesis and GLUT4 expression by exercise. *Comprehensive Physiology, 1*, 921-940 (2011).

9. Richter, E.A. & Hargreaves, M. Exercise, GLUT4, and skeletal muscle glucose uptake. *Physiological Reviews, 93*, 993-1017 (2013).

10. Host, H.H., *et al*. Rapid reversal of adaptive increases in muscle GLUT-4 and glucose transport capacity after training cessation. *Journal of Applied Physiology (Bethesda, Md.: 1985), 84*, 798-802 (1998).

11. McGarrah, R.W., Slentz, C.A. & Kraus, W.E. The effect of vigorous- versus moderate-intensity aerobic exercise on insulin action. *Current Cardiology Reports, 18*, 117 (2016).

12. Ross, R., *et al*. Effects of exercise amount and intensity on abdominal obesity and glucose tolerance in obese adults: a randomized trial. *Annals of Internal Medicine, 162*, 325-334 (2015).

13. Fontana, L., Klein, S. & Holloszy, J.O. Effects of long-term calorie restriction and endurance exercise on glucose tolerance, insulin action, and adipokine production. *Age, 32*, 97-108 (2010).

14. Weiss, E. Washington University School of Medicine CAERIE Group: improvements in glucose tolerance and insulin action induced by increasing energy expenditure or decreasing energy intake: a randomized controlled trial. *American Journal Clinical Nutrition, 84*, 1033-1042 (2006).

15. Slentz, C.A., *et al*. Effects of exercise training alone vs a combined exercise and nutritional lifestyle intervention on glucose homeostasis in prediabetic individuals: a randomised controlled trial. *Diabetologia, 59*, 2088-2098 (2016).

16. *Ibid*.

17. Johansen, M.Y., *et al*. Effect of an intensive lifestyle intervention on glycemic control in patients with type 2 diabetes: a randomized clinical trial. *Journal of the American Medical Association, 318*, 637-646 (2017).

18. Kraus, W.E., *et al*. Physical activity, all-cause and cardiovascular mortality, and cardiovascular disease. *Medicine and Science in Sports and Exercise, 51*, 1270-1281 (2019).

19. Mora, S., *et al*. Physical activity and reduced risk of cardiovascular events: potential mediating mechanisms. *Circulation, 116*, 2110-2118 (2007).

20. Kraus, W.E., *et al*. Effects of the amount and intensity of exercise on plasma lipoproteins. *The New England Journal of Medicine, 347*, 1483-1492 (2002).

21. Mann, S., Beedie, C. & Jimenez, A. Differential effects of aerobic exercise, resistance training and combined exercise modalities on cholesterol and the lipid profile: review, synthesis and recommendations. *Sports Medicine, 44*, 211-221 (2014).

22. Whelton, S.P., *et al*. Effect of aerobic exercise on blood pressure: a meta-analysis of randomized, controlled trials. *Annals of Internal Medicine, 136*, 493-503 (2002).

23. Pescatello, L.S., *et al*. Physical activity to prevent and treat hypertension: a systematic review. *Medicine and Science in Sports and Exercise, 51*, 1314-1323 (2019).

24. Weiss, E.P. & Holloszy, J.O. Improvements in body composition, glucose tolerance, and insulin action induced by increasing energy expenditure or decreasing energy intake. *The Journal of Nutrition, 137*, 1087-1090 (2007).

25. Racette, S.B., *et al*. One year of caloric restriction in humans: feasibility and effects on body composition and abdominal adipose tissue. *The Journals of Gerontology Series A: Biological Sciences and Medical Sciences, 61*, 943-950 (2006).

26. Laborde, S., Mosley, E. & Ueberholz, L. Enhancing cardiac vagal activity: factors of interest for sport psychology. *Progress in Brain Research, 240*, 71-92 (2018).

27. Hautala, A.J., Kiviniemi, A.M. & Tulppo, M.P. Individual responses to aerobic exercise: the role of the autonomic nervous system. *Neuroscience and Biobehavioral Reviews, 33*, 107-115 (2009).

28. Goldsmith, R.L., *et al*. Comparison of 24-hour parasympathetic activity in endurance-trained and untrained young men. *Journal of the American College of Cardiology, 20*, 552-558 (1992).

29. Thompson, P.D., *et al*. Exercise and physical activity in the prevention and treatment of atherosclerotic cardiovascular disease: a statement from the Council on Clinical Cardiology. *Circulation, 107*, 3109-3116 (2003).

30. Sarzynski, M.A., *et al*. Effects of increasing exercise intensity and dose on multiple measures of HDL (High-Density Lipoprotein) function. *Arteriosclerosis, Thrombosis, and Vascular Biology, 38*, 943-952 (2018).

31. McTiernan, A., *et al*. Physical activity in cancer prevention and survival: a systematic review. *Medicine and Science in Sports and Exercise, 51*, 1252-1261 (2019).

32. Moore, S.C., *et al*. Association of leisure-time physical activity with risk of 26 types of cancer in 1.44 million adults. *Journal of the American Medical Association: Internal Medicine, 176*, 816-825 (2016).

33. Holmes, M.D., *et al*. Physical activity and survival after breast cancer diagnosis. *Journal of the American Medical Association, 293*, 2479-2486 (2005).

34. Kenfield, S.A., *et al*. Physical activity and survival after prostate cancer diagnosis in the health professionals follow-up study. *Journal of Clinical Oncology, 29*, 726-732 (2011).

35. Meyerhardt, J.A., *et al.* Physical activity and survival after colorectal cancer diagnosis. *Journal of Clinical Oncology,* 24, 3527-3534 (2006).

36. Zhong, S., *et al.* Association between physical activity and mortality in breast cancer: a meta-analysis of cohort studies. *European Journal of Epidemiology,* 29, 391-404 (2014).

37. Holmes, M.D., *et al.* Physical activity and survival. *Journal of the American Medical Association* (2005).

38. Picon-Ruiz, M., *et al.* Obesity and adverse breast cancer risk and outcome: mechanistic insights and strategies for intervention. *CA: A Cancer Journal for Clinicians,* 67, 378-397 (2017).

39. Longo, V.D. & Fontana, L. Calorie restriction and cancer prevention: metabolic and molecular mechanisms. *Trends in Pharmacological Sciences,* 31, 89-98 (2010).

40. Picon-Ruiz, M., *et al.* Obesity and adverse breast cancer risk and outcome. *CA* (2017).

31. McTiernan, A. Mechanisms linking physical activity with cancer. *Nature Reviews: Cancer,* 8, 205-211 (2008).

42. Jones, L.W., *et al.* Exercise and prognosis on the basis of clinicopathologic and molecular features in early-stage breast cancer: the LACE and pathways studies. *Cancer Research,* 76, 5415-5422 (2016).

43. Asselman, J., *et al.* Marine biogenics in sea spray aerosols interact with the mTOR signaling pathway. *Scientific Reports,* 9, 675 (2019).

44. Hillman, C.H., Erickson, K.I. & Kramer, A.F. Be smart, exercise your heart: exercise effects on brain and cognition. *Nature Reviews: Neuroscience,* 9, 58-65 (2008).

45. Bugg, J.M. & Head, D. Exercise moderates age-related atrophy of the medial temporal lobe. *Neurobiology of Aging,* 32, 506-514 (2011).

46. Erickson, K.I., *et al.* Exercise training increases size of hippocampus and improves memory. *Proceedings of the National Academy of Sciences of the United States of America,* 108, 3017-3022 (2011).

47. Karege, F., *et al.* Decreased serum brain-derived neurotrophic factor levels in major depressed patients. *Psychiatry Research,* 109, 143-148 (2002).

48. Russo-Neustadt, A., Beard, R .C. & Cotman, C.W. Exercise, antidepressant medications, and enhanced brain derived neurotrophic factor expression. *Neuropsychopharmacology,* 21, 679-682 (1999).

49. Szuhany, K.L., Bugatti, M. & Otto, M.W. A meta-analytic review of the effects of exercise on brain-derived neurotrophic factor. *Journal of Psychiatric Research,* 60, 56-64 (2015).

Chapter 13: Starting or improving aerobic-exercise training

1. Richardson, R.S. What governs skeletal muscle VO2max? New evidence. *Medicine and Science in Sports and Exercise,* 32, 100-107 (2000).

2. Rey-Lopez JP, *et al.* Associations of self-reported stair climbing with all-cause and cardiovascular mortality: the Harvard Alumni Health Study. *Preventive Medicine Reports,* 15, 100938 (2019).

3. Skinner, J.S., *et al.* Heart rate versus %VO2max: age, sex, race, initial fitness, and training response – HERITAGE. *Medicine and Science in Sports and Exercise,* 35, 1908-1913 (2003).

4. Tanaka, H., Monahan, K.D. & Seals, D.R. Age-predicted maximal heart rate revisited. *Journal of the American College of Cardiology,* 37, 153-156 (2001).

5. Miller, W.C., Wallace, J.P. & Eggert, K.E. Predicting max HR and the HR-VO2 relationship for exercise prescription in obesity. *Medicine and Science in Sports and Exercise,* 25, 1077-1081 (1993).

6. Karvonen, M.J., Kentala, E. & Mustala, O. The effects of training on heart rate; a longitudinal study. *Annales Medicinae Experimentalis et Biologiae Fenniae,* 35, 307-315 (1957).

7. Davis, J.A. & Convertino, V.A. A comparison of heart rate methods for predicting endurance training intensity. *Medicine and Science in Sports,* 7, 295-298 (1975).

8. Gellish, R.L., *et al.* Longitudinal modeling of the relationship between age and maximal heart rate. *Medicine and Science in Sports and Exercise,* 39, 822-829 (2007).

9. Achten, J., Venables, M.C. & Jeukendrup, A.E. Fat oxidation rates are higher during running compared with cycling over a wide range of intensities. *Metabolism,* 52, 747-752 (2003).

10. Brahler, C.J. & Blank, S.E. VersaClimbing elicits higher VO2max than does treadmill running or rowing ergometry. *Medicine and Science in Sports and Exercise,* 27, 249-254 (1995).

11. Loy, S.F., *et al.* Effects of stairclimbing on VO2max and quadriceps strength in middle-aged females. *Medicine and Science in Sports and Exercise,* 26, 241-247 (1994).

12. Wallick, M.E., *et al.* Physiological responses to in-line skating compared to treadmill running. *Medicine and Science in Sports and Exercise,* 27, 242-248 (1995).

13. Costill, D.L., *et al.* Adaptations to swimming training: influence of training volume. *Medicine and Science in Sports and Exercise,* 23, 371-377 (1991).

14. Almeida, S.A., *et al.* Epidemiological patterns of musculoskeletal injuries and physical training. *Medicine and Science in Sports and Exercise,* 31, 1176-1182 (1999).

15. Jones, B.H., *et al.* Epidemiology of injuries associated with physical training among young men in the army. *Medicine and Science in Sports and Exercise,* 25, 197-203 (1993).

16. Schnohr, P., *et al.* Dose of jogging and long-term mortality: the Copenhagen City Heart Study. *Journal of the American College of Cardiology,* 65, 411-419 (2015).

17. Lee, D.C., *et al.* Leisure-time running reduces all-cause and cardiovascular mortality risk. *Journal of the American College of Cardiology,* 64:472-81 (2014).

18. Hickson, R.C. & Rosenkoetter, M.A. Reduced training frequencies and maintenance of increased aerobic power.

Medicine and Science in Sports and Exercise, 13, 13-16 (1981).

19. Moffatt, R.J., Stamford, B.A. & Neill, R.D. Placement of tri-weekly training sessions: importance regarding enhancement of aerobic capacity. *Research Quarterly,* 48, 583-591 (1977).

20. Hickson, R.C. & Rosenkoetter, M.A. Reduced training frequencies. *Medicine and Science in Sports and Exercise* (1981).

21. Hickson, R.C., *et al.* Reduced training duration effects on aerobic power, endurance, and cardiac growth. *Journal of Applied Physiology: Respiratory, Environmental and Exercise Physiology,* 53, 225-229 (1982).

22. *Ibid.*

23. Pollock, M.L., *et al.* Effects of frequency and duration of training on attrition and incidence of injury. *Medicine and Science in Sports,* 9, 31-36 (1977).

24. American College of Sports Medicine Position Stand. The recommended quantity and quality of exercise for developing and maintaining cardiorespiratory and muscular fitness, and flexibility in healthy adults. *Medicine and Science in Sports and Exercise,* 30, 975-991 (1998).

25. Wisloff, U., *et al.* Superior cardiovascular effect of aerobic interval training versus moderate continuous training in heart failure patients: a randomized study. *Circulation* 115, 3086-3094 (2007).

26. Helgerud, J., *et al.* Aerobic high-intensity intervals improve VO2max more than moderate training. *Medicine and Science in Sports and Exercise,* 39, 665-671 (2007).

27. Wisloff, U., Ellingsen, O. & Kemi, O.J. High-intensity interval training to maximize cardiac benefits of exercise training? *Exercise and Sport Sciences Reviews,* 37, 139-146 (2009).

28. Milanovic, Z., Sporis, G. & Weston, M. Effectiveness of high-intensity interval training (HIT) and continuous endurance training for VO2max improvements: a systematic review and meta-analysis of controlled trials. *Sports Medicine,* 45, 1469-1481 (2015).

29. Viana, R.B., *et al.* Is interval training the magic bullet for fat loss? A systematic review and meta-analysis comparing moderate-intensity continuous training with high-intensity interval training (HIIT). *British Journal of Sports Medicine,* 53, 655-664 (2019).

30. Jelleyman, C., *et al.* The effects of high-intensity interval training on glucose regulation and insulin resistance: a meta-analysis. *Obesity Reviews,* 16, 942-961 (2015).

31. Molmen-Hansen, H.E., *et al.* Aerobic interval training reduces blood pressure and improves myocardial function in hypertensive patients. *European Journal of Preventitive Cardiology,* 19, 151-160 (2012).

32. Guiraud, T., *et al.* Optimization of high intensity interval exercise in coronary heart disease. *European Journal of Applied Physiology,* 108, 733-740 (2010).

33. Little, J.P., *et al.* Low-volume high-intensity interval training reduces hyperglycemia and increases muscle mitochondrial capacity in patients with type 2 diabetes. *Journal of Applied Physiology,* 111, 1554-1560 (2011).

34. Hood, M.S., *et al.* Low-volume interval training improves muscle oxidative capacity in sedentary adults. *Medicine and Science in Sports and Exercise,* 43, 1849-1856 (2011).

35. Kilpatrick, M.W., Greeley, S.J. & Collins, L.H. The impact of continuous and interval cycle exercise on affect and enjoyment. *Research Quarterly for Exercise and Sport,* 86, 244-251 (2015).

36. Allison, M.K., *et al.* Brief intense stair climbing improves cardiorespiratory fitness. *Medicine and Science in Sports and Exercise,* 49, 298-307 (2017).

37. Rogers, M.A., *et al.* Effect of 10 days of physical inactivity on glucose tolerance in master athletes. *Journal of Applied Physiology,* 68, 1833-1837 (1990).

38. *Ibid.*

39. Arem, H., *et al.* Leisure time physical activity and mortality: a detailed pooled analysis of the dose-response relationship. *Journal of the American Medical Association: Internal Medicine,* 175, 959-967 (2015).

40. Schnohr, P., *et al.* Dose of jogging and long-term mortality. *Journal of the American College of Cardiology* (2015).

41. Armstrong, M.E., *et al.* Frequent physical activity may not reduce vascular disease risk as much as moderate activity: large prospective study of women in the United Kingdom. *Circulation,* 131, 721-729 (2015).

42. Shave, R., *et al.* Exercise-induced cardiac troponin elevation: evidence, mechanisms, and implications. *Journal of the American College of Cardiology,* 56, 169-176 (2010).

43. Oxborough, D., *et al.* "Exercise-induced cardiac fatigue" – a review of the echocardiographic literature. *Echocardiography,* 27, 1130-1140 (2010).

44. Mohlenkamp, S., *et al.* Running: the risk of coronary events – prevalence and prognostic relevance of coronary atherosclerosis in marathon runners. *European Heart Journal,* 29, 1903-1910 (2008).

45. La Gerche, A., *et al.* Exercise-induced right ventricular dysfunction and structural remodelling in endurance athletes. *European Heart Journal,* 33, 998-1006 (2012).

46. Andersen, K., *et al.* Risk of arrhythmias in 52 755 long-distance cross-country skiers: a cohort study. *European Heart Journal,* 34, 3624-3631 (2013).

47. Abdulla, J. & Nielsen, J.R. Is the risk of atrial fibrillation higher in athletes than in the general population? A systematic review and meta-analysis. *EP Europace Journal,* 11, 1156-1159 (2009).

48. Mozaffarian, D., *et al.* Physical activity and incidence of atrial fibrillation in older adults: the cardiovascular health study. *Circulation,* 118, 800-807 (2008).

49. Thompson, P.D. Physical fitness, physical activity, exercise training, and atrial fibrillation: first the good news, then the bad. *Journal of the American College of Cardiology,* 66, 997-999 (2015).

50. Breuckmann, F., *et al.* Myocardial late gadolinium enhancement: prevalence, pattern, and prognostic relevance in marathon runners. *Radiology,* 251, 50-57 (2009).

51. Wilson, M., *et al.* Diverse patterns of myocardial fibrosis in lifelong, veteran endurance athletes. *Journal of Applied Physiology (Bethesda, Md.: 1985),* 110, 1622-1626 (2011).

52. Schnohr, P., *et al.* Dose of jogging and long-term mortality. *Journal of the American College of Cardiology* (2015).

53. Armstrong, M.E., *et al.* Frequent physical activity may not reduce vascular disease risk. *Circulation* (2015).

54. Craddock, J.C., Probst, Y.C. & Peoples, G.E. Vegetarian and omnivorous nutrition – comparing physical performance. *International Journal of Sport Nutrition and Exercise Metabolism,* 26, 212-220 (2016).

55. Lynch, H., Johnston, C. & Wharton, C. Plant-based diets: considerations for environmental impact, protein quality, and exercise performance. *Nutrients,* 10, E1841 (2018).

Chapter 14: Fortifying muscles and bones: the science of strength training

1. Raj, I.S., Bird, S.R. & Shield, A.J. Aging and the force-velocity relationship of muscles. *Experimental Gerontology,* 45, 81-90 (2010).

2. Dipietro, L., *et al.* Physical activity, injurious falls, and physical function in aging: an umbrella review. *Medicine and Science in Sports and Exercise,* 51, 1303-1313 (2019).

3. Hunter, G.R., McCarthy, J.P. & Bamman, M.M. Effects of resistance training on older adults. *Sports Medicine (Auckland, N.Z.),* 34, 329-348 (2004).

4. Kim, J.S., Cross, J.M. & Bamman, M.M. Impact of resistance loading on myostatin expression and cell cycle regulation in young and older men and women. *American Journal of Physiology. Endocrinology and Metabolism,* 288, E1110-1119 (2005).

5. Lemmer, J.T., *et al.* Age and gender responses to strength training and detraining. *Medicine and Science in Sports and Exercise,* 32, 1505-1512 (2000).

6. Hunter, G.R., *et al.* Resistance training increases total energy expenditure and free-living physical activity in older adults. *Journal of Applied Physiology,* 89, 977-984 (2000).

7. Pratley, R., *et al.* Strength training increases resting metabolic rate and norepinephrine levels in healthy 50- to 65-yr-old men. *Journal of Applied Physiology,* 76, 133-137 (1994).

8. McCarthy, J.P., *et al.* Compatibility of adaptive responses with combining strength and endurance training. *Medicine and Science in Sports and Exercise,* 27, 429-436 (1995).

9. Sigal, R.J., *et al.* Effects of aerobic training, resistance training, or both on percentage body fat and cardiometabolic risk markers in obese adolescents: the healthy eating aerobic and resistance training in youth randomized clinical trial. *Journal of the American Medical Association: Pediatrics,* 168, 1006-1014 (2014).

10. Sakamoto, K., *et al.* Effects of unipedal standing balance exercise on the prevention of falls and hip fracture among clinically defined high-risk elderly individuals: a randomized controlled trial. *Journal of Orthopaedic Science,* 11, 467-472 (2006).

11. Cadore, E.L., *et al.* Strength and endurance training prescription in healthy and frail elderly. *Aging and Disease,* 5, 183-195 (2014).

12. Seo, D.Y., *et al.* Morning and evening exercise. *Integrative Medicine Research,* 2, 139-144 (2013).

13. Holwerda, A.M., *et al.* Dose-dependent increases in whole-body net protein balance and dietary protein-derived amino accid incorporation into myofibrillar protein during recovery from resistamce exercise in older men. *Journal of Nutrition,* 149, 221–230 (2019).

14. Moore, D.R., *et al.* Protein ingestion to stimulate myofibrillar protein synthesis requires greater relative protein intakes in healthy older versus younger men. *The Journals of Gerontology. Series A, Biological Sciences and Medical Sciences,* 70, 57-62 (2015).

15. Moore, D.R., *et al.* Ingested protein dose response of muscle and albumin protein synthesis after resistance exercise in young men. *American Journal of Clinical Nutrition* 89, 161-168 (2009).

16. Sabatini, D.M., Twenty-five years of mTOR: Uncovering the link from nutrients to growth. *Proceedings of the National Acadamy of Sciences of the USA,* 144, 11818-11825 (2017).

17. Hari, A., *et al.* Exercise-induced improvements in glucose effectiveness are blunted by a high glycemic diet in adults with prediabetes. *Acta diabetologica* 56, 211-217 (2019).

18. Solomon, T.P., *et al.* A low-glycemic diet lifestyle intervention improves fat utilization during exercise in older obese humans. *Obesity,* 21, 2272-2278 (2013).

19. Solomon, T.P., *et al.* Randomized trial on the effects of a 7-d low-glycemic diet and exercise intervention on insulin resistance in older obese humans. *The American Journal of Clinical Nutrition,* 90, 1222-1229 (2009).

20. Fontana, L. & Partridge, L. Promoting health and longevity through diet: from model organisms to humans. *Cell,* 161, 106-118 (2015).

21. Efeyan, A., Zoncu, R. & Sabatini, D.M. Amino acids and mTORC1: from lysosomes to disease. *Trends in Molecular Medicine,* 18, 524-533 (2012).

22. Tang, W.H., *et al.* Intestinal microbial metabolism of phosphatidylcholine and cardiovascular risk. *The New England Journal of Medicine,* 368, 1575-1584 (2013).

Chapter 15: Posture, balance and flexibility: the essential exercises

1. Iannuccilli, J.D., Prince, E.A. & Soares, G.M. Interventional spine procedures for management of chronic low back pain-a primer. *Seminars in Interventional Radiology,* 30, 307-317 (2013).

2. Freburger, J.K., *et al.* The rising prevalence of chronic low back pain. *Archives of Internal Medicine,* 169, 251-258 (2009).

3. Vincent, H.K., *et al.* Musculoskeletal pain, fear avoidance behaviors, and functional decline in obesity: potential interventions to manage pain and maintain

function. *Regional Anesthesia and Pain Medicine,* 38, 481-491 (2013).

4. Grieco, A. Sitting posture: an old problem and a new one. *Ergonomics,* 29, 345-362 (1986).

5. Parker, M. & Johansen, A. Hip fracture. *BMJ,* 333, 27-30 (2006).

6. Pearsaii, D.J. & Reid, J.G. Line of gravity relative to upright vertebral posture. *Clinical Biomechanics,* 7, 80-86 (1992).

7. Opplert, J. & Babault, N. Acute effects of dynamic stretching on muscle flexibility and performance: an analysis of the current literature. *Sports Medicine,* 48, 299-325 (2018).

Chapter 16: Hatha Yoga, Tai Chi and martial arts: East meets West

1. Wolfson, L., *et al.* Balance and strength training in older adults: intervention gains and Tai Chi maintenance. *Journal of the American Geriatrics Society,* 44, 498-506 (1996).

2. Li, F., *et al.* Tai chi and postural stability in patients with Parkinson's disease. *The New England Journal of Medicine,* 366, 511-519 (2012).

3. Li, F., *et al.* Tai chi and fall reductions in older adults: a randomized controlled trial. *The Journals of Gerontology. Series A, Biological Sciences and Medical Sciences,* 60, 187-194 (2005).

4. Voukelatos, A., *et al.* A randomized, controlled trial of tai chi for the prevention of falls: the Central Sydney tai chi trial. *Journal of the American Geriatrics Society,* 55, 1185-1191 (2007).

5. Wang, C., *et al.* A randomized trial of tai chi for fibromyalgia. *The New England Journal of Medicine,* 363, 743-754 (2010).

6. Wang, C., *et al.* Effect of tai chi versus aerobic exercise for fibromyalgia: comparative effectiveness randomized controlled trial. *BMJ,* 360, k851 (2018).

7. Sherman, K.J., *et al.* Comparing yoga, exercise, and a self-care book for chronic low back pain: a randomized, controlled trial. *Annals of Internal Medicine,* 143, 849-856 (2005).

8. Oken, B.S., *et al.* Randomized, controlled, six-month trial of yoga in healthy seniors: effects on cognition and quality of life. *Alternative Therapies in Health and Medicine,* 12, 40-47 (2006).

9. Cramer, H., *et al.* A systematic review and meta-analysis of yoga for low back pain. *The Clinical Journal of Pain,* 29, 450-460 (2013).

10. Tilbrook, H.E., *et al.* Yoga for chronic low back pain: a randomized trial. *Annals of Internal Medicine,* 155, 569-578 (2011).

11. Kiecolt-Glaser, J.K., *et al.* Yoga's impact on inflammation, mood, and fatigue in breast cancer survivors: a randomized controlled trial. *Journal of Clinical Oncology,* 32, 1040-1049 (2014).

12. Hunter, S.D., *et al.* Effects of yoga interventions practised in heated and thermoneutral conditions on endothelium-dependent vasodilatation: the Bikram yoga heart study. *Experimental Physiology,* 103, 391-396 (2018).

13. Kiecolt-Glaser, J.K., *et al.* Yoga's impact on inflammation, mood, and fatigue in breast cancer survivors. *Journal of Clinical Oncology* (2014).

14. Moadel, A.B., *et al.* Randomized controlled trial of yoga among a multiethnic sample of breast cancer patients: effects on quality of life. *Journal of Clinical Oncology,* 25, 4387-4395 (2007).

15. Smith, C., *et al.* A randomised comparative trial of yoga and relaxation to reduce stress and anxiety. *Complementary Therapies in Medicine,* 15, 77-83 (2007).

16. Mustian, K.M., *et al.* Multicenter, randomized controlled trial of yoga for sleep quality among cancer survivors. *Journal of Clinical Oncology,* 31, 3233-3241 (2013).

17. Gothe, N.P., Kramer, A.F. & McAuley, E. The effects of an 8-week Hatha yoga intervention on executive function in older adults. *The Journals of Gerontology. Series A, Biological Sciences and Medical Sciences,* 69, 1109-1116 (2014).

18. Chrousos, G.P. & Gold, P.W. The concepts of stress and stress system disorders. Overview of physical and behavioral homeostasis. *Journal of the American Medical Association,* 267, 1244-1252 (1992).

19. Rozanski, A., Blumenthal, J.A. & Kaplan, J. Impact of psychological factors on the pathogenesis of cardiovascular disease and implications for therapy. *Circulation,* 99, 2192-2217 (1999).

20. Kivimaki, M. & Steptoe, A. Effects of stress on the development and progression of cardiovascular disease. *Nature Reviews: Cardiology,* 15, 215-229 (2018).

21. Yan, L., *et al.* Type 5 adenylyl cyclase disruption increases longevity and protects against stress. *Cell,* 130, 247-258 (2007).

22. Esler, M., *et al.* Overflow of catecholamine neurotransmitters to the circulation: source, fate, and functions. *Physiological Reviews,* 70, 963-985 (1990).

23. Naik, G.S., Gaur, G.S. & Pal, G.K. Effect of modified slow breathing exercise on perceived stress and basal cardiovascular parameters. *International Journal of Yoga,* 11, 53-58 (2018).

24. Bernardi, L., *et al.* Slow breathing increases arterial baroreflex sensitivity in patients with chronic heart failure. *Circulation,* 105, 143-145 (2002).

25. Oneda, B., *et al.* Sympathetic nerve activity is decreased during device-guided slow breathing. *Hypertension Research,* 33, 708-712 (2010).

26. Tracey, K.J. The inflammatory reflex. *Nature,* 420, 853-859 (2002).

27. Borovikova, L.V., *et al.* Vagus nerve stimulation attenuates the systemic inflammatory response to endotoxin. *Nature,* 405, 458-462 (2000).

28. Ghia, J.E., *et al.* The vagus nerve: a tonic inhibitory influence associated with inflammatory bowel disease in a murine model. *Gastroenterology,* 131, 1122-1130 (2006).

29. Seals, D.R., Suwarno, N.O. & Dempsey, J.A. Influence of lung volume on sympathetic nerve discharge in normal humans. *Circulation Research, 67*, 130-141 (1990).

30. Joseph, C.N., *et al.* Slow breathing improves arterial baroreflex sensitivity and decreases blood pressure in essential hypertension. *Hypertension, 46*, 714-718 (2005).

31. Kalyani, B.G., *et al.* Neurohemodynamic correlates of 'OM' chanting: a pilot functional magnetic resonance imaging study. *International Journal of Yoga, 4*, 3-6 (2011).

32. Sadhana Pada, *The Yoga Sutras of Patanjal*, 49-53.

PART V: Prevention

Chapter 17: Take preventative action to stay healthy

1. Venn, A. & Britton, J. Exposure to secondhand smoke and biomarkers of cardiovascular disease risk in never-smoking adults. *Circulation, 115*, 990-995 (2007).

2. Gibbs, K., Collaco, J.M. & McGrath-Morrow, S.A. Impact of tobacco smoke and nicotine exposure on lung development. *Chest, 149*, 552-561 (2016).

3. *Ibid.*

4. Jha, P. & Peto, R. Global effects of smoking, of quitting, and of taxing tobacco. *The New England Journal of Medicine, 370*, 60-68 (2014).

5. Ibid.

6. Thun, M.J., *et al.* 50-year trends in smoking-related mortality in the United States. *The New England Journal of Medicine, 368*, 351-364 (2013).

7. Hecht, S.S. Tobacco carcinogens, their biomarkers and tobacco-induced cancer. *Nature Reviews: Cancer, 3*, 733-744 (2003).

8. Carter, B.D., *et al.* Smoking and mortality – beyond established causes. *The New England Journal of Medicine, 372*, 631-640 (2015).

9. Hackshaw, A., *et al.* Low cigarette consumption and risk of coronary heart disease and stroke: meta-analysis of 141 cohort studies in 55 study reports. *BMJ, 360*, j5855 (2018).

10. Rom, O., *et al.* Cigarette smoking and inflammation revisited. *Respiratory Physiology and Neurobiology, 187*, 5-10 (2013).

11. Burke A., FitzGerald G.A., Oxidative stress and smoking-induced vascular injury, *Progress in Cardiovascular Disease*, Vol 46, Issue 1, 79-90 (2003).

12. Morris, P.B., *et al.* Cardiovascular effects of exposure to cigarette smoke and electronic cigarettes: clinical perspectives from the Prevention of Cardiovascular Disease Section Leadership Council and Early Career Councils of the American College of Cardiology. *Journal of the American College of Cardiology, 66*, 1378-1391 (2015).

13. Smith, C.J., *et al.* IARC carcinogens reported in cigarette mainstream smoke and their calculated log P values. *Food and Chemical Toxicology, 41*, 807-817 (2003).

14. Mineur, Y.S., *et al.* Nicotine decreases food intake through activation of POMC neurons. *Science, 332*, 1330-1332 (2011).

15. Jha, P. & Peto, R. Global effects of smoking, of quitting, and of taxing tobacco. *The New England journal of medicine, 370*, 60-68 (2014).

16. Vineis, P., *et al.* Tobacco and cancer: recent epidemiological evidence. *Journal National Cancer Institute, 96*(2), 99-106 (2004).

17. US Department of Health and Human Services. The Surgeon General's call to action to prevent skin cancer. Office of the Surgeon General. (2014).

18. Holick, M.F. Vitamin D deficiency. *The New England Journal of Medicine, 357*, 266-281 (2007).

19. Hart, P.H., Gorman, S. & Finlay-Jones, J.J. Modulation of the immune system by UV radiation: more than just the effects of vitamin D? *Nature Reviews: Immunology, 11*, 584-596 (2011).

20. Norval, M., Bjorn, L.O. & de Gruijl, F.R. Is the action spectrum for the UV-induced production of previtamin D3 in human skin correct? *Photochemical & Photobiological Sciences, 9*, 11-17 (2010).

21. Zanello, S.B., Jackson, D.M. & Holick, M.F. An immunocytochemical approach to the study of beta-endorphin production in human keratinocytes using confocal microscopy. *Annals of the New York Academy of Sciences, 885*, 85-99 (1999).

22. Lindqvist, P.G., *et al.* Avoidance of sun exposure is a risk factor for all-cause mortality: results from the Melanoma in Southern Sweden cohort. *Journal of Internal Medicine, 276*, 77-86 (2014).

23. Lindqvist, P.G., *et al.* Avoidance of sun exposure as a risk factor for major causes of death: a competing risk analysis of the melanoma in Southern Sweden cohort. *Journal of Internal Medicine, 280*, 375-387 (2016).

24. Matsuoka, L.Y., *et al.* Sunscreens suppress cutaneous vitamin D3 synthesis. *The Journal of Clinical Endocrinology and Metabolism, 64*, 1165-1168 (1987).

25. Holick, M.F. The vitamin D deficiency pandemic: approaches for diagnosis, treatment and prevention. *Reviews in Endocrine & Metabolic Disorders, 18*, 153-165 (2017).

26. Plotnikoff, G.A. & Quigley, J.M. Prevalence of severe hypovitaminosis D in patients with persistent, nonspecific musculoskeletal pain. *Mayo Clinic Proceedings, 78*, 1463-1470 (2003).

27. Turner, M.K., *et al.* Prevalence and clinical correlates of vitamin D inadequacy among patients with chronic pain. *Pain Medicine, 9*, 979-984 (2008).

28. Holick, M.F. The vitamin D deficiency pandemic. *Reviews in Endocrine & Metabolic Disorders* (2017).

29. Lappe, J.M., *et al.* Vitamin D and calcium supplementation reduces cancer risk: results of a randomized trial. *The American Journal of Clinical Nutrition, 85*, 1586-1591 (2007).

30. Wactawski-Wende, J., *et al.* Calcium plus vitamin D supplementation and the risk of colorectal cancer. *The New England Journal of Medicine, 354*, 684-696 (2006).

31. Groves, N.J., McGrath, J.J. & Burne, T.H. Vitamin D as a neurosteroid affecting the developing and adult brain. *Annual Review of Nutrition,* 34, 117-141 (2014).

32. Hoel, D.G., *et al.* The risks and benefits of sun exposure 2016. *Dermato-endocrinology,* 8, e1248325 (2016).

33. Holick, M. Vitamin D: The underappreciated D-lightful hormone that is important for skeletal and cellular health. *Current Opinion in Endocrinology and Diabetes,* 9, 87-98 (2002).

34. Chen, A.C., *et al.* A phase 3 randomized trial of nicotinamide for skin-cancer chemoprevention. *The New England Journal of Medicine,* 373, 1618-1626 (2015).

35. Ombra, M.N., *et al.* Dietary compounds and cutaneous malignant melanoma: recent advances from a biological perspective. *Nutrition and Metabolism* 21, 16:33 (2019).

36. Edelman, E.J. & Fiellin, D.A. In the Clinic. Alcohol Use. *Annals of Internal Medicine,* 164, Itc1-16 (2016).

37. Jensen, T.K., *et al.* Does moderate alcohol consumption affect fertility? Follow up study among couples planning first pregnancy. *BMJ,* 317, 505-510 (1998).

38. Spanagel, R., *et al.* Alcohol consumption and the body's biological clock. *Alcoholism, Clinical and Experimental Research,* 29, 1550-1557 (2005).

39. Wood, A.M., *et al.* Risk thresholds for alcohol consumption: combined analysis of individual-participant data for 599 912 current drinkers in 83 prospective studies. *Lancet,* 391, 1513-1523 (2018).

40. Goldberg, I.J., *et al.* AHA science advisory: wine and your heart: a science advisory for healthcare professionals from the Nutrition Committee, Council on Epidemiology and Prevention, and Council on Cardiovascular Nursing of the American Heart Association. *Circulation,* 103, 472-475 (2001).

41. Gepner, Y., *et al.* Effects of initiating moderate alcohol intake on cardiometabolic risk in adults with type 2 diabetes: a 2-year randomized, controlled trial. *Annals of Internal Medicine,* 163, 569-579 (2015).

42. Davies, M.J., *et al.* Effects of moderate alcohol intake on fasting insulin and glucose concentrations and insulin sensitivity in postmenopausal women: a randomized controlled trial. *Journal of the American Medical Association,* 287, 2559-2562 (2002).

43. Baer, D.J., *et al.* Moderate alcohol consumption lowers risk factors for cardiovascular disease in postmenopausal women fed a controlled diet. *The American Journal of Clinical Nutrition,* 75, 593-599 (2002).

44. Voskoboinik, A., *et al.* Moderate alcohol consumption is associated with atrial electrical and structural changes: Insights from high-density left atrial electroanatomic mapping. *Heart Rhythm,* 16, 251-259 (2019).

45. Voskoboinik, A., *et al.* Regular alcohol consumption is associated with impaired atrial mechanical function in the atrial fibrillation population: a cross-sectional MRI-based study. *JACC: Clinical Electrophysiology,* 4, 1451-1459 (2018).

46. Xin, X., *et al.* Effects of alcohol reduction on blood pressure: a meta-analysis of randomized controlled trials. *Hypertension,* 38, 1112-1117 (2001).

47. Mori, T.A., *et al.* Randomized controlled intervention of the effects of alcohol on blood pressure in premenopausal women. *Hypertension,* 66, 517-523 (2015).

48. Smith-Warner, S.A., *et al.* Alcohol and breast cancer in women: a pooled analysis of cohort studies. *JAMA,* (1998).

49. Giovannucci, E., Alcohol, one-carbon metabolism, and colorectal cancer: recent insights from molecular studies, *American Society of Nutritional Sciences* 2475S-2481S (2004).

50. Garaycoechea, J.I., *et al.* Alcohol and endogenous aldehydes damage chromosomes and mutate stem cells. *Nature,* 553, 171-177 (2018).

51. Sarkola, T., *et al.* Acute effect of alcohol on androgens in premenopausal women. *Alcohol and Alcoholism,* 35, 84-90 (2000).

52. Sarkola, T. & Eriksson, C.J. Testosterone increases in men after a low dose of alcohol. *Alcoholism, Clinical and Experimental Research,* 27, 682-685 (2003).

53. Dorgan, J.F., *et al.* Serum hormones and the alcohol-breast cancer association in postmenopausal women. *Journal of the National Cancer Institute,* 93, 710-715 (2001).

54. Loos, B.G., *et al.* Elevation of systemic markers related to cardiovascular diseases in the peripheral blood of periodontitis patients. *Journal of Periodontology,* 71, 1528-1534 (2000).

55. Noack, B., *et al.* Periodontal infections contribute to elevated systemic C-reactive protein level. *Journal of Periodontology,* 72, 1221-1227 (2001).

56. Amar, S., *et al.* Periodontal disease is associated with brachial artery endothelial dysfunction and systemic inflammation. *Arteriosclerosis, Thrombosis, and Vascular Biology,* 23, 1245-1249 (2003).

57. Beck, J.D., *et al.* Relationship of periodontal disease to carotid artery intima-media wall thickness: the atherosclerosis risk in communities (ARIC) study. *Arteriosclerosis, Thrombosis, and Vascular Biology,* 21, 1816-1822 (2001).

58. Ryden, L., *et al.* Periodontitis increases the risk of a first myocardial infarction: a report from the PAROKRANK Study. *Circulation,* 133, 576-583 (2016).

59. Demmer, R.T., *et al.* The influence of anti-infective periodontal treatment on C-reactive protein: a systematic review and meta-analysis of randomized controlled trials. *PLOS One,* 8, e77441 (2013).

Chapter 18: The importance of health screening

1. Siegel, R.L., Miller, K.D. & Jemal, A. Cancer statistics, 2019. *CA: A Cancer Journal for Clinicians,* 69, 7-34 (2019).

2. Noone, A.M., *et al.* Seer Cancer Statistics Review, 1975-2015, National Cancer Institute, Bethesda, MD. http://seer.cancer.gov/csr/1975_2015/

3. Smith, R.A., *et al.* Cancer screening in the United States, 2019: A review of current American Cancer Society guidelines and current issues in cancer screening. *CA: a cancer journal for clinicians* 69, 184-210 (2019).

4. Siegel, R.L., Miller, K.D. & Jemal, A. Cancer statistics, 2019. *CA* (2019).

5. Bibbins-Domingo, K., *et al.* Screening for colorectal cancer: US Preventive Services Task Force recommendation statement. *Journal of the American Medical Association,* 315, 2564-2575 (2016).

6. Siu, A.L. Screening for breast cancer: US Preventive Services Task Force Recommendation Statement. *Annals of Internal Medicine,* 164, 279-296 (2016).

7. Siegel, R.L., Miller, K.D. & Jemal, A. Cancer statistics, 2019. *CA* (2019).

8. Fenton, J.J., *et al.* US Preventive Services Task Force evidence syntheses, formerly systematic evidence reviews. *Agency for Healthcare Research and Quality* (2018).

9. Loeb, S., *et al.* Uptake of active surveillance for very-low-risk prostate cancer in Sweden. *Journal of the American Medical Association: Oncology,* 3, 1393-1398 (2017).

Part VI: Our minds

Chapter 19: Nourish your mind and train your brain

1. Harburger, L.L., Nzerem, C.K. & Frick, K.M. Single enrichment variables differentially reduce age-related memory decline in female mice. *Behavioral Neuroscience,* 121, 679-688 (2007).

2. Freret, T., *et al.* Rescue of cognitive aging by long-lasting environmental enrichment exposure initiated before median lifespan. *Neurobiology of Aging,* 33, 1005. e1001-1010 (2012).

3. Diamond, M.C., *et al.* Plasticity in the 904-day-old male rat cerebral cortex. *Experimental Neurology,* 87, 309-317 (1985).

4. Thanos, P.K., *et al.* Dopamine D2 gene expression interacts with environmental enrichment to impact lifespan and behavior. *Oncotarget,* 7, 19111-19123 (2016).

5. Wood, N.I., Glynn, D. & Morton, A.J. "Brain training" improves cognitive performance and survival in a transgenic mouse model of Huntington's disease. *Neurobiology of Disease,* 42, 427-437 (2011).

6. Panikkar, R. *Hinduism. The Vedic Experience. Mantramanjari.* Orbis Books (2016).

7. Bailey, C.H. & Kandel, E.R. Structural changes accompanying memory storage. *Annual Review of Physiology,* 55, 397-426 (1993).

8. Yang, G., Pan, F. & Gan, W.B. Stably maintained dendritic spines are associated with lifelong memories. *Nature,* 462, 920-924 (2009).

9. Trachtenberg, J.T., *et al.* Long-term in vivo imaging of experience-dependent synaptic plasticity in adult cortex. *Nature,* 420, 788-794 (2002).

10. Hofer, S.B., *et al.* Experience leaves a lasting structural trace in cortical circuits. *Nature,* 457, 313-317 (2009).

11. Wilbrecht, L., *et al.* Structural plasticity underlies experience-dependent functional plasticity of cortical circuits. *The Journal of Neuroscience,* 30, 4927-4932 (2010).

12. Xu, T., *et al.* Rapid formation and selective stabilization of synapses for enduring motor memories. *Nature,* 462, 915-919 (2009).

13. Yamahachi, H., *et al.* Rapid axonal sprouting and pruning accompany functional reorganization in primary visual cortex. *Neuron,* 64, 719-729 (2009).

14. Schneider, J.S., *et al.* Enriched environment during development is protective against lead-induced neurotoxicity. *Brain Research,* 896, 48-55 (2001).

15. Grutzendler, J., Kasthuri, N. & Gan, W.B. Long-term dendritic spine stability in the adult cortex. *Nature,* 420, 812-816 (2002).

16. Chapman, S.B., *et al.* Neural mechanisms of brain plasticity with complex cognitive training in healthy seniors. *Cerebral Cortex,* 25, 396-405 (2015).

17. Holtmaat, A.J., *et al.* Transient and persistent dendritic spines in the neocortex in vivo. *Neuron,* 45, 279-291 (2005).

18. Xu, T., *et al.* Rapid formation and selective stabilization of synapses. *Nature* (2009).

19. Yamahachi, H., *et al.* Rapid axonal sprouting and pruning. *Neuron* (2009).

20. Lai, G., *et al.* Neural systems for speech and song in autism. *Brain: A Journal of Neurology,* 135, 961-975 (2012).

21. Belleville, S., *et al.* Training-related brain plasticity in subjects at risk of developing Alzheimer's disease. *Brain: A Journal of Neurology,* 134, 1623-1634 (2011).

22. Willis, S.L., *et al.* Long-term effects of cognitive training on everyday functional outcomes in older adults. *Journal of the American Medical Association,* 296, 2805-2814 (2006).

23. Sakai, K.L. Language acquisition and brain development. *Science,* 310, 815-819 (2005).

24. Seinfeld, S., *et al.* Effects of music learning and piano practice on cognitive function, mood and quality of life in older adults. *Frontiers in Psychology,* 4, 810 (2013).

25. Hars, M., *et al.* Effect of music-based multitask training on cognition and mood in older adults. *Age and Ageing,* 43, 196-200 (2014).

26. Sacco, K., *et al.* Motor imagery of walking following training in locomotor attention. The effect of "the tango lesson". *NeuroImage,* 32, 1441-1449 (2006).

27. Schlegel, A., *et al.* The artist emerges: visual art learning alters neural structure and function. *NeuroImage,* 105, 440-451 (2015).

28. Mattson, M.P. & Arumugam, T.V. Hallmarks of brain aging: adaptive and pathological modification by metabolic states. *Cell Metabolism,* 27, 1176-1199 (2018).

29. Mattson, M.P., *et al.* Meal frequency and timing in health and disease. *Proceedings of the National Academy of Sciences,* 111, 16647-16653 (2014).

30. Camandola, S. & Mattson, M.P. Brain metabolism in health, aging, and neurodegeneration. *The EMBO journal* 36, 1474-1492 (2017).

31. Liu, Y., *et al.* SIRT3 mediates hippocampal synaptic adaptations to intermittent fasting and ameliorates deficits in APP mutant mice. *Nature Communications,* 10:1886 (2019).

32. Yang, H., *et al.* Ketone Bodies in Neurological Diseases: Focus on Neuroprotection and Underlying Mechanisms. *Frontiers in Neurology,* 10:585 (2019).

33. Livingston, G., *et al.* Dementia prevention, intervention, and care. *Lancet,* 390, 2673-2734 (2017).

34. Kivipelto, M., Mangialasche, F. & Ngandu, T. Lifestyle interventions to prevent cognitive impairment, dementia and Alzheimer disease. *Nature Reviews: Neurology,* 14, 653-666 (2018).

35. McKee, A.C., *et al.* Chronic traumatic encephalopathy in athletes: progressive tauopathy after repetitive head injury. *Journal of Neuropathology and Experimental Neurology,* 68, 709-735 (2009).

36. Solomon, A., *et al.* Effect of the apolipoprotein E genotype on cognitive change during a multidomain lifestyle intervention: a subgroup analysis of a randomized clinical trial. *Journal of the American Medical Association: Neurology,* 75, 462-470 (2018).

37. Schrijvers, E.M., *et al.* Insulin metabolism and the risk of Alzheimer disease: the Rotterdam Study. *Neurology,* 75, 1982-1987 (2010).

38. Mattson, M.P. & Arumugam, T.V. Hallmarks of brain aging. *Cell Metabolism* (2018).

39. Most, J., *et al.* Calorie restriction in humans: an update. *Ageing Research Reviews,* 39, 36-45 (2017).

40. Mattson, M.P., *et al.* Intermittent metabolic switching, neuroplasticity and brain health. *Nature Reviews: Neuroscience,* 19, 63-80 (2018).

41. Wahl, D., *et al.* Cognitive and behavioral evaluation of nutritional interventions in rodent models of brain aging and dementia. *Clinical Interventions in Aging,* 12, 1419-1428 (2017).

42. Botchway, B.O.A., *et al.* Nutrition: Review on the Possible Treatment for Alzheimer's Disease. *Journal of Alzheimer's Disease,* 61:867–883 (2018).

43. Petersson, S.D. & Philippou, E. Mediterranean diet, cognitive function, and dementia: a systematic review of the evidence. *Advances in Nutrition,* 7, 889-904 (2016).

44. Tosti, V., Bertozzi, B. & Fontana, L. Health benefits of the mediterranean diet: metabolic and molecular mechanisms. *The Journals of Gerontology: Series A,* 73, 318-326 (2017).

45. Stigger, F.S., *et al.* Effects of Exercise on Inflammatory, Oxidative, and Neurotrophic Biomarkers on Cognitively Impaired Individuals Diagnosed With Dementia or Mild Cognitive Impairment: A Systematic Review and Meta-Analysis. *The Journals of Gerontology Series A Biological Sciences Medical Sciences,* 74:616–624 (2019).

46. Lautenschlager, N.T., *et al.* Effect of physical activity on cognitive function in older adults at risk for Alzheimer disease: a randomized trial. *Journal of the American Medical Association,* 300, 1027-1037 (2008).

47. Blumenthal, J.A., *et al.* Lifestyle and neurocognition in older adults with cognitive impairments: A randomized trial. *Neurology,* 92, e212-e223 (2019).

48. Mavros, Y., *et al.* Mediation of cognitive function improvements by strength gains after resistance training in older adults with mild cognitive impairment: outcomes of the study of mental and resistance training. *Journal of the American Geriatrics Society,* 65, 550-559 (2017).

49. Colcombe, S.J., *et al.* Aerobic exercise training increases brain volume in aging humans. *The Journals of Gerontology. Series A, Biological Sciences and Medical Sciences,* 61, 1166-1170 (2006).

50. Colcombe, S.J., *et al.* Cardiovascular fitness, cortical plasticity, and aging. *Proceedings of the National Academy of Sciences of the United States of America,* 101, 3316-3321 (2004).

51. Erickson, K.I., *et al.* Exercise training increases size of hippocampus and improves memory. *Proceedings of the National Academy of Sciences of the United States of America,* 108, 3017-3022 (2011).

52. Erickson, K.I., *et al.* Aerobic fitness is associated with hippocampal volume in elderly humans. *Hippocampus,* 19, 1030-1039 (2009).

53. Stranahan, A.M., *et al.* Voluntary exercise and caloric restriction enhance hippocampal dendritic spine density and BDNF levels in diabetic mice. *Hippocampus,* 19, 951-961 (2009).

54. Kobilo, T., Yuan, C. & van Praag, H. Endurance factors improve hippocampal neurogenesis and spatial memory in mice. *Learning & Memory,* 18, 103-107 (2011).

55. Lautenschlager, N.T., *et al.* Effect of physical activity on cognitive function. *Journal of the American Medical Association* (2008).

56. Moon, H.Y., *et al.* Running-Induced Systemic Cathepsin B Secretion Is Associated with Memory Function. *Cell Metabolism,* 24:332–340 (2016).

57. Ju, Y.E., *et al.* Sleep quality and preclinical Alzheimer disease. *Journal of the American Medical Association Neurology,* 70, 587-593 (2013).

58. Shan, Z., *et al.* Sleep duration and risk of type 2 diabetes: a meta-analysis of prospective studies. *Diabetes Care,* 38, 529-537 (2015).

59. Buxton, O.M., *et al.* Adverse metabolic consequences in humans of prolonged sleep restriction combined with circadian disruption. *Science Translational Medicine,* 4, 129ra143 (2012).

60. Buxton, O.M., *et al.* Sleep restriction for 1 week reduces insulin sensitivity in healthy men. *Diabetes,* 59, 2126-2133 (2010).

61. Sutherland, K., *et al.* Prediction in obstructive sleep apnoea: diagnosis, comorbidity risk, and treatment outcomes. *Expert Review of Respiratory Medicine,* 12, 293-307 (2018).

62. Rodriguez, J.C., Dzierzewski, J.M. & Alessi, C.A. Sleep problems in the elderly. *The Medical Clinics of North America*, 99, 431-439 (2015).

63. Wilbrecht, L., *et al.* Structural plasticity underlies experience-dependent functional plasticity of cortical circuits. *The Journal of Neuroscience*, 30, 4927-4932 (2010).

Chapter 20: Rest and sleep quality

1. Enqin, Z., Health Preservation and Rehabilitation, Publishing House of Shanghai College of Traditional Chinese Medicine. (1988).

2. *Ibid.*

1. Montagna, P., *et al.* Familial and sporadic fatal insomnia. *Lancet: Neurology*, 2, 167-176 (2003).

2. Ohayon, M.M., *et al.* Meta-analysis of quantitative sleep parameters from childhood to old age in healthy individuals: developing normative sleep values across the human lifespan. *Sleep*, 27, 1255-1273 (2004).

3. Xie, L., *et al.* Sleep drives metabolite clearance from the adult brain. *Science*, 342, 373-377 (2013).

4. Baharav, A., *et al.* Fluctuations in autonomic nervous activity during sleep displayed by power spectrum analysis of heart rate variability. *Neurology*, 45, 1183-1187 (1995).

5. Trinder, J., *et al.* Autonomic activity during human sleep as a function of time and sleep stage. *Journal of Sleep Research*, 10, 253-264 (2001).

6. Carrington, M., *et al.* The influence of sleep onset on the diurnal variation in cardiac activity and cardiac control. *Journal of Sleep Research*, 12, 213-221 (2003).

7. Born, J., *et al.* Effects of sleep and circadian rhythm on human circulating immune cells. *Journal of Immunology*, 158, 4454-4464 (1997).

8. Westermann, J., *et al.* System consolidation during sleep – a common principle underlying psychological and immunological memory formation. *Trends in Neurosciences*, 38, 585-597 (2015).

9. Bryant, P.A., Trinder, J. & Curtis, N. Sick and tired: does sleep have a vital role in the immune system? *Nature Reviews: Immunology*, 4, 457-467 (2004).

10. Diekelmann, S. & Born, J. The memory function of sleep. *Nature Reviews: Neuroscience*, 11, 114-126 (2010).

11. Plihal, W. & Born, J. Effects of early and late nocturnal sleep on declarative and procedural memory. *Journal of Cognitive Neuroscience*, 9, 534-547 (1997).

12. Yang, G., *et al.* Sleep promotes branch-specific formation of dendritic spines after learning. *Science (New York, N.Y.)*, 344, 1173-1178 (2014).

13. Berry, J.A., *et al.* Sleep facilitates memory by blocking dopamine neuron-mediated forgetting. *Cell*, 161, 1656-1667 (2015).

14. Plihal, W. & Born, J. Effects of early and late nocturnal sleep on memory. *Journal of Cognitive Neuroscience* (1997).

15. Durmer, J.S. & Dinges, D.F. Neurocognitive consequences of sleep deprivation. *Seminars in Neurology*, 25, 117-129 (2005).

16. Van Someren, E.J., *et al.* Slow brain oscillations of sleep, resting state, and vigilance. *Progress in Brain Research*, 193, 3-15 (2011).

17. Marshall, L. & Born, J. The contribution of sleep to hippocampus-dependent memory consolidation. *Trends in Cognitive Sciences*, 11, 442-450 (2007).

18. Landsness, E.C., *et al.* Sleep-dependent improvement in visuomotor learning: a causal role for slow waves. *Sleep*, 32, 1273-1284 (2009).

19. Wagner, U., *et al.* Sleep inspires insight. *Nature*, 427, 352-355 (2004).

20. Klimesch, W. EEG alpha and theta oscillations reflect cognitive and memory performance: a review and analysis. *Brain Research: Brain Research Reviews*, 29, 169-195 (1999).

21. Craig, M., *et al.* Wakeful rest promotes the integration of spatial memories into accurate cognitive maps. *Hippocampus*, 26, 185-193 (2016).

22. Musiek, E.S., Xiong, D.D. & Holtzman, D.M. Sleep, circadian rhythms, and the pathogenesis of Alzheimer disease. *Experimental & Molecular Medicine*, 47, e148 (2015).

23. Kang, J.E., *et al.* Amyloid-beta dynamics are regulated by orexin and the sleep-wake cycle. *Science*, 326, 1005-1007 (2009).

24. Roh, J.H., *et al.* Potential role of orexin and sleep modulation in the pathogenesis of Alzheimer's disease. *The Journal of Experimental Medicine*, 211, 2487-2496 (2014).

25. Ooms, S., *et al.* Effect of 1 night of total sleep deprivation on cerebrospinal fluid beta-amyloid 42 in healthy middle-aged men: a randomized clinical trial. *Journal of the American Medical Association: Neurology*, 71, 971-977 (2014).

26. Ju, Y.S., *et al.* Slow wave sleep disruption increases cerebrospinal fluid amyloid-beta levels. *Brain: A Journal of Neurology*, 140, 2104-2111 (2017).

27. Holth, J.K., *et al.* The sleep-wake cycle regulates brain interstitial fluid tau in mice and CSF tau in humans. *Science (New York, N.Y.)*, 363, 880-884 (2019).

28. Mander, B.A., *et al.* beta-amyloid disrupts human NREM slow waves and related hippocampus-dependent memory consolidation. *Nature Neuroscience*, 18, 1051-1057 (2015).

29. Kim, J.H., *et al.* Sleep duration and mortality in patients with coronary artery disease. *The American Journal of Cardiology*, 123, 874-881 (2019).

30. Tasali, E., *et al.* Slow-wave sleep and the risk of type 2 diabetes in humans. *Proceedings of the National Academy of Sciences of the United States of America*, 105, 1044-9 (2008).

31. Spiegel, K., *et al.* Brief communication: sleep curtailment in healthy young men is associated with decreased leptin levels, elevated ghrelin levels, and increased hunger and appetite. *Annals of Internal Medicine*, 141, 846-50 (2004).

32. Pires, G.N., *et al.* Effects of acute sleep deprivation on state anxiety levels: a systematic review and meta-

analysis. *Sleep Medicine,* 24, 109-118 (2016).

33. Tsuno, N., Besset, A. & Ritchie, K. Sleep and depression. *The Journal of Clinical Psychiatry,* 66, 1254-69 (2005).

34. Ratcliff, R. & Van Dongen, H.P. Diffusion model for one-choice reaction-time tasks and the cognitive effects of sleep deprivation. *Proceedings of the National Academy of Sciences of the United States of Americ*a, 108, 11285-90 (2011).

35. Durmer, J.S. & Dinges, D.F. Neurocognitive consequences of sleep deprivation. *Seminars in Neurology,* 25, 117-29 (2005).

36. Webb, W.A., HW. *Measurement and characteristics of nocturnal sleep.* Grune and Stratton (1969).

37. Colrain, I.M., *et al.* Sleep evoked delta frequency responses show a linear decline in amplitude across the adult lifespan. *Neurobiology of Aging,* 31, 874-883 (2010).

38. Webb, W.B. & Agnew, H.W., Jr. Sleep stage characteristics of long and short sleepers. *Science (New York, N.Y.),* 168, 146-147 (1970).

39. Hartmann, E., Baekeland, F. & Zwilling, G.R. Psychological differences between long and short sleepers. *Archives of General Psychiatry,* 26, 463-468 (1972).

40. Heo, J.Y., *et al.* Effects of smartphone use with and without blue light at night in healthy adults: a randomized, double-blind, cross-over, placebo-controlled comparison. *Journal of Psychiatric Research,* 87, 61-70 (2017).

41. Lyall, L.M., *et al.* Association of disrupted circadian rhythmicity with mood disorders, subjective wellbeing, and cognitive function: a cross-sectional study of 91,105 participants from the UK Biobank. *Lancet: Psychiatry,* 5, 507-514 (2018).

42. Kubitz, K.A., *et al.* The effects of acute and chronic exercise on sleep. A meta-analytic review. *Sports Medicine (Auckland, N.Z.),* 21, 277-291 (1996).

43. Dworak, M., *et al.* Increased slow wave sleep and reduced stage 2 sleep in children depending on exercise intensity. *Sleep Medicine,* 9, 266-272 (2008).

44. Kalak, N., *et al.* Daily morning running for 3 weeks improved sleep and psychological functioning in healthy adolescents compared with controls. *The Journal of Adolescent Health,* 51, 615-622 (2012).

45. Naylor, E., *et al.* Daily social and physical activity increases slow-wave sleep and daytime neuropsychological performance in the elderly. *Sleep,* 23, 87-95 (2000).

46. Yamanaka, Y., *et al.* Morning and evening physical exercise differentially regulate the autonomic nervous system during nocturnal sleep in humans. *American Journal of Physiology: Regulatory, Integrative and Comparative Physiology,* 309, R1112-1121 (2015).

47. Mustian, K.M., *et al.* Multicenter, randomized controlled trial of yoga for sleep quality among cancer survivors. *Journal of Clinical Oncology,* 31, 3233-3241 (2013).

48. Patra, S. & Telles, S. Positive impact of cyclic meditation on subsequent sleep. *Medical Science Monitor: International Medical Journal of Experimental and Clinical Research,* 15, Cr375-381 (2009).

49. Ferrarelli, F., *et al.* Experienced mindfulness meditators exhibit higher parietal-occipital EEG gamma activity during NREM sleep. *PLOS One,* 8, e73417 (2013).

50. Dentico, D., *et al.* Short meditation trainings enhance non-REM sleep low-frequency oscillations. *PLOS One,* 11, e0148961 (2016).

51. Huber, R., Ghilardi, M.F., Massimini, M. & Tononi, G. Local sleep and learning. *Nature* 430, 78-81 (2004).

52. Hanlon, E.C., *et al.* Effects of skilled training on sleep slow wave activity and cortical gene expression in the rat. *Sleep,* 32, 719-729 (2009).

53. Pugin, F., *et al.* Local increase of sleep slow wave activity after three weeks of working memory training in children and adolescents. *Sleep,* 38, 607-614 (2015).

54. Papalambros, N.A., *et al.* Acoustic enhancement of sleep slow oscillations and concomitant memory improvement in older adults. *Frontiers in Human Neuroscience,* 11, 109 (2017).

55. Zhou, J., *et al.* Pink noise: effect on complexity synchronization of brain activity and sleep consolidation. *Journal of Theoretical Biology,* 306, 68-72 (2012).

Chapter 21: Mindfulness meditation: learning to live in the present

1. Nhất Hạnh, Mobi Ho, and Mai Vo-Dinh. *The miracle of mindfulness: an introduction to the practice of meditation.* Beacon Press. (1987).

2. Aurelius, M., *Meditations.* Penguin Classics. (2006).

3. Enqin, Z., *Health Preservation and Rehabilitation,* Publishing House of Shanghai College of Traditional Chinese Medicine. (1988).

4. Nyklicek, I. & Kuijpers, K.F. Effects of mindfulness-based stress reduction intervention on psychological well-being and quality of life: is increased mindfulness indeed the mechanism? *Annals of Behavioral Medicine,* 35, 331-340 (2008).

5. Speca, M., *et al.* A randomized, wait-list controlled clinical trial: the effect of a mindfulness meditation-based stress reduction program on mood and symptoms of stress in cancer outpatients. *Psychosomatic Medicine,* 62, 613-622 (2000).

6. Friis, A.M., *et al.* Kindness matters: a randomized controlled trial of a mindful self-compassion intervention improves depression, distress, and HbA1c among patients with diabetes. *Diabetes Care,* 39, 1963-1971 (2016).

7. Teasdale, J.D., Segal, Z. & Williams, J.M. How does cognitive therapy prevent depressive relapse and why should attentional control (mindfulness) training help? *Behaviour Research and Therapy,* 33, 25-39 (1995).

8. Black, D.S., *et al.* Mindfulness meditation and improvement in sleep quality and daytime impairment among older adults with sleep disturbances: a

randomized clinical trial. *Journal of the American Medical Association: Internal Medicine,* 175, 494-501 (2015).

9. Kabat-Zinn, J., *et al.* Effectiveness of a meditation-based stress reduction program in the treatment of anxiety disorders. *The American Journal of Psychiatry,* 149, 936-943 (1992).

10. Gong, H., *et al.* Mindfulness meditation for insomnia: a meta-analysis of randomized controlled trials. *Journal of Psychosomatic Research,* 89, 1-6 (2016).

11. Kristeller, J.L. & Hallett, C.B. An exploratory study of a meditation-based intervention for binge eating disorder. *Journal of Health Psychology,* 4, 357-363 (1999).

12. Cash, E., *et al.* Mindfulness meditation alleviates fibromyalgia symptoms in women: results of a randomized clinical trial. *Annals of Behavioral Medicine,* 49, 319-330 (2015).

13. Karege, F., *et al.* Decreased serum brain-derived neurotrophic factor levels in major depressed patients. *Psychiatry research* 109, 143-148 (2002).

14. Russo-Neustadt, A., Beard, R.C. & Cotman, C.W. Exercise, antidepressant medications, and enhanced brain derived neurotrophic factor expression. *Neuropsychopharmacology,* 21, 679-682 (1999).

15. Szuhany, K.L., Bugatti, M. & Otto, M.W. A meta-analytic review of the effects of exercise on brain-derived neurotrophic factor. *Journal of psychiatric research* 60, 56-64 (2015).

16. Flook, L., *et al.* Promoting prosocial behavior and self-regulatory skills in preschool children through a mindfulness-based Kindness Curriculum. *Developmental Psychology,* 51, 44-51 (2015).

17. Tang, Y.Y., *et al.* Short-term meditation training improves attention and self-regulation. *Proceedings of the National Academy of Sciences of the United States of America,* 104, 17152-17156 (2007).

18. Tang, Y.Y., *et al.* Short-term meditation training improves attention and self-regulation. *Proceedings of the National Academy of Sciences USA,* 104, 17152-17156 (2007).

19. Tang, Y.Y., *et al.* Short-term meditation induces white matter changes in the anterior cingulate. *Proceedings of the National Academy of Sciences of the United States of America,* 107, 15649-15652 (2010).

20. Slagter, H.A., Davidson, R.J. & Lutz, A. Mental training as a tool in the neuroscientific study of brain and cognitive plasticity. *Frontiers in Human Neuroscience,* 5, 17 (2011).

21. Lutz, A., *et al.* Attention regulation and monitoring in meditation. *Trends in Cognitive Sciences,* 12, 163-169 (2008).

22. Baer, R.A. Self-focused attention and mechanisms of change in mindfulness-based treatment. *Cognitive Behaviour Therapy,* 38 (Suppl. 1), 15-20 (2009).

23. Moore, A. & Malinowski, P. Meditation, mindfulness and cognitive flexibility. *Consciousness and Cognition,* 18, 176-186 (2009).

24. Lutz, A., *et al.* Mental training enhances attentional stability: neural and behavioral evidence. *The Journal of Neuroscience,* 29, 13418-13427 (2009).

25. Goldin, P.R. & Gross, J.J. Effects of mindfulness-based stress reduction (MBSR) on emotion regulation in social anxiety disorder. *Emotion,* 10, 83-91 (2010).

26. Gu, J., *et al.* How do mindfulness-based cognitive therapy and mindfulness-based stress reduction improve mental health and wellbeing? A systematic review and meta-analysis of mediation studies. *Clinical Psychology Review,* 37, 1-12 (2015).

27. Nolenhoeksema, S. & Morrow, J. Effects of rumination and distraction on naturally-occurring depressed mood. *Cognition & Emotion,* 7, 561-570 (1993).

28. Killingsworth, M.A. & Gilbert, D.T. A wandering mind is an unhappy mind. *Science,* 330, 932 (2010).

29. Perestelo-Perez, L., *et al.* Mindfulness-based interventions for the treatment of depressive rumination: Systematic review and meta-analysis. *International Journal of Clinical and Health Psychology: IJCHP,* 17, 282-295 (2017).

30. Farb, N.A., *et al.* Minding one's emotions: mindfulness training alters the neural expression of sadness. *Emotion,* 10, 25-33 (2010).

31. Moore, A. & Malinowski, P. Meditation. *Consciousness and Cognition* (2009).

32. Zeidan, F., *et al.* Mindfulness meditation improves cognition: evidence of brief mental training. *Consciousness and Cognition,* 19, 597-605 (2010).

33. Carson, J.W., *et al.* Mindfulness-based relationship enhancement. *Behaviour Therapy,* 35, 471-494 (2004).

34. Krasner, M.S., *et al.* Association of an educational program in mindful communication with burnout, empathy, and attitudes among primary care physicians. *Journal of the American Medical Association,* 302, 1284-1293 (2009).

35. Van Dam, N.T., *et al.* Self-compassion is a better predictor than mindfulness of symptom severity and quality of life in mixed anxiety and depression. *Journal of Anxiety Disorders,* 25, 123-130 (2011).

36. Fortney, L., *et al.* Abbreviated mindfulness intervention for job satisfaction, quality of life, and compassion in primary care clinicians: a pilot study. *Annals of Family Medicine,* 11, 412-420 (2013).

37. Enqin, Z., *Health Preservation and Rehabilitation,* Publishing House of Shanghai College of Traditional Chinese Medicine. (1988).

38. Kivimaki, M. & Steptoe, A. Effects of stress on the development and progression of cardiovascular disease. *Nature Reviews: Cardiology,* 15, 215-229 (2018).

39. Crestani, C.C. Emotional stress and cardiovascular complications in animal models: a review of the influence of stress type. *Frontiers in Physiology,* 7, 251 (2016).

40. Williams, J.E., *et al.* Anger proneness predicts coronary heart disease risk: prospective analysis from the atherosclerosis risk in communities (ARIC) study. *Circulation,* 101, 2034-2039 (2000).

41. Yusuf, S., *et al.* Effect of potentially modifiable risk factors associated with myocardial infarction in 52 countries (the INTERHEART study): case-control study. *Lancet,* 364, 937-952 (2004).

42. Enqin, Z. *Health Preservation and Rehabilitation,* Publishing House of Shanghai College of Traditional Chinese Medicine. (1988).

43. Aurelius, M., *Meditations.* Penguin Classics. (2006).

44. Esler, M., *et al.* Overflow of catecholamine neurotransmitters to the circulation: source, fate, and functions. *Physiological Reviews,* 70, 963-985 (1990).

45. Chrousos, G.P. & Gold, P.W. The concepts of stress and stress system disorders. Overview of physical and behavioral homeostasis. *Journal of the American Medical Association,* 267, 1244-1252 (1992).

46. Kivimaki, M. & Steptoe, A. Effects of stress on the development and progression of cardiovascular disease. *Nature Reviews: Cardiology,* 15, 215-229 (2018).

47. Ho, D., *et al.* Adenylyl cyclase type 5 deficiency protects against diet-induced obesity and insulin resistance. *Diabetes,* 64, 2636-2645 (2015).

48. Yan, L., *et al.* Type 5 adenylyl cyclase disruption increases longevity and protects against stress. *Cell,* 130, 247-258 (2007).

49. De Lorenzo, M.S., *et al.* Reduced malignancy as a mechanism for longevity in mice with adenylyl cyclase type 5 disruption. *Aging Cell,* 13, 102-110 (2014).

50. Tindle, H.A., *et al.* Optimism, cynical hostility, and incident coronary heart disease and mortality in the Women's Health Initiative. *Circulation,* 120, 656-662 (2009).

51. Brown, K.W. & Ryan, R.M. The benefits of being present: mindfulness and its role in psychological well-being. *Journal of Personality and Social Psychology,* 84, 822-848 (2003).

52. *Ibid.*

53. Li, P., *et al.* The peptidergic control circuit for sighing. *Nature* 530, 293-297 (2016).

Chapter 22: Family, happiness and a future without fear

1. The *I Ching,* or, *Book of Changes,* (Princeton University Press; 3rd edition, 1967).

2. House, J.S., Landis, K.R. & Umberson, D. Social relationships and health. *Science,* 241, 540-545 (1988).

3. Fiske, A.P. Using individualism and collectivism to compare cultures – a critique of the validity and measurement of the constructs: comment on Oyserman *et al.* (2002). *Psychological Bulletin,* 128, 78-88 (2002).

4. Blumenthal, J.A., *et al.* Psychosocial factors and coronary disease: a national multicenter clinical trial (ENRICHD) with a North Carolina focus. *North Carolina Medical Journal,* 58, 440-444 (1997).

5. Rozanski, A., Blumenthal, J.A. & Kaplan, J. Impact of psychological factors on the pathogenesis of cardiovascular disease and implications for therapy. *Circulation,* 99, 2192-2217 (1999).

6. Cohen, S., *et al.* Social ties and susceptibility to the common cold. *Journal of the American Medical Association,* 277, 1940-1944 (1997).

7. Kiecolt-Glaser, J.K., *et al.* Hostile marital interactions, proinflammatory cytokine production, and wound healing. *Archives of General Psychiatry,* 62, 1377-1384 (2005).

8. Herlitz, J., *et al.* The feeling of loneliness prior to coronary artery bypass grafting might be a predictor of short-and long-term postoperative mortality. *European Journal of Vascular and Endovascular Surgery,* 16, 120-125 (1998).

9. Bierhaus, A., *et al.* A mechanism converting psychosocial stress into mononuclear cell activation. *Proceedings of the National Academy of Sciences of the United States of America,* 100, 1920-1925 (2003).

10. Lutgendorf, S.K., *et al.* Social support, psychological distress, and natural killer cell activity in ovarian cancer. *Journal of Clinical Oncology,* 23, 7105-7113 (2005).

11. Chuang-tzu. *Chuang-tzu* (Chinese-English Bilingual Edition), Foreign Language Teaching and Research Press, (2012).

12. Diamond, A. & Lee, K. Interventions shown to aid executive function development in children 4 to 12 years old. *Science,* 333, 959-964 (2011).

13. Friedman, N.P., *et al.* Not all executive functions are related to intelligence. *Psychological Science,* 17, 172-179 (2006).

14. The *I Ching,* or, *Book of Changes,* (Princeton University Press; 3rd edition, 1967).

15. Chuang-tzu. *Chuang-tzu (Chinese-English Bilingual Edition).* Foreign Language Teaching and Research Press (2012).

16. Greenberg, P.E., *et al.* The economic burden of adults with major depressive disorder in the United States (2005 and 2010). *The Journal of Clinical Psychiatry,* 76, 155-162 (2015).

17. Nietzsche, W., Kaufmann, W. (translator), *The Gay Science,* Vintage Books (1974).

18. The *I Ching,* or, *Book of Changes,* (Princeton University Press; 3rd edition, 1967).

19. Ricard, M. *Happiness: A Guide to Developing Life's Most Important Skill.* Little, Brown and Company (2007).

20. Liu, B., *et al.* Does happiness itself directly affect mortality? The prospective UK Million Women Study. *Lancet,* 387, 874-881 (2016).

21. Palomar-Garcia, M.A., *et al.* Modulation of functional connectivity in auditory-motor networks in musicians compared with nonmusicians. *Cerebral Cortex,* 27, 2768-2778 (2017).

22. Kleber, B., *et al.* Voxel-based morphometry in opera singers: Increased gray-matter volume in right somatosensory and auditory cortices. *NeuroImage,* 133, 477-483 (2016).

23. Shaffer, J. Neuroplasticity and clinical practice: building brain power for health. *Frontiers in Psychology,* 7, 1118 (2016).

24. *The I Ching, or, Book of Changes*, (Princeton University Press; 3rd edition, 1967).

25. Bertozzi, B., Tosti, V. & Fontana, L. Beyond calories: an integrated approach to promote health, longevity, and well-being. *Gerontology,* 63, 13-19 (2017).

26. Nisbet, E.K., Zelenski, J.M. & Murphy, S.A. Happiness is in our nature: exploring nature relatedness as a contributor to subjective well-being. *Journal of Happiness Studies,* 12, 303-322 (2011).

27. Hartig, T., *et al.* Tracking restoration in natural and urban field settings. *Journal of Environmental Psychology,* 23, 109-123 (2003).

28. Ueshiba, M. *The Art Of Peace. Teachings of the Founder of Aikido Pocket Classic*, Shambhala Pocket Classics (1993).

29. Holt, N.J., Using the experience-sampling method to examine the psychological mechanisms by which participatory art improves wellbeing. *Perspect Public Health,* 138(1), 55-65, (2018).

30. Singer, T., Klimencki, O.M., Empathy and compassion. *Current Biology,* 22;24(18) R875-R878, (2014).

31. Paulson, S., *et al.* The power of meaning: the quest for an existential roadmap. *Annual of the New York Academy of Science,* 1432(1), 10-28, (2018).

32. Chuang-tzu. *Chuang-tzu (Chinese-English Bilingual Edition).* Foreign Language Teaching and Research Press (2012).

33. Spinoza, B. *The Philosophy of Spinoza.* Edited by Joseph Ratner. SophiaOmni Press, 2014.

34. Kolb, D.F., R. *Toward an applied theory of experiential learning,* (John Wiley, 1975).

35. Holman, D., Pavlica, K. & Thorpe, R. Rethinking Kolb's theory of experiential learning in management education – The contribution of social constructionism and activity theory. *Manage. Learn.* 28, 135-148 (1997).

36. Edmondson, A. & Moingeon, B. From organizational learning to the learning organization. *Manage. Learn.* 29, 5-20 (1998).

Part VII: Our world

Chapter 23: A healthy sustainable environment to live in

1. Weigel, S., Kuhlmann, J. & Huhnerfuss, H. Drugs and personal care products as ubiquitous pollutants: occurrence and distribution of clofibric acid, caffeine and DEET in the North Sea. *The Science of the Total Environment,* 295, 131-141 (2002).

2. Landrigan, P.J., *et al.* The Lancet Commission on pollution and health. *Lancet,* 391:462-512 (2018).

3. Zhang, S., *et al.* Simultaneous quantification of polycyclic aromatic hydrocarbons (PAHs), polychlorinated biphenyls (PCBs), and pharmaceuticals and personal care products (PPCPs) in Mississippi river water, in New Orleans, Louisiana, USA. *Chemosphere,* 66, 1057-1069 (2007).

4. Kolpin, D.W., *et al.* Pharmaceuticals, hormones, and other organic wastewater contaminants in U.S. streams, 1999-2000: a national reconnaissance. *Environmental Science & Technology,* 36, 1202-1211 (2002).

5. Fent, K., Weston, A.A. & Caminada, D. Ecotoxicology of human pharmaceuticals. *Aquatic Toxicology,* 76, 122-159 (2006).

6. Oldenkamp, R., Beusen, A.H.W. & Huijbregts, M.A.J. Aquatic risks from human pharmaceuticals-modelling temporal trends of carbamazepine and ciprofloxacin at the global scale. *Environmental Research Letters,* 14, 11 (2019).

7. Meinshausen, M., *et al.* Greenhouse-gas emission targets for limiting global warming to 2 degrees C. *Nature,* 458, 1158-1162 (2009).

8. Vermeulen S.J., Campbell B.M., Ingram J.S.I., Climate change and food systems. Annual Revue Environmental Resources, 37, 195-222 (2012).

9. Fontana, L., *et al.* Energy efficiency as a unifying principle for human, environmental and global health. *F1000 Research,* 2: 101 (2013).

10. Willett, W., *et al.* Food in the anthropocene: the EAT-Lancet Commission on healthy diets from sustainable food systems. *Lancet,* 393(10170) 447-492 (2019).

11. Fontana, L., Atella, V. & Kammen, D.M. Energy efficiency. *F1000Research* (2013).

12. Lovins, A.B., Lovins, L.H. & Hawken, P. A road map for natural capitalism. *Harvard Business Review,* 77, 145-158, 211 (1999).

Chapter 24 Pollution is making us sick

1. Anderson, J.O., Thundiyil, J.G. & Stolbach, A. Clearing the air: a review of the effects of particulate matter air pollution on human health. *Journal of Medical Toxicology,* 8, 166-175 (2012).

2. Pope, C.A., 3rd, *et al.* Lung cancer, cardiopulmonary mortality, and long-term exposure to fine particulate air pollution. *Journal of the American Medical Association,* 287, 1132-1141 (2002).

3. Atkinson, R.W., *et al.* Epidemiological time series studies of PM2.5 and daily mortality and hospital admissions: a systematic review and meta-analysis. *Thorax,* 69, 660-665 (2014).

4. Gauderman, W.J., *et al.* Effect of exposure to traffic on lung development from 10 to 18 years of age: a cohort study. *Lancet* 369, 571-577 (2007).

5. Pope, C.A., 3rd, *et al.* Lung cancer, cardiopulmonary mortality, and fine particulate air pollution. *Journal of the American Medical Association* (2002).

6. Krewski, D., *et al.* Extended follow-up and spatial analysis of the American Cancer Society study linking particulate air pollution and mortality. *Research Report (Health Effects Institute),* 5-114 (2009).

7. Lelieveld, J., *et al.* The contribution of outdoor air pollution sources to premature mortality on a global scale. *Nature,* 525, 367-371 (2015).

8. WHO's urban ambient air pollution database – update 2016, World Health Organization, (2016).

9. Stanek, L.W., *et al.* Attributing health effects to apportioned components and sources of particulate

matter: an evaluation of collective results. *Atmospheric Environment,* 45, 5655-5663 (2011).

10. Erisman J.W., Schaap, M., The need for ammonia abatement with respect to secondary PM reductions in Europe. *Environmental Pollution,* 129(1) 159-163 (2004).

11. Behera, S.N., *et al.* Ammonia in the atmosphere: a review on emission sources, atmospheric chemistry and deposition on terrestrial bodies. *Environmental Science and Pollution Research International,* 20, 8092-8131 (2013).

12. Carnevale, C., Pisoni, E. & Volta, M. A non-linear analysis to detect the origin of PM10 concentrations in Northern Italy. *The Science of the Total Environment,* 409, 182-191 (2010).

13. Tsimpidi, A.P., Karydis, V.A. & Pandis, S.N. Response of inorganic fine particulate matter to emission changes of sulfur dioxide and ammonia: the eastern United States as a case study. *Journal of the Air & Waste Management Association (1995),* 57, 1489-1498 (2007).

14. Pinder, R.W., Adams, P.J. & Pandis, S.N. Ammonia emission controls as a cost-effective strategy for reducing atmospheric particulate matter in the Eastern United States. *Environmental Science & Technology,* 41, 380-386 (2007).

15. Food and Agricultural Organization (FAO): Meat Market Review. Oct 2018. http://www.fao.org/3/CA2129EN/ca2129en.pdf

16. USDA: Livestock Slaughter 2018 Summary https://downloads.usda.library.cornell.edu/usda-esmis/files/rx913p88g/fn107f118/1257b8885/lstk0120.pdf

17. USDA: Poultry Slaughter 2018 Summary https://downloads.usda.library.cornell.edu/usda-esmis/files/pg15bd88s/p8418w155/7p88cq28g/pslaan19.pdf

18. Sutton, M.A., *et al.* Too much of a good thing. *Nature,* 472, 159-161 (2011).

19. The World Bank: Fertilizer consumption (kilograms per hectare of arable land) http://data.worldbank.org/indicator/AG.CON.FERT.ZS

20. US EPA. Pesticides Industry Sales and Usage: 2008–2012. https://www.epa.gov/sites/production/files/2017-01/documents/pesticides-industry-sales-usage-2016_0.pdf

21. Hubbard, R.K., Newton, G.L. & Hill, G.M. Water quality and the grazing animal. *Journal of Animal Science,* 82, E255-263 (2004).

22. Carpenter, S.R., *et al.* Nonpoint pollution of surface waters with phosphorus and nitrogen. *Ecological Applications,* 8, 559-568 (1998).

23. Sims, J.T., Simard, R.R. & Joern, B.C. Phosphorus loss in agricultural drainage: historical perspective and current research. *Journal of Environmental Quality,* 27, 277-293 (1998).

24. Cantor, K.P., *et al.* Drinking water source and chlorination byproducts. I. Risk of bladder cancer. *Epidemiology,* 9, 21-28 (1998).

25. Richardson, S.D. Disinfection by-products and other emerging contaminants in drinking water. *Trac-Trends in Analytical Chemistry,* 22, 666-684 (2003).

26. Krasner, S.W., *et al.* Occurrence of a new generation of disinfection byproducts. *Environmental Science & Technology,* 40, 7175-7185 (2006).

27. Kopittke, P.M., *et al.* Soil and the intensification of agriculture for global food security. *Environmental Pollution,* 132:105078 (2019).

28. Sarmah, A.K., Meyer, M.T. & Boxall, A.B. A global perspective on the use, sales, exposure pathways, occurrence, fate and effects of veterinary antibiotics (VAs) in the environment. *Chemosphere,* 65, 725-759 (2006).

29. Casey, J.A., *et al.* High-density livestock operations, crop field application of manure, and risk of community-associated methicillin-resistant Staphylococcus aureus infection in Pennsylvania. *Journal of the American Medical Association Internal Medicine,* 173, 1980-1990 (2013).

30. Fleming-Dutra, K.E., *et al.* Prevalence of inappropriate antibiotic prescriptions among US ambulatory care visits, 2010-2011. *Journal of the American Medical Association,* 315, 1864-1873 (2016).

31. Martinez, J.L. Environmental pollution by antibiotics and by antibiotic resistance determinants. Environ Pollut., 157:2893-902 (2009).

32. Han, R.W., *et al.* Simultaneous determination of 38 veterinary antibiotic residues in raw milk by UPLC-MS/MS. *Food chemistry* 181, 119-126 (2015).

33. Rokka, M., *et al.* The residue levels of narasin in eggs of laying hens fed with unmedicated and medicated feed. *Molecular Nutrition & Food Research,* 49, 38-42 (2005).

34. Hawken, P.L., Amory; Lovins, L Hunter *Natural Capitalism: Creating the Next Industrial Revolution,* (US Green Building Council; 1st edition, 2000).

35. Vermeulen S.J., Campbell B.M., Ingram J.S.I., Climate change and food systems. Annual Revue Environmental Resources, 37, 195-222 (2012).

36. Fontana, L., *et al.* Energy efficiency as a unifying principle for human, environmental and global health. *F1000 Research,* 2: 101 (2013).

37. Willett, W., *et al.* Food in the anthropocene: the EAT-Lancet Commission on healthy diets from sustainable food systems. *Lancet,* 393(10170) 447-492 (2019).

38. Tilman, D., *et al.* Agricultural sustainability and intensive production practices. *Nature,* 418, 671-677 (2002).

39. Hansen, J., *et al.* Global warming in the twenty-first century: an alternative scenario. *Proceedings of the National Academy of Sciences of the United States of America,* 97, 9875-9880 (2000).

Chapter 25: Securing the future

1 Fontana, L., Atella, V. & Kammen, D.M. Energy efficiency. *F1000Research* (2013).

2. Pimentel, D. & Pimentel, M. Sustainability of meat-based and plant-based diets and the environment. *The American Journal of Clinical Nutrition,* 78, 660s-663s (2003).

3. *Ibid.*

4. Horrigan, L., Lawrence, R.S. & Walker, P. How sustainable agriculture can address the environmental and human health harms of industrial agriculture. *Environmental Health Perspectives,* 110, 445-456 (2002).

5. Tilman, D., *et al.* Agricultural sustainability and intensive production practices. *Nature* (2002).

6. Watts, N., Amann, M., *et al.* The 2019 report of the The Lancet Countdown on health and climate change: ensuring that the health of a child born today is not defined by a changing climate. *Lancet,* 394, 1836-1878 (2019).

Appendix: What gets measured, gets done: track your progress

1. Fontana, L. & Hu, F.B. Optimal body weight for health and longevity: bridging basic, clinical, and population research. *Aging Cell,* 13, 391-400 (2014).

2. Fontana, L., Partridge, L. & Longo, V.D. Extending healthy life span – from yeast to humans. *Science,* 328, 321-326 (2010).

3. Fontana, L., Klein, S. & Holloszy, J.O. Effects of long-term calorie restriction and endurance exercise on glucose tolerance, insulin action, and adipokine production. *Age,* 32, 97-108 (2010).

4. Calnan, D.R. & Brunet, A. The FoxO code. *Oncogene,* 27:2276-88 (2008).

5. Kaptoge, S., *et al.* C-reactive protein concentration and risk of coronary heart disease, stroke, and mortality: an individual participant meta-analysis. *Lancet,* 375, 132-140 (2010).

6. Fontana, L., *et al.* Visceral fat adipokine secretion is associated with systemic inflammation in obese humans. *Diabetes,* 56, 1010-1013 (2007).

7. Pearson, T.A., *et al.* Markers of inflammation and cardiovascular disease: application to clinical and public health practice: a statement for healthcare professionals from the Centers for Disease Control and Prevention and the American Heart Association. *Circulation,* 107, 499-511 (2003).

8. Fontana, L., *et al.* Long-term calorie restriction is highly effective in reducing the risk for atherosclerosis in humans. *Proceedings of the National Academy of Sciences,* 101, 6659-6663 (2004).

9. Franceschi, C., *et al.* Inflammaging: a new immune-metabolic viewpoint for age-related diseases. *Nature Reviews: Endocrinology,* 14, 576-590 (2018).

10. Emerging Risk Factors Collaboration, Kaptoge, S., *et al.* C-reactive protein concentration and risk of coronary heart disease, stroke, and mortality: an individual participant meta-analysis. *Lancet,* 375:132-40 (2010).

11. Lloyd-Jones, D.M., *et al.* Lifetime risk of developing coronary heart disease. *Lancet,* 353, 89-92 (1999).

12. Libby, P. & Hansson, G.K. From Focal Lipid Storage to Systemic Inflammation: JACC Review Topic of the Week. *Journal of the American College of Cardiology,* 74:1594-1607 (2019).

13. O'Keefe, J.H., Cordain, L., Harris, W.H., Moe, R.M. & Vogel, R. Optimal low-density lipoprotein is 50 to 70 mg/dl - Lower is better and physiologically normal. *Journal of the American College of Cardiology,* 43, 2142-2146 (2004).

14. Wilson, P.W.F., *et al.* Systematic review for the 2018 AHA/ACC/AACVPR/AAPA/ABC/ACPM/ADA/ AGS/APhA/ASPC/NLA/PCNA guideline on the management of blood cholesterol: a report of the American College of Cardiology/ American Heart Association Task Force on Clinical Practice Guidelines. *Circulation,* 139, e1144-e1161 (2019).

15. Rosenson, R.S., *et al.* The Evolving Future of PCSK9 Inhibitors. *Journal of the American College of Cardiology,* 72:314-329 (2018).

16. Goldstein, J.L. & Brown, M.S. A century of cholesterol and coronaries: from plaques to genes to statins. *Cell,* 161, 161-172 (2015).

17. Mills, G.L. & Taylaur, C.E. The distribution and composition of serum lipoproteins in eighteen animals. *Comparative Biochemistry and Physiology. B, Comparative Biochemistry,* 40, 489-501 (1971).

18. Chapman, M.J. & Goldstein, S. Comparison of the serum low density lipoprotein and of its apoprotein in the pig, rhesus monkey and baboon with that in man. *Atherosclerosis,* 25, 267-291 (1976).

19. Kwiterovich, P.O., Jr., Levy, R.I. & Fredrickson, D.S. Neonatal diagnosis of familial type-II hyperlipoproteinaemia. *Lancet,* 1, 118-121 (1973).

20. O'Keefe, J.H., *et al.* Optimal low-density lipoprotein. *Journal of the American College of Cardiology,* (2004).

21. Arnett, D.K., *et al.* 2019 ACC/AHA Guideline on the primary prevention of cardiovascular disease: executive summary – report of the American College of Cardiology/ American Heart Association Task Force on Clinical Practice Guidelines. *Journal of the American College of Cardiology,* 74, 1376-1414 (2019).

22. *Ibid.*

23. Kathiresan, S. A PCSK9 missense variant associated with a reduced risk of early-onset myocardial infarction. *The New England Journal of Medicine,* 358, 2299-2300 (2008).

24. Goldstein, J.L. & Brown, M.S. A century of cholesterol and coronaries. *Cell* (2015).

25. Rader, D.J. & Hovingh, G.K. HDL and cardiovascular disease. *Lancet,* 384, 618-625 (2014).

26. Barter, P., *et al.* HDL cholesterol, very low levels of LDL cholesterol, and cardiovascular events. *The New England Journal of Medicine,* 357, 1301-1310 (2007).

27. *Ibid.*

28. McGillicuddy, F.C., *et al.* Inflammation impairs reverse cholesterol transport in vivo. *Circulation,* 119, 1135-1145 (2009).

29. Walldius, G., *et al.* The apoB/apoA-I ratio is better than the cholesterol ratios to estimate the balance between plasma proatherogenic and antiatherogenic lipoproteins and to predict coronary risk. *Clinical Chemistry and Laboratory Medicine,* 42, 1355-1363 (2004).

30. van Deventer, H.E., *et al*. Non-HDL cholesterol shows improved accuracy for cardiovascular risk score classification compared to direct or calculated LDL cholesterol in a dyslipidemic population. *Clinical Chemistry,* 57, 490-501 (2011).

31. Toh, R. Assessment of HDL cholesterol removal capacity: toward clinical application. *Journal of Atherosclerosis and Thrombosis,* 26, 111-120 (2019).

32. Emerging risk factors collaboration. Sarwar, N., *et al*. Diabetes mellitus, fasting blood glucose concentration, and risk of vascular disease: a collaborative meta-analysis of 102 prospective studies. *Lancet,* 375, 2215-2222 (2010).

33. Emerging Risk Factors Collaboration, Di Angelantonio, E., *et al*. Glycated hemoglobin measurement and prediction of cardiovascular disease. *JAMA*, 311:1225-33 (2014).

34. Tirosh, A., *et al*. Normal fasting plasma glucose levels and type 2 diabetes in young men. *The New England journal of medicine* 353, 1454-1462 (2005).

35. Simons, L.A., Friedlander, Y., McCallum, J. & Simons, J. Fasting plasma glucose in non-diabetic elderly women predicts increased all-causes mortality and coronary heart disease risk. *Australian and New Zealand journal of medicine* 30, 41-47 (2000).

36. Tanne, D., Koren-Morag, N. & Goldbourt, U. Fasting plasma glucose and risk of incident ischemic stroke or transient ischemic attacks: a prospective cohort study. *Stroke* 35, 2351-2355 (2004).

37. Weykamp, C. HbA1c: a review of analytical and clinical aspects. *Annals of laboratory medicine* 33, 393-400 (2013).

38. Tirosh, A., *et al*. Normal fasting plasma glucose levels and type 2 diabetes in young men. *The New England journal of medicine* 353, 1454-1462 (2005).

39. Lewington, S., Clarke, R., Qizilbash, N., Peto, R. & Collins, R. Age-specific relevance of usual blood pressure to vascular mortality: a meta-analysis of individual data for one million adults in 61 prospective studies. *Lancet* 360, 1903-1913 (2002).

40. *Ibid*.

41. Whelton, P.K., *et al*. 2017 ACC/AHA/AAPA/ABC/ACPM/AGS/APhA/ASH/ASPC/NMA/PCNA Guideline for the Prevention, Detection, Evaluation, and Management of High Blood Pressure in Adults: Executive Summary: A Report of the American College of Cardiology/American Heart Association Task Force on Clinical Practice Guidelines. *Hypertension,* 71, 1269-1324 (2018).

42. *Ibid*.

43. Williams, C.J., *et al*. Genes to predict VO2max trainability: a systematic review. *BMC genomics* 18, 831 (2017).

44. Fitzgerald, M.D., Tanaka, H., Tran, Z.V. & Seals, D.R. Age-related declines in maximal aerobic capacity in regularly exercising vs. sedentary women: A meta-analysis. *J. Appl. Physiol.* 83, 160-165 (1997).

ACKNOWLEDGEMENTS

This book would not be possible without the love and support of my mother Antonietta, my dear son Lorenzo, my sisters Anita and Liliana, and my wife Laura.

There are many others who have given me their help and encouragement in this journey. Critical support came from my uncle Francesco Iozzi and my dear friends Tadd and Debbie Ottman, My-Anh Tran-Dang, Annie Gottlieb, Juniper Pennypacker, Peter Cistulli, Tom Carnahan and Ted Bakewell.

A special thank you goes to my publisher, Pam Brewster, who worked closely with me for almost a year crafting this book for the public.

In the development of my research program I have many to acknowledge, they include my mentor and dear friend, Dr John Otto Holloszy, but also doctors Samuel Klein, Timothy Meyer, Edward Weiss, Dennis Villareal, Sandor J Kovács, Philip Stein and Ali Ehsani.

I have also to thank the many postdoctoral fellows, PhD students, research dietitians, technicians and coordinators who were critical to my lab's success.

Finally, I would like to thank the many outstanding international research partners and collaborators, including Frank Hu, Gokhan Hotamisligil and James Mitchell (Harvard Medical School), Jeffery I Gordon (Washington University in St.Louis), David Sabatini (Massachusetts Institute of Technology), Linda Partridge (Max Planck Institute of Aging), Mark Mattson and Rafael De Cabo (National Institute on Aging), Marco De Maria (Groningen University), Ana Maria Cuervo, Yousin Suh and Derek Huffman (Albert Einstein College of Medicine), Pinchas Cohen and Valter Longo (University of Southern California), Dudley Lamming (Wisconsin University), Roberto Pili (Indiana University), William E Kraus (Duke University), Janko Nikolich-Žugich (University of Tucson, Arizona), Brian Kennedy (National University of Singapore), John R Speakman (Chinese Academy of Sciences), Piero Ruggenenti and Giuseppe Remuzzi (Mario Negri Nord), Stephen Simpson, Peter Cistulli, and Stephen Fuller (University of Sydney).